T0358932

Medically Complex Patients

Editors

ROBERT B. SCHONBERGER
STANLEY H. ROSENBAUM

ANESTHESIOLOGY CLINICS

www.anesthesiology.theclinics.com

Consulting Editor
LEE A. FLEISHER

December 2016 • Volume 34 • Number 4

ELSEVIER

1600 John F. Kennedy Boulevard • Suite 1800 • Philadelphia, Pennsylvania, 19103-2899

http://www.theclinics.com

ANESTHESIOLOGY CLINICS Volume 34, Number 4
December 2016 ISSN 1932-2275, ISBN-13: 978-0-323-47734-5

Editor: Katie Pfaff
Developmental Editor: Kristen Helm

Anesthesiology Clinics (ISSN 1932-2275) is published quarterly by Elsevier Inc., 360 Park Avenue South, New York, NY 10010-1710. Months of issue are March, June, September, and December. Periodicals postage paid at New York, NY and at additional mailing offices. Subscription prices are $100.00 per year (US student/resident), $330.00 per year (US individuals), $400.00 per year (Canadian individuals), $596.00 per year (US institutions), $753.00 per year (Canadian institutions), $225.00 per year (Canadian and foreign student/resident), $455.00 per year (foreign individuals), and $753.00 per year (foreign institutions). To receive student and resident rate, orders must be accompanied by name of affiliated institution, date of term, and the *signature* of program/residency coordinator on institutions letterhead. Orders will be billed at individual rate until proof of status is received. Foreign air speed delivery is included in all *Clinics'* subscription prices. All prices are subject to change without notice. POSTMASTER: Send address changes to *Anesthesiology Clinics,* Elsevier Health Sciences Division, Subscription Customer Service, 3251 Riverport Lane, Maryland Heights, MO 63043. Customer Service (orders, claims, online, change of address): Elsevier Health Sciences Division, Subscription Customer Service, 3251 Riverport Lane, Maryland Heights, MO 63043. **Tel:1-800-654-2452 (U.S. and Canada); 314-447-8871 (outside U.S. and Canada). Fax: 314-447-8029. E-mail: journalscustomerservice-usa@elsevier.com (for print support); journalsonlinesupport-usa@elsevier.com (for online support).**

Reprints. For copies of 100 or more of articles in this publication, please contact the Commercial Reprints Department, Elsevier Inc., 360 Park Avenue South, New York, NY 10010-1710. Tel.: 212-633-3874; Fax: 212-633-3820; E-mail: reprints@elsevier.com.

Anesthesiology Clinics, is also published in Spanish by McGraw-Hill Inter-americana Editores S. A., P.O. Box 5-237, 06500 Mexico D. F., Mexico.

Anesthesiology Clinics, is covered in *MEDLINE/PubMed (Index Medicus), Current Contents/Clinical Medicine, Excerpta Medica, ISI/BIOMED,* and *Chemical Abstracts.*

Contributors

CONSULTING EDITOR

LEE A. FLEISHER, MD, FACC, FAHA
Robert D. Dripps Professor and Chair of Anesthesiology and Critical Care, Professor of Medicine, Perelman School of Medicine, University of Pennsylvania, Philadelphia, Pennsylvania

EDITORS

ROBERT B. SCHONBERGER, MD, MHS
Assistant Professor; Associate Director for Clinical Research, Department of Anesthesiology, Yale School of Medicine, New Haven, Connecticut

STANLEY H. ROSENBAUM, MA, MD
Professor of Anesthesiology, Internal Medicine, and Surgery; Director, Division of Perioperative and Adult Anesthesia; Vice Chairman for Academic Affairs, Department of Anesthesiology, Yale School of Medicine, New Haven, Connecticut

AUTHORS

ABED ABUBAIH, MD
Attending Anesthesiologist, Department of Anesthesiology and Critical Care Medicine, Hadassah – Hebrew University Medical Center, Hebrew University – Hadassah School of Medicine, Jerusalem, Israel

JULIANNE AHDOUT, MD
Resident Physician, Department of Anesthesiology, Cedars-Sinai Medical Center, Los Angeles, California

BISHWAJIT BHATTACHARYA, MD, FACS
Assistant Professor of Surgery, Section of General Surgery, Trauma & Surgical Critical Care, Department of Surgery, Yale School of Medicine, New Haven, Connecticut

TRICIA E. BRENTJENS, MD
Associate Professor of Anesthesiology at CUMC, Department of Anesthesiology, College of Physicians and Surgeons, Columbia University, New York, New York

DANIEL R. BROWN, MD, PhD
Professor of Anesthesiology; Director, Multidisciplinary Critical Care Practice, Department of Anesthesiology and Critical Care, Mayo Clinic, Rochester, Minnesota

RYAN CHADHA, MD
Clinical Fellow, Department of Anesthesiology, College of Physicians and Surgeons, Columbia University, New York, New York

KIMBERLY A. DAVIS, MD, MBA, FACS, FCCM
Vice Chairman of Clinical Affairs; Chief of the Section of General Surgery, Trauma, & Surgical Critical Care; Professor, Department of Surgery; Trauma Medical Director; Surgical Director, Quality and Performance Improvement, Yale-New Haven Hospital, Yale School of Medicine, New Haven, Connecticut

GERALDINE C. DIAZ, DO
Clinical Associate, Department of Anesthesiology/Critical Care, University of Chicago, Chicago, Illinois

JORDAN E. GOLDHAMMER, MD
Assistant Professor, Department of Anesthesiology, Sidney Kimmel Medical College, Thomas Jefferson University, Philadelphia, Pennsylvania

MAZYAR JAVIDROOZI, MD, PhD
Department of Anesthesiology and Critical Care Medicine, Englewood Hospital and Medical Center, TeamHealth Research Institute, Englewood, New Jersey

GARY J. KAML, MD, FACS
Assistant Professor of Surgery, Section of General Surgery, Trauma, & Surgical Critical Care, Department of Surgery, Yale School of Medicine, New Haven, Connecticut

BENJAMIN A. KOHL, MD
Professor, Department of Anesthesiology, Sidney Kimmel Medical College, Thomas Jefferson University, Philadelphia, Pennsylvania

GREGG P. LOBEL, MD
Department of Anesthesiology and Critical Care Medicine, Englewood Hospital and Medical Center, TeamHealth Research Institute, Englewood, New Jersey

LINDA L. MAERZ, MD, FACS, FCCM
Associate Professor of Surgery and Anesthesiology, Section of General Surgery, Trauma & Surgical Critical Care, Department of Surgery, Yale School of Medicine, New Haven, Connecticut

ADRIAN A. MAUNG, MD, FACS, FCCM
Associate Professor of Surgery, Section of General Surgery, Trauma & Surgical Critical Care, Department of Surgery, Yale School of Medicine, New Haven, Connecticut

SARA E. NEVES, MD
Instructor, Department of Anesthesia, Critical Care, and Pain Medicine, Beth Israel Deaconess Medical Center, Harvard Medical School, Boston, Massachusetts

MICHAEL NUROK, MBChB, PhD
Medical Director, Cardiac Surgery Intensive Care Unit; Medical Director, Cedars-Sinai Medical Center, Los Angeles, California

MICHAEL F. O'CONNOR, MD
Professor of Anesthesiology, Department of Anesthesiology/Critical Care, University of Chicago, Chicago, Illinois

MISTY A. RADOSEVICH, MD
Instructor of Anesthesiology, Department of Anesthesiology and Critical Care, Mayo Clinic, Rochester, Minnesota

JOHN F. RENZ, MD, PhD
Professor, Department of Surgery, University of Chicago, Chicago, Illinois

NICHOLAS SADOVNIKOFF, MD
Department of Anesthesiology, Perioperative and Pain Medicine, Brigham & Women's Hospital, Boston, Massachusetts

RADWAN SAFA, MD, PhD
Department of Anesthesiology, Perioperative and Pain Medicine, Brigham & Women's Hospital, Boston, Massachusetts

ARYEH SHANDER, MD
Department of Anesthesiology and Critical Care Medicine, Englewood Hospital and Medical Center, TeamHealth Research Institute, Englewood, New Jersey

CHARLES WEISSMAN, MD
Professor and Chair, Department of Anesthesiology and Critical Care Medicine, Hadassah – Hebrew University Medical Center, Hebrew University – Hadassah School of Medicine, Jerusalem, Israel

MICHAEL M. WOLL, MD, FACS
Clinical Fellow, Surgical Critical Care, Section of General Surgery, Trauma & Surgical Critical Care, Department of Surgery, Yale School of Medicine, New Haven, Connecticut

Contents

Foreword: The Patient with Multimorbidities: Does 1 + 1 Always Simply Equal 2?   xiii

Lee A. Fleisher

Preface: Medically Complex Patients   xv

Robert B. Schonberger and Stanley H. Rosenbaum

Anesthetic Management of the Adult Patient with Concomitant Cardiac and Pulmonary Disease   633

Misty A. Radosevich and Daniel R. Brown

Several common diseases of the cardiac and pulmonary systems and the interactions of the two in disease and anesthetic management are discussed. Management of these disease processes in isolation is reviewed and how the management of one organ system impacts another is then explored. For example, in a patient with acute lung injury and right heart failure, lung-protective ventilation may directly conflict with strategies to minimize right heart afterload. Such challenging clinical scenarios require appreciation of each disease entity, their appropriate management, and the balance between competing priorities.

Anesthesia for the Patient with Concomitant Hepatic and Renal Impairment   645

Tricia E. Brentjens and Ryan Chadha

Hepatic and renal disease are common comorbidities in patients presenting for intermediate- and high-risk surgery. With the evolution of perioperative medicine, anesthesiologists are encountering more patients who have significant hepatic and renal disease, both acute and chronic in nature. It is important that anesthesiologists have an in-depth understanding of the physiologic derangements seen with hepatic and renal disease to evaluate and manage these patients appropriately. Perioperative management requires an understanding of the physiologic perturbations associated with each disease process. This article elucidates the goals in the management and treatment of this complex patient population.

Coexisting Cardiac and Hematologic Disorders   659

Jordan E. Goldhammer and Benjamin A. Kohl

Patients with concomitant cardiac and hematologic disorders presenting for noncardiac surgery are challenging. Anemic patients with cardiac disease should be approached in a methodical fashion. Transfusion triggers and target should be based on underlying symptomatology. The approach to anticoagulation management in patients with artificial heart valves, cardiac devices, or severe heart failure in the operative setting must encompass a complete understanding of the rationale of a patient's therapy as well as calculate the risk of changing this regimen. This article focuses on common disorders and discusses strategies to optimize care in patients with coexisting cardiac and hematologic disease.

Surgical Critical Care for the Trauma Patient with Cardiac Disease   669

Michael M. Woll and Linda L. Maerz

The elderly population is rapidly increasing in number. Therefore, geriatric trauma is becoming more prevalent. All practitioners caring for geriatric trauma patients should be familiar with the structural and functional changes naturally occurring in the aging heart, as well as common preexisting cardiac diseases in the geriatric population. Identification of the shock state related to cardiac dysfunction and targeted assessment of perfusion and resuscitation are important when managing elderly patients. Finally, management of cardiac dysfunction in the trauma patient includes an appreciation of the inherent effects of trauma on cardiac function.

Surgical Critical Care for the Patient with Sepsis and Multiple Organ Dysfunction   681

Gary J. Kaml and Kimberly A. Davis

Sepsis and multiple organ dysfunction syndrome (MODS) is common in the surgical intensive care unit. Sepsis involves infection and the patient's immune response. Timely recognition of sepsis and swift application of evidence-based interventions is critical to the success of therapy. This article reviews the nature of the septic process, existing definitions of sepsis, and current evidence-based treatment strategies for sepsis and MODS. An improved understanding of the process of sepsis and its relation to MODS has resulted in clinical definitions and scoring systems that allow for the quantification of disease severity and guidelines for treatment.

Anesthesia for Patients with Concomitant Cardiac and Renal Dysfunction   697

Radwan Safa and Nicholas Sadovnikoff

Renal disease and cardiovascular disease are commonly encountered in the same patient. The dynamic interactions between renal disease and cardiovascular disease have an impact on perioperative management. Renal failure is an independent risk factor for cardiovascular disease and the link between the two disease states remains to be fully elucidated.

Anesthesia for Patients with Anemia   711

Aryeh Shander, Gregg P. Lobel, and Mazyar Javidroozi

Anemia is a common and often ignored condition in surgical patients. Anemia is usually multifactorial and iron deficiency and inflammation are commonly involved. An exacerbating factor in surgical patients is iatrogenic blood loss. Anemia has been repeatedly shown to be an independent predictor of worse outcomes. Patient blood management (PBM) provides a multimodality framework for prevention and management of anemia and related risk factors. The key strategies in PBM include support of hematopoiesis and improving hemoglobin level, optimizing coagulation and hemostasis, use of interdisciplinary blood conservation modalities, and patient-centered decision making throughout the course of care.

Anesthesia Patients with Concomitant Cardiac and Hepatic Dysfunction 731

Julianne Ahdout and Michael Nurok

Anesthesia and surgery in patients with hepatic and cardiac dysfunction poses a challenge for anesthesiologists. It is imperative to optimize these patients perioperatively. Cirrhosis is associated with a wide range of cardiovascular abnormalities. Cirrhotic cardiomyopathy is characterized by blunted contractile responsiveness or systolic incompetence, and/or diastolic dysfunction. In liver disease, anesthetic drug distribution, metabolism, and elimination may be altered. Among patients with liver disease, propofol is a reasonable anesthetic choice and cisatracurium is the preferred neuromuscular blocker. Regional anesthesia should be used whenever appropriate if not contraindicated by coagulopathy, because it reduces the need for systemic analgesia.

Anesthesia for Patients with Traumatic Brain Injuries 747

Bishwajit Bhattacharya and Adrian A. Maung

Traumatic brain injury (TBI) represents a wide spectrum of disease and disease severity. Because the primary brain injury occurs before the patient enters the health care system, medical interventions seek principally to prevent secondary injury. Anesthesia teams that provide care for patients with TBI both in and out of the operating room should be aware of the specific therapies and needs of this unique and complex patient population.

Anesthesia for Patients with Concomitant Sepsis and Cardiac Dysfunction 761

Abed Abubaih and Charles Weissman

Anesthesiologists faced with a patient with sepsis and concurrent cardiac dysfunction must be cognizant of the patient's cardiac status and cause of the cardiac problem to appropriately adapt physiologic and metabolic monitoring and anesthetic management. Anesthesia in such patients is challenging because the interaction of sepsis and cardiac dysfunction greatly complicates management. Intraoperative anesthesia management requires careful induction and maintenance of anesthesia; optimizing intravascular volume status; avoiding lung injury during mechanical ventilation; and close monitoring of arterial blood gases, serum lactate concentrations, and hematology renal and electrolyte parameters. Such patients have increased mortality because of their inability to adequately compensate for the cardiovascular changes caused by sepsis.

Anesthesia for Patients with Peripheral Vascular Disease and Cardiac Dysfunction 775

Sara E. Neves

Patients with vascular disease and cardiac dysfunction present particular challenges to the anesthesiologist. They are hemodynamically brittle, at high risk of morbidity and mortality during surgery, and often carry additional comorbidities that increase their complexity and risk. Those with peripheral vascular disease should be assumed to have coronary artery disease and tend to have other systemic vascular problems. Poor cardiac function further worsens perfusion in an already compromised peripheral vascular system. Care of these patients requires judicious monitoring, an anesthetic that optimizes hemodynamic function, and avoidance of particularly likely complications such as perioperative myocardial ischemia, stroke, and bleeding.

Anesthesia for Patients with Concomitant Hepatic and Pulmonary Dysfunction   797

Geraldine C. Diaz, Michael F. O'Connor, and John F. Renz

Hepatic function and pulmonary function are interrelated with failure of one organ system affecting the other. With improved therapies, patients with concomitant hepatic and pulmonary failure increasingly enjoy a good quality of life and life expectancy. Therefore, the prevalence of such patients is increasing with more presenting for both emergent and elective surgical procedures. Hypoxemia requires a thorough evaluation in patients with end-stage liver disease. The most common etiologies respond to appropriate therapy. Portopulmonary hypertension and hepatopulmonary syndrome are associated with increased perioperative morbidity and mortality. It is incumbent on the anesthesiologist to understand the physiology of liver failure and its early effect on pulmonary function to ensure a successful outcome.

Index   809

ANESTHESIOLOGY CLINICS

FORTHCOMING ISSUES

March 2017
Obstetric Anesthesia
Robert R. Gaiser and Onyi Onuoha,
Editors

June 2017
Pharmacology
Alan D. Kaye, *Editor*

September 2017
Anesthesia Outside of the Operating Room
Mark S. Weiss and Wendy L. Gross,
Editors

RECENT ISSUES

September 2016
Advances in Neuroscience in Anesthesia and Critical Care
W. Andrew Kofke, *Editor*

June 2016
Pain Management
Perry G. Fine and Michael A. Ashburn,
Editors

March 2016
Preoperative Evaluation
Debra Domino Pulley and
Deborah C. Richman, *Editors*

THE CLINICS ARE AVAILABLE ONLINE!
Access your subscription at:
www.theclinics.com

Foreword

The Patient with Multimorbidities: Does 1 + 1 Always Simply Equal 2?

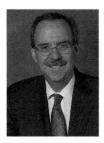

Lee A. Fleisher, MD, FACC, FAHA
Consulting Editor

Over the past several decades, anesthesiologists, surgeons, and others have developed strategies to care for the patient with medical conditions. These have taken the form of review papers or formal Guidelines like those produced by the American Heart Association/American College of Cardiology. Yet patients frequently have more than one medical condition, and some of the conditions have unique interactions or require contrary management approaches. In such circumstances, the simple addition of the recommendations may not be simple arithmetic. In this issue of *Anesthesiology Clinics*, the authors have evaluated some unique combinations of medical conditions that anesthesiologists might face, and provide outstanding advice on management.

This issue was proposed by a leader in thought in this arena and previous editor on this topic, Stanley H. Rosenbaum, MA, MD. Dr Rosenbaum is a Professor of Anesthesiology, Internal Medicine and Surgery at the Yale School of Medicine. He is the Vice-Chair for Academic Affairs and the Director of the Division of Perioperative and Adult Anesthesia within the Department of Anesthesiology. He received the Lifetime Achievement Award from the Society of Critical Care Anesthesiologists in 2011. He is joined by Robert B. Schonberger, MD, MHS, a cardiac anesthesiologist and clinical informatics researcher at the Yale School of Medicine, where he is an Assistant Professor of Anesthesiology. Dr Schonberger is an NIH-funded researcher and has focused on the integration of surgical care and long-term cardiovascular risk reduction, the analysis of bias within large administrative datasets, and new techniques to minimize gaseous microemboli during extracorporeal support. Together, they have edited

Anesthesiology Clin 34 (2016) xiii–xiv
http://dx.doi.org/10.1016/j.anclin.2016.09.002
1932-2275/16/© 2016 Published by Elsevier Inc.

anesthesiology.theclinics.com

an issue that provides a guide to the current state-of-the-art, science, and care around the issues of the medically complex patient.

Lee A. Fleisher, MD, FACC, FAHA
Perelman School of Medicine
University of Pennsylvania
3400 Spruce Street, Dulles 680
Philadelphia, PA 19104, USA

E-mail address:
Lee.Fleisher@uphs.upenn.edu

Preface

Medically Complex Patients

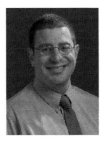 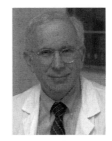

Robert B. Schonberger, MD, MHS   Stanley H. Rosenbaum, MA, MD
Editors

Life is complex, and caring for patients in the face of medical complexity is what physicians do every day. But what exactly do we mean by medical complexity? For the present issue of *Anesthesiology Clinics*, we have conceived of complexity as arising out of the interactions of multiple physiologic systems. Specifically, how should we care for patients who have dysfunction in multiple organ systems and for whom the demands of those organ systems appear to conflict?

The old adage that cardiologists like patients "dry" and nephrologists like them "wet" must seem strangely unfocused to the non-medical person. But, while it is intuitively obvious that our bodies perform best when they are treated as an appropriately integrated whole, the reality of our patients' diseases offers daily and persistent challenges to this unified vision. For the complex medical patient, sometimes the body is divided against itself, and the anesthesiologist or other critical care physician must prioritize, temporize, and compromise to shepherd a person safely through the perioperative care episode.

Each of the following articles approaches one aspect of medical complexity for the anesthesiologist. Although it is true that "hard cases make bad law," in the critical care environment, it is the hard cases that bring out our best. We thank each of

Anesthesiology Clin 34 (2016) xv–xvi
http://dx.doi.org/10.1016/j.anclin.2016.09.001
1932-2275/16/© 2016 Elsevier Inc. All rights reserved.

anesthesiology.theclinics.com

the authors for taking on some very hard cases; we hope they will teach you as they have taught us.

Robert B. Schonberger, MD, MHS
Department of Anesthesiology
Yale School of Medicine
333 Cedar Street, TMP-3
New Haven, CT 06520, USA

Stanley H. Rosenbaum, MA, MD
Division of Perioperative & Adult Anesthesia
Department of Anesthesiology
Yale School of Medicine
333 Cedar Street
New Haven, CT 06520, USA

E-mail addresses:
robert.schonberger@yale.edu (R.B. Schonberger)
stanley.rosenbaum@yale.edu (S.H. Rosenbaum)

Anesthetic Management of the Adult Patient with Concomitant Cardiac and Pulmonary Disease

Misty A. Radosevich, MD*, Daniel R. Brown, MD, PhD

KEYWORDS

- Anesthesia • Obstructive lung disease • COPD • Asthma • Restrictive lung disease
- Pulmonary hypertension • Systolic heart failure • Diastolic heart failure

KEY POINTS

- Balancing the demands of concurrent heart and lung disease during the administration of anesthesia can be challenging, but understanding the physiology behind each disease process allows for thoughtful management of each and minimizes the adverse effects resulting from such coexisting conditions.
- Management of left heart failure and valvular lesions in the setting of lung disease focuses on reducing forces that contribute to increased pulmonary venous pressure and possible resultant pulmonary congestion or edema.
- Right ventricular (RV) failure is intimately tied to the status of the pulmonary system, and management efforts are best directed at reducing or avoiding excessive RV afterload imposed by the pulmonary vasculature and thoracic pressures.
- Management of patients with pulmonary disease resulting in cor pulmonale similarly includes efforts to, where possible, reduce pulmonary vascular resistance (PVR), including avoiding hypoxia, hypercarbia, high positive end-expiratory pressure (PEEP), high intrathoracic pressure, pain, hypothermia, and N_2O.
- Many factors interact to affect the clinical picture of patients with concomitant heart and lung disease. It follows that anesthetic management requires careful attention to multiple interacting forces to optimize intraoperative care.

INTRODUCTION

Anesthesiologists are increasingly faced with complex patients suffering from multiple comorbidities and often of advanced age. As the population ages, many disease processes develop or progress. Many of these aging individuals seek medical care,

Department of Anesthesiology and Critical Care, Mayo Clinic, 200 First Street Southwest, Rochester, MN 55905, USA
* Corresponding author.
E-mail address: Radosevich.Misty@mayo.edu

Anesthesiology Clin 34 (2016) 633–643
http://dx.doi.org/10.1016/j.anclin.2016.06.001   **anesthesiology.theclinics.com**

including procedures requiring anesthetic care. In some cases, the appropriate management or natural course of one disease has important consequences for a concomitant condition and, subsequently, optimal management. These interactions make the delivery of anesthesia challenging for providers. Such competing priorities may be seen in patients with concomitant heart and lung disease, and this review describes interactions of the heart and lung in disease and outlines key points in management of specific scenarios.

CARDIOVASCULAR DISEASE AND EFFECTS ON THE PULMONARY SYSTEM
Heart Failure

Left heart systolic dysfunction
The etiology of left ventricular (LV) failure or dysfunction is commonly due to ischemia or infarction related to coronary artery disease (CAD) but may also be secondary to toxins, radiation, infections, congenital diseases, chronic valvular disease, or idiopathic in nature.

The basic abnormality in left heart failure is a reduction in cardiac output (CO) that leads to an imbalance between systemic oxygen delivery and metabolic needs of the body. Extensive compensatory mechanisms characterize heart failure and have important implications in disease management. Increased sympathetic outflow, activation of the renin-angiotensin-aldosterone system, and antidiuretic hormone secretion represent the efforts of the body to maintain CO in the setting of reduced systolic function. Chronic management focuses on reducing the maladaptive effects of these compensatory mechanisms (LV remodeling, elevated systemic vascular resistance [SVR], and fluid retention).

Fluid retention can become maladaptive and result in reduced pulmonary vascular compliance secondary to vascular congestion or pulmonary edema associated with elevated filling pressures, which are transmitted to the pulmonary venous system. Concomitant lung disease, such as chronic obstructive pulmonary disease (COPD), reduces pulmonary reserve in these patients. Even modest degrees of pulmonary edema or reductions in vital capacity related to low pulmonary vascular compliance and vascular congestion may lead to respiratory distress or failure.

Anesthetic management of patients with LV systolic dysfunction takes into consideration the compensatory mechanisms in place, which may be currently maintaining a patient's hemodynamics. Induction of anesthesia may reduce the sympathetic outflow on which these patients rely and precipitate decompensation, emphasizing the importance of careful titration of induction agents.

Maintenance of anesthesia should include avoiding LV volume overload by judicious fluid management. Fluid management may be challenging and relies on clinical judgment and context. Titrating fluid administration to balance ongoing losses and fluid shifts related to capillary leak is ideally guided by trending filling pressures or other measures of intravascular volume, if available. Miscalculation of fluid management may lead to pulmonary edema and/or progressive systolic dysfunction. Excessive reductions in myocardial contractility are limited by reducing doses of volatile agents and maintaining coronary perfusion pressure (CPP). Measures to reduce afterload (without compromising CPP) and avoidance of sudden and significant increases in SVR have a favorable impact on myocardial work. Although the afterload reduction related to volatile agents and intravenous anesthetics is favorable to the failing left heart, It should be considered that intravenous fluids administered in the setting of anesthetic-induced vasodilation may not be tolerated as preoperative SVR returns when anesthetic agents are discontinued. With a return to baseline SVR, a relative state of volume overload and subsequent decompensation with pulmonary congestion or edema may develop.

At the extremes of heart failure, patients may require mechanical support with an intra-aortic balloon pump or ventricular assist device.

Management
1. Judicious fluid management
2. Maintaining adequate coronary perfusion pressure (CPP)
3. Minimizing anesthetic-associated myocardial depression, for example, careful selection and titration of intravenous and volatile agents
4. Avoiding sudden and excessive increases in SVR as may be seen with induction, incision, or light anesthesia

Diastolic dysfunction

Heart failure with preserved ejection fraction, or diastolic dysfunction, is an increasingly appreciated condition and is notable because patients with this condition may be even more prone than those with systolic heart failure to pulmonary complications related to commonly encountered perioperative events, such as tachycardia and volume shifts. Management of this population differs from that for systolic dysfunction in important ways that have an impact on their anesthetic management.

The principal abnormality in diastolic dysfunction is a noncompliant LV and may often present with a reduced LV chamber size. The physical changes of the ventricle commonly result from compensatory ventricular remodeling in the setting of several conditions, including long-standing systemic hypertension and aortic stenosis, impaired relaxation due to myocardial ischemia, or genetically mediated as in hypertrophic cardiomyopathies. Volume management takes into consideration the stiff ventricle in these conditions. Inadequate preload can compromise CO by underfilling the LV and exacerbating LV outflow tract obstruction in those with hypertrophic cardiomyopathy. Likewise, venodilation is not well tolerated if venous return is decreased enough to result in reduced ventricular preload. Due to the poorly compliant nature of the LV in diastolic dysfunction, adequate filling during diastole is time dependent. Tachycardia and arrhythmias are poorly tolerated because diastolic time is disproportionately reduced with increasing heart rates. Atrial fibrillation is particularly problematic due to the loss of atrial kick, which becomes a greater and greater contributor to LV diastolic filling as ventricular compliance declines.

The pulmonary complications seen with diastolic dysfunction are those related to elevated LV and atrial filling pressures, which are transmitted to the pulmonary venous system. Such pressure increases may precipitate pulmonary vascular congestion, reduced pulmonary compliance, and pulmonary edema. Flash pulmonary edema can occur in the setting of sudden increases in LV diastolic pressures, including myocardial ischemia, hypertensive emergencies, and acute aortic and mitral regurgitation. Again, as in LV systolic dysfunction or failure, patients with concomitant lung disease may lack the pulmonary reserve to compensate for increases in pulmonary vascular volume or the development of edema and an associated decrease in pulmonary compliance. Management of such complications requires treatment of the underlying cause, that is, rate and rhythm control in rapid atrial fibrillation, reperfusion of an occluded coronary artery, urgent control of blood pressure in hypertensive emergencies, and afterload reduction until early surgical repair can be undertaken in acute valvular dysfunction.

Management
1. Maintain normal sinus rhythm, avoid tachycardia.
2. Avoid hypovolemia but avoid excessive preload.

3. Avoid significant reductions in SVR.
4. Maintain adequate CPP in the setting of increased LV diastolic pressure.

Right ventricular dysfunction

Discussion regarding heart failure has commonly focused on LV dysfunction. The clinical significance of right ventricular (RV) dysfunction, however, is increasingly appreciated. Of particular importance to an anesthesia provider is the interaction of the pulmonary vasculature and intrathoracic pressures as they affect the right heart.

Right heart dysfunction/failure is frequently associated with left heart failure. There are several other conditions, however, that may precipitate RV dysfunction, including chronic lung disease, acute respiratory distress syndrome (ARDS), pulmonary embolus (PE), tricuspid or pulmonary valve regurgitation or stenosis, sleep-disordered breathing syndromes, pulmonary hypertension (PH), and RV ischemia/infarction. Right heart failure has been reported to occur in up to 20% to 50% of LV assist device cases.[1]

Pulmonary physiology and disease can have important consequences for the RV and thus are important to appreciate in managing RV failure. Acute and chronic lung disease may precipitate changes in PVR and increase RV afterload with or without reduction in RV stroke volume. Relevant factors related to pulmonary disease include hypoxia, development of auto-PEEP, and hypercapnia, including permissive hypercapnia associated with lung-protective ventilation strategies. Application of high PEEP and high intrathoracic pressure further contribute to increased RV workload. Minimizing the aforementioned variables reduces stress on the RV and facilitate forward stroke volume and maintenance of CO in these patients. As in LV failure, at the extremes of right heart failure, patients may require mechanical circulatory support.

Management
1. Avoid hypoxia, application of high PEEP, development of auto-PEEP, high tidal volumes, and hypercapnia.
2. Be cautious with the application of lung-protective ventilation strategies because the associated hypercapnia may adversely affect the RV. Monitor $Paco_2$ and avoid sudden increases in this parameter.

Lung-protective ventilation and right heart dysfunction/failure

Several studies[2,3] and meta-analyses[3,4] have suggested reduced pulmonary complications with the use of lung-protective ventilation strategies in patients without ARDS undergoing mechanical ventilation. These studies include patients undergoing general anesthesia and requiring short-term mechanical ventilation. The implication of this is that low tidal volume, lung-protective ventilation could be applied to all comers, including those for whom the consequences of this strategy may be unfavorable due to the frequently associated hypercapnia with this strategy. Such patients include those with RV dysfunction or baseline increases in PVR (pulmonary hypertension, pulmonary embolism, LV dysfunction, and mitral valve disease). The significance of low tidal volume ventilation and possibly high PEEP ventilation strategies include, as in ARDS, permissive hypercapnia and potentially compression of alveolar vessels with high PEEP strategies. Potential consequences of these changes are an increase in RV afterload due to increased PVR and reduced RV systolic function. Observations from severe ARDS patients report hypercapnia-induced increases in PVR do result in RV systolic dysfunction.[5] High PEEP and a restrictive fluid management strategy may further disadvantage the RV by reducing venous return and RV preload.

Moreover, the direct myocardial depressant effect of hypercarbia and acidosis may also impair RV performance.

Despite these concerns, the presence of right heart dysfunction does not exclude these patients from a low tidal volume, lung-protective ventilation strategy. The demonstrated outcomes benefit of lung-protective ventilation with low tidal volumes is a strong motivating factor for the development of strategies to support the right heart and limit RV dysfunction associated with this technique to facilitate this method of ventilation. Suggested management includes increased respiratory rates to eliminate CO_2 as long as auto-PEEP is avoided. The potential impact of increased shear stress with increased respiratory rate requires further investigation but is a potential concern. Another approach is the gradual introduction of lung protective ventilation to limit hypercapnia, especially acute hypercapnia.[5] Other suggested strategies in the setting of RV dysfunction/failure aim to minimize plateau pressures and PEEP.[6] Tracheal gas insufflation may be a useful technique to reduce RV afterload because this method has been shown to enable a reduction in Pa_{CO_2} by as much as 15%,[7] and facilitate a decrease in inspiratory pressure by approximately 5 cm H_2O (when using pressure controlled ventilation) without increasing Pa_{CO_2}.[8]

Management
1. Caution must be applied when using lung-protective ventilation strategies in patients with right heart dysfunction or failure because permissive hypercapnia increases the workload of the RV and may simultaneously depress contractility.
   a. Titrate respiratory rate to Pa_{CO_2}.
   b. Gradually apply a lung-protective ventilation strategy as tolerated and avoid sudden, acute increases in CO_2.
   c. Minimize PEEP and plateau pressures to avoid further increases in PVR against which the RV must work.

Valvular Disease

Stenotic valve lesions
Mitral stenosis Mitral stenosis is most commonly related to rheumatic heart disease but is also seen in rheumatoid arthritis, systemic lupus erythematosus, carcinoid heart disease, or due to severe valvular calcification or congenital stenosis.

Symptomatic mitral stenosis is frequently associated with dyspnea and poor exercise tolerance. Shortness of breath may be due to either reduced CO related to flow limitation created by the stenotic lesion and/or transmission of elevated left atrial (LA) pressures to the pulmonary vasculature, producing reduced pulmonary compliance and vital capacity. Pulmonary function can be adversely affected in these patients with increases in CO, tachycardia, and atrial arrhythmias. Increases in CO associated with fluid administration, pregnancy, anemia, fever, and sepsis are poorly tolerated as the transvalvular gradient increases and LA pressure rises, further straining the upstream pulmonary vasculature. Likewise, tachycardia reduces available time for LA emptying and increases end-diastolic volume and pressure. Atrial fibrillation develops in approximately 50% of these patients, increasing in incidence with age and LA diameter.[9] This arrhythmia further compromises function through loss of atrial contraction because coordinated atrial activity is often needed to overcome the pressure gradient across the mitral valve. As in other conditions raising LA pressure, elevated pulmonary venous pressures result and predispose to reduced pulmonary compliance, edema and potentially RV dysfunction. Persistently elevated pulmonary venous pressures may in severe cases cause pulmonary capillary rupture and subsequent hemoptysis.

Aortic stenosis The aortic stenosis lesion is commonly seen in elderly patients due to calcification of the aortic valve or in younger patients related to a bicuspid aortic valve. In the developing world, aortic stenosis (AS) may be found as a sequela of rheumatic heart disease. Although symptoms related to the AS may include dyspnea, the primary driver for symptoms is flow limitation created by the stenotic valve and subsequently reduced CO. The pulmonary system is not prominently affected in AS unless heart failure or mitral valve disease develop as a consequence of the disease.

Management
1. Maintain normal sinus rhythm; specifically, avoid tachycardia and loss of atrial contraction.
2. Avoid sudden and significant increases in CO.
3. Avoid precipitants of pulmonary vasoconstriction in those with evidence of RV dysfunction.

Regurgitant valve lesions
Mitral regurgitation As in mitral stenosis, symptoms of mitral regurgitation (MR) are related to either reduced forward stroke volume, increased pulmonary venous pressure, or a combination of the two. The causes of MR are more diverse than those related to mitral stenosis, including papillary muscle or chordae tendineae rupture related to ischemia or trauma, valvular destruction in the setting of endocarditis, mitral valve prolapse, myxomatous degeneration, and functional abnormality related to a dilated LV.

The pulmonary manifestations are, as in mitral stenosis, those related to increased pulmonary venous pressure, reduced pulmonary compliance, and pulmonary artery hypertension. Acute mitral insufficiency as in trauma or ischemia/infarction can rapidly produce pulmonary edema because the left atrium is suddenly exposed to high pressure and volume from regurgitant flow. This elevated pressure is transmitted back to the pulmonary system and acute, or flash, pulmonary edema ensues. The left atrium in chronic MR undergoes compensatory dilation to accommodate the regurgitant volume associated with the incompetent valve and, therefore, is associated with lower pressures, effectively protecting the pulmonary vasculature.

Principles of management in mitral regurgitation involve reducing SVR to promote forward systemic flow and reducing LV volume to improve valve coaptation. Heart rate is best maintained in the high-normal range (80–100 bpm) to reduce regurgitant time and ventricular overfilling, which promotes mitral annular dilation and reduces valvular coaptation. Fluid management should avoid excessive volume administration that would further dilate the LV. The dilated ventricle may benefit, however, from modest preload augmentation and may be necessary in those with reduced ventricular function or those with volume depletion. In acute, severe decompensation, intra-aortic balloon counterpulsation may be of benefit by improving forward flow, reducing regurgitant fraction, and improving CPP. To the same end, mechanical circulatory support devices may be considered as well.

Aortic regurgitation Aortic regurgitation (AR) may be acute or chronic in nature and symptoms related to the disease depend on the acuity of the regurgitation.

Acute AR may develop secondary to endocarditis, trauma, or aortic dissection. The hemodynamic consequences of acute AR are related to an acute reduction in effective forward stroke volume and subsequent cardiogenic shock. Pulmonary consequences are related to rapid increases in LV end-diastolic volume and pressure and the precipitation of pulmonary edema. This state is similar in clinical presentation and management as in acute MR in that interventions aim to reduce afterload, maintain compensatory increases in HR, and appropriate volume management. Consideration may be given to augmentation of contractility as well.

The indolent nature of chronic AR leads to adaptation by the LV, which accommodates the increased end-diastolic volumes associated with the lesion. With time, however, the LV dilation associated with AR leads to systolic dysfunction and mitral valve annular dilation with subsequent MR. These changes can have upstream effects on the pulmonary vascular system, as seen in LV failure and chronic MR, such as pulmonary vascular congestion, edema, and vascular remodeling resulting in pulmonary hypertension.

Tricuspid regurgitation Tricuspid regurgitation is most often a functional defect related to annular dilation in the setting of RV dilation but may be secondary to a primary valve lesion related to causes such as endocarditis, mechanical trauma (pacemaker leads and catheters), carcinoid syndrome, or drug-induced valve disease. When severe, the hemodynamic consequences of this lesion are related to right heart failure from volume overload and reduced forward flow. Systemic effects include edema, ascites, and hepatic and renal venous congestion. These effects are exacerbated by increases in PVR. Management of severe tricuspid regurgitation includes avoidance of elevations in PVR to reduce RV afterload and the pressure gradient across the tricuspid valve driving regurgitation, maintenance of a high-normal heart rate to reduce systolic and regurgitant time, and careful volume management because hypovolemia further reduces the already decreased forward stroke volume, although hypervolemia may worsen annular dilation and hence regurgitation.

Management
1. Maintain low-normal SVR (or PVR in the case of tricuspid regurgitation) to facilitate forward flow.
2. Maintain high-normal heart rate, ideally 80 bpm to 100 bpm.
3. Avoid hypovolemia and consider modest volume administration to augment ventricular function and forward stroke volume.
4. Recognize potential for RV dysfunction related to pulmonary hypertension and avoid conditions that increase PVR.
5. Consider intra-aortic balloon counterpulsation or mechanical circulatory support devices in acute decompensated MR.

PULMONARY DISEASE AND EFFECTS ON THE CARDIOVASCULAR SYSTEM
Obstructive Lung Disease

Management of patients with obstructive pulmonary processes frequently involves issues related to hyperinflation/intrinsic PEEP and the subsequent increase in intrathoracic lung volume and pressure. The physiology of such air trapping relates to loss of elasticity of lung parenchyma, reduced structural integrity of airways, bronchoconstriction, and excess secretions.

Ventilator management considerations include avoidance of dynamic hyperinflation with its attendant risks of hemodynamic impairment and barotrauma by using

1. Low inspiratory/expiratory (I:E) ratios
2. Adequate inspiratory flow to meet the low I:E ratio and patient demand without excessively increasing peak airway pressure
3. Limiting respiratory rate and tidal volumes to facilitate adequate expiration time

The cardiovascular effects of COPD include negative effects on right, and subsequently left, ventricular filling as the pressure drop facilitating venous return and RV filling is reduced. This may be exacerbated by hypovolemia or vasodilating agents, such as anesthetic gases or some induction agents. Further impairment in ventricular filling occurs due to extrinsic pressure on the heart, in effect reducing diastolic compliance. Moreover, the pressure related to hyperinflation may be transmitted to pulmonary vessels and increase PVR, leading to increased RV afterload. Clinically, these interactions can produce systemic hypotension. Alveolar dead space increases as areas of hyperinflation compress capillaries and $Paco_2$ rises. Subsequent acidosis may lead to further increases in PVR as well as electrolyte disturbances and resultant arrhythmias.[10] Long-standing severe lung disease may cause right heart failure (cor pulmonale) in 20% to 30% of patients with COPD.[11] These patients are often managed with diuretics and may have associated electrolyte disturbances or volume depletion, the latter being worrisome in this preload-dependent state.

This population is predisposed to atrial and ventricular arrhythmias not only secondary to medication-induced electrolyte disturbances but also due to hypoxia, hypercapnia, increased sympathetic nervous system activity, and comorbidities, such as ischemic heart disease, and medications (β-agonists and theophylline). Chronic treatment often involves addressing the underlying disease and comorbid conditions: for example, supplemental oxygen; ventilation support (noninvasive or invasive); and reducing bronchoconstriction to improve oxygenation, ventilation, and respiratory-related pH alterations.

Anesthetic management includes reducing RV afterload with oxygen administration and avoidance of hypercarbia and other causes of increased PVR. Careful volume management is important to avoid septal shifting and impaired LV filling. Hypovolemia should be avoided, however, as the failing RV relies on preload to maintain contractility. RV CPP must be maintained and use of norepinephrine may be necessary to avoid a downward spiral of RV dilation, causing myocardial ischemia, with ischemia causing further RV dysfunction. Furthermore, in a hemodynamically unstable patient, inotropic therapy may be necessary (eg, dobutamine and milrinone).

A special consideration in the patient with cor pulmonale is permissive hypercapnia, a common consequence of lung-protective ventilation strategies in ARDS. This is especially relevant because several studies are suggesting benefit in using a lung-protective ventilation strategy in all ventilated patients even in the absence of lung injury (discussed previously).

Management
1. Avoiding hyperinflation/auto-PEEP
   a. Preoperative disease optimization
   b. Careful attention to ventilator management: low I:E ratios, limiting respiratory rate and tidal volumes to facilitate adequate expiration time
2. Cor pulmonale
   a. Reducing RV afterload with oxygen, avoidance of hypercarbia and other causes of increased PVR
   b. Careful volume management: avoiding hypervolemia-associated distension of the RV and septal shift-mediated impairment of LV filling; avoiding hypovolemia in the preload-dependent failing RV
   c. Inotropic therapy may be necessary (eg, dobutamine or milrinone)

3. Arrhythmias
   a. Therapy is targeted at the underlying disease. Reduce sympathetic outflow by treating hypoxia, hypercapnia, and acid-base disturbances. Caution with use of β-blockers in moderate–severe COPD

Restrictive Lung Disease

Restrictive lung disease represents a category with a substantial number of conditions, most frequently divided into extrinsic and intrinsic disease. Intrinsic processes include acute and chronic conditions, such as pulmonary edema related to CHF or ARDS, re-expansion of a previously collapsed lung, sarcoidosis, and pulmonary fibrosis related to interstitial lung disease, to name a few. Extrinsic processes include those related to the chest wall, such as obesity, scoliosis, ankylosing spondylitis, large burn scar, pleural effusion, diaphragm paralysis/dysfunction, and neuromuscular diseases.

Cardiovascular effects of restrictive lung disease may be seen in conditions, such as pulmonary fibrosis, due to progressive changes of the pulmonary vasculature (eg, loss of vessels and remodeling of vessel walls) that cause increased PVR and, later, pulmonary hypertension (defined as mean pulmonary arterial pressure >25 mm Hg at rest) and right heart failure. With time, these changes may become fixed and unresponsive to interventions such as supplemental oxygen and medical therapy. Management of this cardiopulmonary interaction is similar to that outlined for obstructive lung disease, for example, avoidance of precipitants of increased PVR, such as hypoxia, hypercapnia, acidosis, hypothermia, and nitrous oxide (N_2O). In the setting of right heart failure and low CO related to pulmonary hypertension, pulmonary vasodilator therapy may be helpful if a reversible component of pulmonary hypertension is present. Such agents include inhaled nitric oxide (NO), inhaled or intravenous prostanoids, milrinone, and dobutamine (the latter 2 have the added benefit of positive inotropy but also potential systemic vasodilation).

Management
1. Avoid precipitants of increased PVR: hypoxia, hypercapnia, acidosis, hypothermia and N_2O, and high PEEP and tidal volumes.
2. Consider pulmonary vasodilator therapy: inhaled NO, inhaled or intravenous prostanoids, milrinone, and dobutamine (the latter 2 have the added benefit of positive inotropy).

Obstructive Sleep Apnea and Obesity Hypoventilation Syndrome

Obstructive sleep apnea (OSA) has been identified as an independent risk factor for several cardiovascular diseases, including myocardial ischemia, systemic and pulmonary hypertension (PH), arrhythmias, CHF, and stroke.[12] This condition is associated with recurrent periods of arterial hypoxemia and hypercarbia which, when chronic, may lead to pulmonary hypertension (World Health Organization [WHO] group 3) and eventual right heart dysfunction or failure. More recently, left heart dysfunction and elevated pulmonary venous pressures have been implicated as a cause of pulmonary hypertension in this group.[13]

Obesity hypoventilation syndrome (OHS) is associated not only with episodes of arterial hypoxia but also more prolonged hypercarbia, which contributes to the process of PH. Similarly, systemic hypertension is frequent in these patients and often associated with LV hypertrophy, LV dysfunction, and elevated pulmonary venous pressures. Long-standing pulmonary venous and arterial hypertension leads to remodeling of the pulmonary vessels and eventual dysfunction of the RV.

Although the treatment of these conditions is best done well in advance of the perioperative period, patients may present for urgent or emergent surgery with concomitant nonoptimized or undiagnosed OSA/OHS. Management with regard to the cardiovascular implications of these conditions includes consideration of common coexisting diseases, such as obesity, diabetes mellitus, hypertension, and, as a corollary, increased risk for CAD and cardiovascular events with severe OSA.[14]

Heart failure as a consequence of severe OSA has been suggested by several studies, which have demonstrated improvement in cardiac function with CPAP therapy.[15,16] Causal or not, at the least, patients with OSA have a high association with both systolic and diastolic heart failure.[17] Suggested mechanisms for heart failure include nocturnal hypertension and decreased intrathoracic pressure due to inspiratory efforts against upper airway obstruction, which the LV must overcome to effectively contract.[18] In addition to the commonly associated diagnoses of hypertension and diabetes in OSA patients, which may contribute to CAD, OSA may directly cause CAD due to systemic inflammation, sympathetic nervous system activation associated with hypoxic and hypercarbic events, and endothelial dysfunction.[18] CAD may further impair myocardial function due to ischemia, especially in a hypertrophied or dilated ventricle as is often seen in heart failure.

Management includes maintaining adequate CPP, avoiding excessive afterload and minimizing ventricular distention due to excessive preload. Being cognizant of the potential for pulmonary hypertension in this population and avoiding factors that promote increases in PVR improve RV performance and CO. Postoperative management should include minimizing respiratory depressants, extubation when fully awake, maintenance of an upright position, and institution of noninvasive positive pressure ventilation to maintain airway patency if necessary (using a patient's own equipment if available).

Management
1. Maintain adequate CPP and avoid excessive afterload and ventricular distention with excessive preload.
2. In the OHS with known or possible PH, avoid factors that promote increases in PVR.
3. Avoid postoperative hypoventilation: minimize respiratory depressants, extubate when fully awake, maintain upright position, and institute noninvasive positive pressure ventilation to maintain airway patency if necessary.

SUMMARY

Balancing the demands of concurrent heart and lung disease during the administration of anesthesia can be challenging, but understanding the physiology behind each disease process allows for optimal patient care by balancing management priorities. Management of left heart failure and valvular lesions in the setting of lung disease focuses on reducing forces that contribute to increased pulmonary venous pressure and possible resultant pulmonary congestion or edema. RV failure is intimately tied to the status of the pulmonary system and management efforts are best directed at reducing or avoiding excessing RV afterload imposed by the pulmonary vasculature and intrathoracic pressures. Management of patients with pulmonary disease resulting in cor pulmonale similarly includes efforts to, where possible, reduce PVR, including avoiding hypoxia, hypercarbia, high PEEP and intrathoracic pressure, pain, hypothermia, and N_2O. Often there are competing priorities in patients with concomitant heart and lung disease and optimal anesthetic management requires careful prioritization and continuous reassessment.

REFERENCES

1. Argiriou M, Kolokotron SM, Sakellaridis T, et al. Right heart failure post left ventricular assist device implantation. J Thorac Dis 2014;6(Suppl 1):S52–9.
2. Futier E, Constantin JM, Paugam-Burtz C, et al. A trial of intraoperative low-tidal-volume ventilation in abdominal surgery. N Engl J Med 2013;369(5):428–37.
3. Neto AS, Simonis FD, Barbas CS, et al. Lung-protective ventilation with low tidal volumes and the occurrence of pulmonary complications in patients without acute respiratory distress syndrome: a systematic review and individual patient data analysis. Crit Care Med 2015;43(10):2155–63.
4. Hemmes SN, Serpa Neto A, Schultz MJ. Intraoperative ventilatory strategies to prevent postoperative pulmonary complications: a meta-analysis. Curr Opin Anaesthesiol 2013;26(2):126–33.
5. Zochios V, Jones N. Acute right heart syndrome in the critically ill patient. Heart Lung Vessel 2014;6(3):157–70.
6. Repesse X, Charron C, Vieillard-Baron A. Right ventricular failure in acute lung injury and acute respiratory distress syndrome. Minerva Anestesiol 2012;78(8): 941–8.
7. Ravenscraft SA, Burke WC, Nahum A, et al. Tracheal gas insufflation augments CO_2 clearance during mechanical ventilation. Am Rev Respir Dis 1993;148(2): 345–51.
8. Hoffman LA, Miro AM, Tasota FJ, et al. Tracheal gas insufflation. Limits of efficacy in adults with acute respiratory distress syndrome. Am J Respir Crit Care Med 2000;162(2 Pt 1):387–92.
9. Diker E, Aydogdu S, Ozdemir M, et al. Prevalence and predictors of atrial fibrillation in rheumatic valvular heart disease. Am J Cardiol 1996;77(1):96–8.
10. Edrich T, Sadovnikoff N. Anesthesia for patients with severe chronic obstructive pulmonary disease. Curr Opin Anaesthesiol 2010;23(1):18–24.
11. Naeije R. Pulmonary hypertension and right heart failure in chronic obstructive pulmonary disease. Proc Am Thorac Soc 2005;2(1):20–2.
12. Bradley TD, Floras JS. Obstructive sleep apnoea and its cardiovascular consequences. Lancet 2009;373(9657):82–93.
13. Kholdani C, Fares WH, Mohsenin V. Pulmonary hypertension in obstructive sleep apnea: is it clinically significant? A critical analysis of the association and pathophysiology. Pulm Circ 2015;5(2):220–7.
14. Marin JM, Carrizo SJ, Vicente E, et al. Long-term cardiovascular outcomes in men with obstructive sleep apnoea-hypopnoea with or without treatment with continuous positive airway pressure: an observational study. Lancet 2005;365(9464): 1046–53.
15. Kaneko Y, Floras JS, Usui K, et al. Cardiovascular effects of continuous positive airway pressure in patients with heart failure and obstructive sleep apnea. N Engl J Med 2003;348(13):1233–41.
16. Arias MA, Garcia-Rio F, Alonso-Fernandez A, et al. Obstructive sleep apnea syndrome affects left ventricular diastolic function: effects of nasal continuous positive airway pressure in men. Circulation 2005;112(3):375–83.
17. Wang H, Parker JD, Newton GE, et al. Influence of obstructive sleep apnea on mortality in patients with heart failure. J Am Coll Cardiol 2007;49(15):1625–31.
18. Gottlieb DJ, Yenokyan G, Newman AB, et al. Prospective study of obstructive sleep apnea and incident coronary heart disease and heart failure: the sleep heart health study. Circulation 2010;122(4):352–60.

Anesthesia for the Patient with Concomitant Hepatic and Renal Impairment

Tricia E. Brentjens, MD*, Ryan Chadha, MD

KEYWORDS

- Acute versus chronic hepatic failure • Acute versus chronic renal failure
- RIFLE criteria • Intraoperative organ protection • Model for end-stage liver disease
- Liver and kidney transplantation

KEY POINTS

- Hepatic and renal disease are prevalent in the general population and must be managed appropriately by anesthesiologists.
- Preoperative optimization, intraoperative end-organ protection, and an anesthetic plan to control physiologic derangement are the cornerstones of an effective management strategy.
- Evaluation of these patients must include an understanding of their current disease pathophysiology (with pharmacologic and nonpharmacologic treatment), risk stratification, and a detailed preoperative evaluation.
- The ultimate treatment of end-stage hepatic or renal disease is organ transplantation.

INTRODUCTION

Hepatic and renal disease are becoming common comorbidities in patients presenting for intermediate and high-risk surgery. Reasons for this development are an aging population, better long-term survival of patients, and continuously improving outcomes after surgery, and with critical care medicine.[1] With the evolution of perioperative medicine, anesthesiologists are encountering more patients who have significant hepatic and renal disease, acute and chronic in nature. Acute hepatic failure is usually defined as deterioration of liver function in an 8- to 28-day time period, whereas chronic liver disease is defined as more than 6 months in duration. Similarly, acute renal failure and acute kidney injury are defined as a decrease in function over 7 days, and chronic renal failure presents over months to years. Renal disease has been further defined by the RIFLE criteria (**Table 1**).[2]

Department of Anesthesiology, College of Physicians and Surgeons, Columbia University, 622 West 168th Street-PH 5, New York, NY 10032, USA
* Corresponding author.
E-mail address: tb164@cumc.columbia.edu

Anesthesiology Clin 34 (2016) 645–658
http://dx.doi.org/10.1016/j.anclin.2016.06.002   **anesthesiology.theclinics.com**

Table 1
RIFLE criteria

Stage	GFR Criteria	Urine Output Criteria
Risk	Increased Cr × 1.5 or GFR decrease >25%	UOP <0.5 mL/kg/h × 6 h
Injury	Increased Cr × 2 or GFR decrease >50%	UOP <0.5 mL/kg/h × 12 h
Failure	Increased Cr × 3 or GFR decrease >75% OR Cr >4 mg/dL or acute rise >0.5 mg/dL	UOP <0.3 mL/kg/h × 24 h OR Anuria × 12 h
Loss of function	Persistent ARF × 4 wk	
ESRD	ESRD for >3 mo	

Abbreviations: ARF, acute renal failure; Cr, creatinine; ESRD, end-stage renal disease; GFR, glomerular filtration rate; UOP, urine output.

Data from Wagener G, Brentjens T. Renal disease: the anesthesiologist's perspective. Anesthesiol Clin 2006;24:523–47.

It is important that anesthesiologists have an in-depth understanding of the physiologic derangements seen with hepatic and renal disease to evaluate and manage these patients appropriately. Perioperative management requires an understanding of the physiologic perturbations associated with each disease process. This article elucidates the goals in the management and treatment of this complex patient population.

PATIENT EVALUATION OVERVIEW
Etiologies, Clinical Signs, and Systems-Based Physiology of Hepatic and Renal Disease

Hepatic and renal disease have different etiologies, clinical signs, and physiologic characteristics. Causes of acute liver failure are most commonly acetaminophen toxicity followed by acute viral hepatitis, whereas chronic hepatic disease is most commonly secondary to hepatitis B or C and alcoholism. Rare causes include primary biliary cirrhosis, Wilson disease, and hemochromatosis.[3] Acute renal failure is usually classified as prerenal (caused by a state of hypoperfusion, such as hypovolemia or sepsis), intrarenal (nephrotoxic substances, such as contrast, aminoglycosides, or nonsteroidal anti-inflammatory drugs), or postrenal (obstruction caused by kidney stones, benign prostatic hypertrophy, or bladder neck obstruction). Chronic kidney disease is secondary to systemic conditions, such as diabetes mellitus, hypertension, or rare glomerular diseases.[2] **Box 1** reviews the clinical signs of both diseases.

The physiologic characteristics of hepatic disease involve several perturbations to multiple organ systems. The cardiovascular system develops a hyperdynamic state caused by low systemic vascular resistance secondary to the lack of hepatic clearance of vasodilatory substances. Another comorbidity of significance is portopulmonary hypertension, found in 0.4% to 2.5% of patients with cirrhosis. This is

Box 1
Clinical signs of hepatic and renal disease

Hepatic Disease
Jaundice, fatigue, asterixis, ascites, gynecomastia, spider angiomata, palmar erythema

Renal Disease
Fatigue, numbness, nausea, abdominal pain, hypertension, edema, difficulty urinating, discoloration of urine

defined by a mean pulmonary artery pressure greater than 25 mm Hg and a pulmonary vascular resistance greater than 240 dynexsxcm̄-5. Patients with alcoholic, amyloid, and Wilson liver disease are prone to the development of cirrhotic cardiomyopathy, which is a state of systolic and diastolic dysfunction.[4] The pulmonary system is prone to the development of restrictive physiology, which can be secondary to the presence of large volume ascites, pleural effusions, and/or hepatic hydrothorax. A unique pathology is hepatopulmonary syndrome involving a state of pulmonary vasodilation leading to orthodeoxia (hypoxia while sitting up, improves on lying down), and platypnea (dyspnea while sitting up, improving on lying down).[1]

Fluid retention is common in the patients with cirrhosis and is caused by low systemic vascular resistance and splanchnic vasodilation, hypoalbuminemia, portal hypertension, and secondary hyperaldosteronism. Electrolyte abnormalities common in hepatic disease include hyponatremia and hypokalemia. Hyponatremia is secondary to fluid overload or nonosmotic hypersecretion of arginine vasopressin from the pituitary. Hypokalemia is caused by hyperaldosteronism and diuretic use. These patients frequently have a metabolic alkalosis, which is caused by intravascular volume depletion.[5] The most severe renal complication is hepatorenal syndrome, which is defined by a high plasma creatinine and a low urine sodium concentration in the absence of intrinsic renal disease. Hepatorenal syndrome is a rapidly progressive manifestation of end-stage liver disease and associated with a mortality of 50% within a month of onset.[6]

The gastrointestinal manifestations of hepatic disease include a risk of aspiration caused by increased intra-abdominal pressure secondary to ascites and a bleeding risk caused by presence of gastric and esophageal varices. Malnutrition is common secondary to poor protein intake and decreased albumin levels. Neurologically, this patient population is at risk for hepatic encephalopathy, a neuropsychiatric complication associated with high ammonia levels but with an incompletely understood pathogenesis. Symptoms can range from mild confusion to coma. Hematologic derangements include decreased synthesis of coagulation factors, dysfunctional platelets and thrombocytopenia, and dysfibrinogenemia, which put the patient at risk for bleeding. Conversely, decreased levels of protein C and S, and antithrombin increase the risk for thrombotic events.[5]

Similarly, renal disease leads to significant multiorgan dysfunction. Significant systemic hypertension may be present requiring multiple agents for adequate control. Left ventricular hypertrophy and diastolic dysfunction are prevalent, with poor tolerance of myocardial ischemia and high risk for volume overload. Hyperlipidemia promotes accelerated atherosclerosis and arteriovenous fistulas can lead to high-output cardiac failure. Common electrolyte disturbances found in renal disease include a moderate compensated anion gap acidosis, hyperkalemia (which can be triggered by catabolic stress, potassium-sparing diuretics, acidosis, and red blood cell transfusion), and significant derangements in magnesium and phosphate handling.[6]

Gastrointestinal derangements are important to consider in this population. Protein malnutrition is common, and uremia can lead to decreased gastric emptying with increased risk of aspiration. Neurologic manifestations range from drowsiness to myoclonus and seizures. Distal sensorimotor neuropathy and autonomic neuropathy are common in patients undergoing dialysis. In terms of hematologic function, normocytic anemia is secondary to decreased erythropoietin and chronic blood loss, and uremic coagulopathy can result in defective release of von Willebrand factor and significant platelet dysfunction.

Risk Stratification

Acute hepatitis has been associated with poor perioperative outcomes. Nonemergency procedures should be postponed until patients have recovered from their acute liver injury. Chronic liver disease is risk stratified using two scoring systems: the Child-Turcotte-Pugh and the Model for End-Stage Liver Disease score (**Table 2**). Patients in Child-Turcotte-Pugh class A tolerate surgery well, whereas those in class B (especially for cardiac surgery and abdominal surgery including hepatic resection) and class C are at high risk. The 90-day mortality in Child-Turcotte-Pugh class A, B, and C was found to be 2%, 22%, and 55%, respectively. However, the variability in assignments of scores has limited its usage.[7] The Model for End-Stage Liver Disease score has been validated in predicting outcome in nontransplant surgery. A score of 15 represents one possible cutoff for a significant increase in poor outcomes.[4] Also, the type of surgical procedure influences perioperative outcomes, because abdominal, laparotomy, cholecystectomy, cardiac, bariatric, and emergent procedures are associated with significant increases in mortality.[1]

Renal disease has been validated in numerous studies as a risk factor for serious postoperative complications. A creatinine value of 2 mg/dL has been found to be an independent risk factor for cardiac complications, and a predictor for postoperative renal failure.[8] Acute kidney injury has been implicated in multiple studies as a risk factor for postoperative mortality after noncardiac and cardiac surgery, emphasizing the importance of postponing nonemergent procedures until any potentially reversible kidney injury has resolved.[9,10]

Preoperative Evaluation

Finally, the appropriate preoperative evaluation must be performed to show the current physiologic state of the patient. **Box 2** reviews an approach to this evaluation.[5,9,11–13]

MANAGEMENT GOALS

The management of hepatic and renal disease spans the perioperative period. After appropriate preoperative evaluation and risk stratification of their current condition, goals include optimization, intraoperative organ protection, and perioperative anesthetic physiologic management.

Table 2
The Child-Turcotte-Pugh score and the Model for End-Stage Liver Disease score

Characteristic	1 Point	2 Points	3 Points
Ascites	None	Controlled	Refractory
Encephalopathy	Absent	Controlled	Dense
Albumin (g/L)	>3.5	2.8–3.5	<2.8
Bilirubin (mg/dL)	<2	2.0–3.0	>3
INR	<1.7	1.7–2.3	>2.3

Abbreviations: CTP, Child-Turcotte-Pugh; INR, international normalized ratio.
CTP class A: 5–6 points, 4% 3-month mortality. CTP class B: 7–9 points, 14% 3-month mortality. CTP class C: 10–15 points, 51% 3-month mortality.
Model for End Stage Liver Disease score = $(.957 \times \log e \, [\text{serum Cr (mg/dL)}] + .378 \times \log e \, [\text{serum bilirubin (mg/dL)}] + 1.120 \times \log e \, [\text{INR}]) \times 10$.
Minimum for all values is 1, and maximum value for creatinine is 4.

Box 2
Preoperative evaluation for chronic hepatic and renal disease

1. Detailed preoperative history and physical
   a. Hepatic disease: cause of cirrhosis, recent exacerbation (variceal bleed, infections, worsening encephalopathy), signs of end-stage liver disease (encephalopathy, coagulopathy, varices, ascites), date of most recent paracentesis, presence of hepatopulmonary and hepatorenal syndromes.
   b. Renal disease: cause of renal disease, acute versus chronic renal failure, if currently on dialysis date of last session, dialysis access.

2. Laboratory testing
   a. Complete blood count with differential.
   b. Coagulation profile including fibrinogen.
   c. Comprehensive metabolic panel including liver function tests.
   d. Type and screen, especially in the setting of previous transfusion, to rule out the presence of antibodies.

3. Cardiac testing
   a. Hepatic disease: depending on the American Heart Association risk stratification of the patient and surgery, appropriate cardiac testing should be performed. Dobutamine stress and/or a nuclear stress test reveal most coronary artery disease and cardiomyopathy. In the setting of elevated right ventricular systolic pressure, a right heart catheterization is recommended to assess degree of pulmonary hypertension.
   b. Renal disease: depending on the American Heart Association risk stratification of the patient and surgery, appropriate cardiac testing should be performed. Nuclear stress versus dobutamine stress is able to assess for potential coronary artery disease. Coronary computed tomography scan may be another consideration in the setting of significant coronary artery calcification.

4. Assessment of liver function: although liver function tests and abdominal ultrasound studies can indicate liver disease, they are not able to quantify the severity of disease. Indocyanine green clearance and lidocaine clearance have been used to better assess the degree of functional hepatic tissue.

Preoperative Optimization

Optimization of hepatic disease is multifocal, regardless of whether the patient is suffering from acute or chronic liver disease.

- Active conditions triggering an exacerbation must be stabilized.
  - Gastrointestinal bleed secondary to varices
  - Infection
  - Volume overload
  - Electrolyte abnormalities; most importantly hyponatremia. Several studies have found hyponatremia to be associated with a significant risk of postoperative mortality, and this risk is increased in patients with liver disease.[14]
- Encephalopathy should be monitored closely and treated aggressively. A sudden change in mental status should raise concern for cerebral edema or elevated ammonia levels.
- Treatment of coagulopathy must be balanced versus risk of thrombosis.
- End-organ conditions, such as hepatorenal, hepatopulmonary, and cirrhotic cardiomyopathy, must be treated supportively because the only treatment is transplantation.[4]

The optimization of patients with renal disease is relative to their need for dialysis.

- Dialysis-dependent patients should receive dialysis ideally the day of or day before surgery to achieve the most physiologic fluid, electrolyte, and acid-base status.
- Patients with acute renal failure may benefit from interventions to maintain urine output because nonoliguric renal failure has been shown to have better renal outcomes than oliguric renal failure.[15]
- In the setting of severe anemia, correcting to a physiologic hematocrit may be appropriate.[5]

Intraoperative Organ Protection

Although a rare event, perioperative liver failure is associated with significant morbidity and mortality, especially in patients with liver disease. In addition to underlying cirrhosis, risk factors include significant intraoperative blood loss and age greater than 70 years. Intraoperative liver protection involves preserving hepatic blood flow while minimizing hepatic venous congestion. Avoidance of ischemia and edema in the liver are of higher importance during hepatic resection, where the degree of ischemia-reperfusion injury plays a significant role in outcome.[16]

In patients with renal disease not requiring renal-replacement therapy, it is important to preserve remaining renal function. Maintenance of oxygen delivery and minimizing oxygen demand to the kidneys is critical, as is the suppression of renovascular constriction and promotion of renal vasodilation. Although preoperative angiotensin-converting enzyme inhibitors are a matter of continued investigation, their role in long-term kidney disease is central. Maintenance of tubular flow is also recommended because common practice is to maintain urine output greater than 0.5 mL/kg/h. Renal injury is common in vascular, cardiac, and transplant procedures and many practitioners institute pharmacologic renal-protection strategies with diuretic and inotropic drugs despite the lack of supporting data.[17]

Perioperative Anesthetic Physiologic Management

In terms of anesthetic technique, regional anesthesia is often not an option because of coagulopathy and thrombocytopenia so general anesthesia is the most common choice. Induction considerations include rapid sequence induction because of the presence of ascites with the addition of reverse Trendelenburg to minimize desaturation by increasing functional residual capacity. Premedication should be avoided in the setting of encephalopathy to reduce risk of aspiration. Propofol is a good choice for an induction agent because of its rapid clearance secondary to lipid solubility. However, it should be used judiciously because it depresses the circulation through inhibition of reflex tachycardia and vasodilation. Maintenance of anesthesia is traditionally with volatile agents, isoflurane having the smallest effect on hepatic blood flow. In patients with increased intracranial pressures, maintenance with intravenous anesthetics, such as propofol, may reduce cerebral blood flow.[5,18]

Intraoperative management for patients with hepatic disease includes the choice of appropriate monitoring. Invasive blood pressure monitoring is recommended in intermediate- and high-risk surgery because of the likelihood of hemorrhage and altered hemodynamics during surgery. Central access is often required for the administration of vasopressors and inotropes. Pulmonary artery catheter placement may be helpful to monitor volume status to prevent hepatic congestion.

There are significant alterations in drug metabolism with hepatic disease. In terms of neuromuscular blockade, the duration of action of succinylcholine may be prolonged because of decreased pseudocholinesterase levels. Rocuronium is dependent on biliary metabolism and vecuronium is metabolized to 3-hydroxyvecuronium, which is active at the neuromuscular junction, so the effect of both may be prolonged. Cistatracurium is metabolized by Hoffman degradation, so it is minimally affected. For analgesic management, acetaminophen should be used with caution because of its liver metabolism and potential toxicity. Opioids with the exception of remifentanyl are all dependent on hepatic biotransformation and should be dosed accordingly.[18]

In patients with renal disease, venous access may be difficult because of the presence of arteriovenous fistulas and grafts. Intraoperative monitoring may include invasive blood pressure monitoring because of the high incidence of cardiomyopathy and coronary artery disease in this population. The choice of anesthetic depends on the procedure. Regional anesthesia is an attractive option, with the caveat that many patients take antiplatelet medications that could preclude its use. If general anesthesia is chosen, full stomach precautions should be considered for patients with diabetes and autonomic neuropathy. For induction, succinylcholine is an option, but should be avoided when the potassium is elevated. During the maintenance of anesthesia, it should be noted that positive pressure ventilation, hypoxia, and hypercarbia lead to decreases in renal blood flow.[8]

As with hepatic disease, there are alterations in pharmacology in patients with renal disease. Rocuronium and vecuronium are 30% dependent on renal excretion so their duration of action may be prolonged. Cisatracurium and atracurium are both metabolized by Hoffman degradation and thus are unaffected by renal disease. Nonsteroidal anti-inflammatory agents are often avoided because of the risk of worsening renal failure. Fentanyl and hydromorphone are the preferred narcotic agents because morphine and meperidine have active metabolites that accumulate in renal disease. Sevoflurane has been shown to produce elevated fluoride levels in combination with CO_2 absorbents, creating Compound A, which has resulted in renal failure in animal models. However, this has never been demonstrated to have clinical relevance in human studies.[19]

PHARMACOLOGIC STRATEGIES FOR MANAGEMENT

There are several pharmacologic means of optimizing patients with hepatic disease before surgery.

- In the setting of acute upper gastrointestinal bleeding, proton pump inhibitors (eg, pantoprazole, esmoprazole, omeprazole) are commonly used.[20] β-Blocker therapy (eg, nadolol or propranolol) can prevent rebleeding from varices by reducing portal pressure.
- Common infections seen in patients with hepatic disease are spontaneous bacterial peritonitis, bacteremia caused by gut flora translocation, and pneumonia. These are most commonly caused by gram-negative pneumococcus, which depending on resistances can be treated with pencillins (eg, piperacillin-tazobactam), cephalosporins (eg, ceftriaxone), or carbapenems (eg, meropenem, imipenem).[21]
- Ascites is treated with diuretics (furosemide and spironolactone), which often render patients hypovolemic. Spironolactone has a half-life of 2 to 3 days, so this is sometimes stopped preoperatively to prevent intraoperative hyperkalemia.[6]
- Hyponatremia is the most common electrolyte abnormality found in hepatic disease. Although nonpharmacologic strategies are more commonly used in management, hypertonic saline is a consideration in patients with neurologic symptoms.

- Hepatic encephalopathy should be treated with lactulose orally or rectally and titrated to approximately three bowel movements daily. Older therapies, such as neomycin or metronidazole, have been found to be ineffective or harmful in recent studies.[12]
- Coagulopathy is managed with vitamin K intravenously.[12] Prothrombin complex concentrate has been used to reverse coagulopathy in patients with cirrhosis; however, there are concerns of thrombotic events associated with its use.[22]

There are pharmacologic means of optimizing patients with renal disease for surgical procedures. In patients with prerenal azotemia, infusions of crystalloid and colloid solutions can improve tubular flow. Anemia is managed with erythropoietin or its various derivatives, with the caveat that this must be initiated 2 to 4 weeks before surgery. In patients with worsening acute renal failure not on dialysis, the anesthesiologist can use diuretic infusions, such as furosemide, to improve management of fluid balance. Although renal outcomes may be improved, there has been no clear mortality benefit demonstrated.[23]

End-organ protection of the liver can be attempted pharmacologically. Sevoflurane and propofol have been showed to attenuate ischemic reperfusion injury[24] Animal studies have demonstrated that dexmedetomidine and remifentanil have been associated with lesser degrees of ischemic reperfusion injury than control groups.[25,26] This has not been validated in human studies. Maintenance of hemodynamics with vasopressor infusions, such as norepinephrine, vasopressin, and phenylephrine, and inotropic infusions, such as epinephrine, can help maintain perfusion to the diseased liver.

Several pharmacologic agents confer end organ protections for patients with renal disease. Renovascular constriction is prevented with the use of angiotensin-converting enzyme inhibitors. Renal-protective strategies have been explored in vascular, cardiac, and transplant surgery. Administration of furosemide, mannitol, dopamine, and fenoldopam have all been studied, with no definitive therapy found to consistently and reproducibly improve outcomes.[27]

NONPHARMACOLOGIC STRATEGIES FOR MANAGEMENT

Nonpharmacologic optimization of patients with hepatic disease consists of

- Management of variceal bleeding through endoscopic interventions.
- Management of ascites with large-volume paracentesis.
- Coagulopathy can be treated with blood products including fresh frozen plasma and cryoprecipitate.[7]
- Hyponatremia is typically corrected slowly (<12 mEq over 24 hours) with fluid restriction.

Nonpharmacologic optimization of patients with renal disease consists of

- Renal-replacement therapy for the treatment of fluid balance, electrolyte imbalances, and correction of acidosis.
- In patients not requiring renal-replacement therapy, fluid and sodium restriction prevents fluid overload, and potassium restriction prevents hyperkalemia.[28]

Most of the nonpharmacologic means of end-organ protection in patients with hepatic disease are based on intraoperative surgical technique during hepatic surgery. Minimizing portal vein and/or hepatic artery clamping time, and intermittent clamping can reduce the risk of postoperative liver failure. Intermittent hepatic vascular clamping has also been proven in animal models to confer a degree of ischemic preconditioning.[29] In patients undergoing extensive liver resections, preoperative portal vein embolization can allow for hypertrophy of the remaining liver to preserve remaining liver function.[30] Use of low central venous pressures also reduces the risk of liver congestion and blood loss intraoperatively. Finally, avoidance of hypotension, hypoxia, hypocarbia, and hypercarbia are important because they all reduce portal vein flow.

In renal disease, hypercarbia and hypoxia reduce renal blood flow. Avoidance of nephrotoxic substances (**Box 3**) also prevents further damage to compromised kidneys.[31] Establishing a surgical plan with the surgeon that minimizes vascular clamping that compromises kidney flow also confers some protection on patients with renal disease not on dialysis. This has been found to be beneficial in aortic and urologic surgery.

SELF-MANAGEMENT STRATEGIES

Several studies have established that patients with hepatic and renal disease poorly manage their conditions, so it is important that there is an emphasis on self-management in the perioperative period.[32] It has also been shown that patients who are aware of their disease are more effectively able to manage it.[33] In patients with liver disease, the importance of compliance with medications for prophylaxis against bleeding and infection, avoidance of hepatotoxic substances, such as alcohol and acetaminophen, and sodium and fluid restriction are critical. Similarly, in patients with renal disease, compliance with dialysis, the avoidance of nephrotoxic substances, and appropriate management of the underlying disease are important. Management under the consultation of a hepatologist and nephrologist is advised.

EVALUATION, ADJUSTMENT, AND RECURRENCE

Despite appropriate preparation and management in the perioperative period, patients with hepatic and renal disease are at high risk for significant postoperative complications. Postoperatively, hemorrhage, sepsis, liver failure, fluid overload, and hepatorenal syndrome are the most common complications in patients with hepatic disease.[34] Similarly, studies have shown that postoperative mortality in patients with chronic renal disease progressing to dialysis dependent renal failure is 26%.[35]

PHARMACOLOGIC AND NONPHARMACOLOGIC THERAPIES
Hepatic Disease

There are several pharmacologic and nonpharmacologic strategies to treat the various physiologic derangements of hepatic disease. The cardiovascular system is typically in a vasodilatory state and can be managed with vasopressor infusions, such as

---

Box 3
Common nephrotoxic substances used in the perioperative period

Antibiotics: aminoglycosides, cephalosporins, vancomycin

Antihypertensives: angiotensin-converting enzyme inhibitors, angiotensin receptor blockers

Nonsteroidal anti-inflammatory agents

Immunosuppressants: cyclosporine, tacrolimus

Contrast dyes

phenylephrine and norepinephrine. Vasopressin is often depleted in patients with end-stage liver disease, so it may be especially beneficial in this patient population.[36] Portopulmonary hypertension is managed with pulmonary vasodilators including oxygen, nitric oxide, prostaglandin analogues, phosphodiesterase inhibitors, and endothelin receptor antagonists. Right ventricular inotropic support is provided with such agents as dobutamine and milrinone.[37] Pharmacologic interventions for restrictive lung physiology include diuresis with furosemide and spironolactone. This lung physiology may also improve with large-volume paracentesis. Hepatic hydrothorax is typically not drained because of likelihood of reaccumulation and is often treated with diuresis. Hepatopulmonary syndrome has no effective pharmacologic treatment with the only treatment being liver transplantation.

In terms of fluid and electrolyte balance, hyponatremia is traditionally managed non-pharmacologically with sodium and fluid restriction. However, severe cases with neurologic manifestations must be treated with 3% normal saline, and not corrected more than 12 mEq/24 hours. A new class of drugs known as vaptams have been used to help treat hyponatremia. Although the only known treatment of hepatorenal syndrome is liver transplantation, the use of terlipressin, a vasopressin analogue, and 25% albumin have been shown to be potentially effective.[6] Transjugular intrahepatic portosystemic shunt (TIPS) has also been shown to improve renal function in patients with hepatorenal syndrome. Depending on the hemodynamics of the patient, continuous venovenous hemodialysis and intermittent hemodialysis are options if renal-replacement therapy in necessitated.

Precipitating factors for hepatic encephalopathy include hypovolemia, hypoglycemia, gastrointestinal bleeding, renal failure, active infection, and sedative medications. Hepatic encephalopathy is often managed with lactulose, ideally titrated to three bowel movements a day. However, nonpharmacologic interventions are critical to avoid potential precipitating factors. Coagulopathy is managed with the use of such agents as vitamin K or Prothrombin Complex Concentrate, and fresh frozen plasma or cryoprecipitate. Platelets are transfused rarely because most are consumed via hypersplenism. Management of esophageal varices is typically prophylaxis with β-blockers, propranolol, and nadolol. In the setting of active bleeding, varices are treated with endoscopic banding, a Sengstein-Blakemore tube may be placed in extreme situations to attenuate hemorrhage. Ascites is treated with diuretics, large-volume paracentesis, and nonpharmacologically with sodium and fluid restriction. In intractable cases, a TIPS can be considered. In obstructive jaundice, sodium deoxycholate acts as a bile salt to help detoxify bacterial endotoxin and reduce risk of endotoxemia.[6]

Renal Disease

Patients with renal disease often have concomitant cardiopulmonary abnormalities. Coronary artery disease is managed with the use of calcium and phosphate binders, because they are beneficial in reducing the incidence of vessel calcification. Statin therapy can slow the rate of atherosclerosis. Renovascular hypertension is not uncommonly difficult to control. Multiple agents including β-blockers, angiotensin-converting enzyme inhibitors, calcium-channel blockers, α_2-agonists, and diuretics may be required for treatment of hypertension. Aldosterone receptor blockers should be used with caution because of the risk of hyperkalemia. Left ventricular hypertrophy and diastolic dysfunction are managed with tight blood pressure control and aggressive fluid management with diuretics to help prevent volume overload. The cornerstone of nonpharmacologic management of cardiopulmonary disease associated with renal disease is sodium and fluid restriction. In more advanced renal disease, dialysis is more effective in managing overall fluid balance.

Renal disease is characterized by chronic metabolic acidosis, hyperkalemia, and hyperphosphatemia. Pharmacologically, oral sodium bicarbonate tablets are used to manage metabolic acidosis caused by low bicarbonate. A two-fold approach is often used to treat hyperkalemia. First, insulin, bicarbonate, and β-agonists are used to move potassium into the intracellular space. Next, potassium is excreted using diuretic therapy or potassium binders, such as sodium kayexalate. Phosphate is managed with the use of oral phosphate binders. Nonpharmacologic management of acidosis, hyperkalemia, and fluid balance is most effectively achieved with dialysis. In the setting of acute renal failure with hemodynamic instability, continuous venovenous hemodialysis may be more effective. Symptoms related to sensory neuropathy secondary to renal disease are managed with such agents as gabapentin, pregabalin, and duloxetine. Progression of this neuropathy is prevented with appropriate pressure point padding. Severe neurologic symptoms secondary to uremia can usually be reversed with initiation of dialysis. In regards to the hematologic consequences of renal disease, anemia is often treated with erythropoietin and the administration of desmopressin can help platelet adhesion.[5]

SURGICAL TREATMENT OPTIONS

In the setting of severe hepatic and renal disease, surgical treatments are considered. In patients with portal hypertension and intractable ascites or continuing variceal bleeding, TIPS is considered to help reduce portal pressures as seen in **Fig. 1**.[38]

However, the TIPS procedure is temporizing and does not halt disease progression. For patients with end-stage liver disease, the only curative surgical treatment is liver transplantation. The most common indication for liver transplantation in the United States is cirrhosis secondary to hepatitis C. Donor organs can come from cadaveric and living donor sources. Traditionally, contraindications to liver transplantation

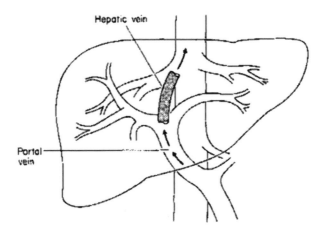

Fig. 1. Transjugular intrahepatic portosystemic shunt. (*From* McCormick PA, Dick R, Burroughs AK. Review article: the transjugular intrahepatic portosystemic shunt (TIPS) in the treatment of portal hypertension. Aliment Pharmacol Ther 1994;8:273–82; with permission.)

include severe cardiopulmonary disease including portopulmonary hypertension, septic shock, severe neurologic injury, active alcohol or drug use, or lack of family/social support.

Patients with certain forms of renal disease may be responsive to surgical treatment. Patients with known renal artery stenosis undergo stenting to reverse existing renal disease. Patients with obstruction within their kidney, ureter, or bladder leading to renal failure undergo urologic procedures to treat the obstruction. Renal transplantation is a known cure for patients with all forms of kidney pathology. The most common indication is diabetes mellitus. Similar to liver transplantation, donor organs come from deceased or living donors.

TREATMENT, RESISTANCE, AND COMPLICATIONS

With major abdominal organ transplantation, there are significant complications that can occur in the early postoperative and late postoperative period that are associated with a high morbidity and mortality.[39]

Liver Transplantation
- Early complications
  - Surgical complications
    - Postoperative bleeding
    - Hepatic artery thrombosis
    - Portal vein thrombosis
    - Bile duct leak
  - Primary nonfunction of the graft
  - Acute rejection
  - Infection
- Late complications
  - Chronic rejection
  - Chronic renal failure
  - Recurrent liver disease and cirrhosis

Renal Transplantation
- Early complications
  - Surgical complications
    - Thrombosis
    - Ureter necrosis leading to urine leak
  - Acute rejection
- Late complications
  - Chronic rejection
  - Infection (usually viral)
  - Malignancy (usually lymphoma)

EVALUATION OF OUTCOME AND LONG-TERM RECOMMENDATIONS

Because of the advent of safer surgical techniques and advances in immunosuppression, liver and kidney transplantation has become associated with increased survival rates. Mortality for liver transplantation at 1 year is 85%, and 75% at 5 years.[39] Similarly, with renal transplant, 1-year survival is 95% and 5-year survival is 85%.[39] With increased morbidity and prolonged hospitalizations associated with the hemodialysis of chronic kidney disease and chronic liver disease, more patients are opting to be listed for organ transplantation.

SUMMARY

Patients with concomitant hepatic and renal disease are becoming more prevalent in the perioperative setting. Through effective risk stratification, preoperative evaluation, and an understanding of their physiology, successful outcomes are maximized. Management goals consist of preoperative optimization of the patient, intraoperative end-organ protection, and appropriate modification of the anesthetic because of the physiologic abnormalities found in hepatic and renal disease. Pharmacologic and non-pharmacologic strategies, including patient self-management, should be used to help in management. However, it must be recognized that these patients are at high risk for morbidity and mortality postoperatively, and that transplantation is the only proven therapy for these end-organ diseases.

REFERENCES

1. Hoetzel A, Ryan H, Schmidt R. Anesthestic considerations for the patient with liver disease. Curr Opin Anaesthesiol 2012;25:340–7.
2. Wagener G, Brentjens T. Renal disease: the anesthesiologist's perspective. Anesthesiol Clin 2006;24:523–47.
3. Patel T. Surgery in the patient with liver disease. Mayo Clin Proc 1999;74:593–9.
4. Kiamanesh D, Rumley J, Moitra VK. Monitoring and managing hepatic disease in anaesthesia. Br J Anaesth 2013;111(Suppl 1):i50–61.
5. Sladen R. Perioperative care for the patient with renal or hepatic disease. New York: Wolters Kluwer; 2001. p. 99–103.
6. Wagener G. Liver anesthesia and critical care medicine. New York: Springer Science; 2012.
7. Leung, CCH, Young, KK. Clinical aspects of hepatic disease. Anaesth Intensive Care Med 2015;16:11–3.
8. Craig RG, Hunter JM. Recent developments in the perioperative management of adult patients with chronic kidney disease. Br J Anaesth 2008;101(3):296–310.
9. McBride WT, Gilliland H. Acute Renal Failure. Surgery 2009;27:11.
10. Borthwick E, Ferguson A. Perioperative acute kidney: risk factors, recognition, management, and management. BMJ 2010;341:c3365.
11. Yao F. Yao and Artusio' anesthesiology: problem oriented patient management. New York: Wolters-Kluwer; 2011.
12. Muilenburg D, Singh A, Torzilli G, et al. Surgery in the patient with liver disease. Med Clin North Am 2009;93:1065–81.
13. Fleisher L, Fleischmann K, Auerbach A, et al. 2014 ACC/AHA guideline on perioperative cardiovascular evaluation and management of patients undergoing noncardiac surgery. J Am Coll Cardiol 2014;64(22):e77–137.
14. Leung A, McAlister F, Rogers S, et al. Preoperative hyponatremia and perioperative complications. Arch Intern Med 2012;172:1474–81.
15. Morgan D, Ho K. Comparison of nonoliguric and oliguric severe acute kidney injury according to the RIFLE criteria. Nephron Clin Pract 2010;115:59–65.
16. Serracino-Inglott F, Habib NA, Mathie RT. Hepatic ischemia-reperfusion injury. Am J Surg 2001;181:160–6.
17. Agarwal RC, Jain R, Yadava A. Prevention of perioperative renal failure. Indian J Anaesth 2008;52:38–43.
18. Mcclain R, Ramakrishna H, Aniskevich S III, et al. Anesthetic pharmacology and perioperative considerations for the end-stage liver disease patient. Curr Clin Pharmacol 2015;10:35–46.

658 Brentjens & Chadha

19. Croinin D, Shorten G. Anesthesia and renal disease. Curr Opin Anaesthesiol 2002;15:359–63.
20. Lodato F, Azzaroli F, Di Girolamo M, et al. Proton pump inhibitors in cirrhosis: tradition or evidence based practice. World J Gastroenterol 2008;14:2980–5.
21. Wyke RJ. Bacterial infections complicating liver disease. Baillieres Clin Gastroenterol 1989;3:187–210.
22. Soresen B, Spahn D, Innerhofer P, et al. Clinical review: prothrombin complex concentrates-evaluation of safety and thrombogenicity. Crit Care 2011;15:201.
23. Ahmed US, Iqbal HI, Akbar SR. Furosemide in acute kidney injury: a vexed issue. Austin J Nephrol Hypertens 2014;5:1025.
24. Pandey C, Nath S, Pandey V, et al. Perioperative ischaemia-induced liver injury and protection strategies: an expanding horizon for anesthesiologists. Indian J Anaesth 2013;57:223–9.
25. Sahin T, Begec Z, Toprak H, et al. The effects of dexmedetomidine on liver ischemia-reperfusion injury in rats. J Surg Res 2013;183:385–90.
26. Yang L, Lao K, Liu Y, et al. Remifentanil preconditioning reduce hepatic ischemia reperfusion injury in rats via inducible nitric oxide synthase expression. Anesthesiology 2011;114:1036–47.
27. Jarnberg P. Renal protection strategies in the perioperative period. Best Pract Res Clin Anaesthesiol 2004;18:645–60.
28. Rang ST, West NL, Howard J, et al. Anaesthesia for chronic renal disease and renal transplantation. EAU-EBU Update Series 2006;4:246.
29. Chouillard E, Gumbs A, Cerqui D. Vascular clamping in liver surgery: physiology, indications, and techniques. Ann Surg Innov Res 2010;4:2.
30. Clavien P, Petrowsky H, DeOliveira M, et al. Strategies for safer liver surgery and partial liver transplantation. N Engl J Med 2007;356:1545–59.
31. Jones D, Lee HT. Perioperative renal protection. Best Pract Res Clin Anaesthesiol 2008;22:193–208.
32. Volk M, Fisher N, Fontana R. Patient knowledge about disease self-management in cirrhosis. Am J Gastroenterol 2013;108(3):302–5.
33. Lau-Walker M, Presky J, Webzell I, et al. Patients with alcohol-related liver disease-beliefs about their illness and factors that influence their self-management. J Adv Nurs 2016;72(1):173–85.
34. Millwala F, Nguyen G, Thuluvath P. Outcomes of patients with cirrhosis undergoing non-hepatic surgery: risk assessment and management. World J Gastroenterol 2007;30:4056–63.
35. Hsu CY, Chertow GM, McCulloch CE, et al. Nonrecovery of kidney function and death after acute on chronic renal failure. Clin J Am Soc Nephrol 2009;4:891–8.
36. Wagener G, Kovalevskaya G, Minhaz M. Vasopressin deficiency and vasodilatory state in end-stage liver disease. J Cardiothorac Vasc Anesth 2011;25:665–70.
37. Runo J. Liver transplantation for portopulmonary hypertension. Clin Liver Dis 2014;4:74–6.
38. McCormick P, Dick R, Burroughs A. Review article: the transjugular intrahepatic portosystemic shunt (TIPS) in the treatment of portal hypertension. Aliment Pharmacol Ther 1994;8:273–82.
39. Coventry B. Cardiothoracic, vascular, renal, and transplant surgery. London: Springer-Verlag; 2014.

Coexisting Cardiac and Hematologic Disorders

Jordan E. Goldhammer, MD*, Benjamin A. Kohl, MD

KEYWORDS

- Cardiac manifestations of sickle cell disease • Perioperative transfusion threshold
- Essential thrombocytosis • Idiopathic thrombotic purpura
- Perioperative anticoagulation management of artificial heart valves
- Perioperative anticoagulation management of ventricular assist devices
- Anticoagulation management of severe heart failure

KEY POINTS

- Patients with concomitant cardiac and hematologic disorders presenting for noncardiac surgery are challenging to even the most experienced anesthesiologists.
- Anemic patients with cardiac disease should be approached in a methodical fashion.
- Transfusion triggers and target should be based on underlying symptomatology, with a focus on end-organ perfusion and oxygenation.
- The approach to anticoagulation management in patients with artificial heart valves, cardiac devices, or severe heart failure in the operative setting must encompass a complete understanding of the rationale of a patient's therapy as well as calculate the risk of changing this regimen.
- This article focuses on several of the more common disorders and discusses strategies to optimize care in patients with coexisting cardiac and hematologic disease.

INTRODUCTION

Patients with concomitant cardiac and hematologic disorders presenting for noncardiac surgery are challenging to even the most experienced anesthesiologists. Understanding the rationale of a patient's therapy and calculating the risk of changing this regimen in the perioperative period are essential. This article focuses on several of the more common disorders and discusses strategies to optimize care in patients with coexisting cardiac and hematologic disease.

Department of Anesthesiology, Sidney Kimmel Medical College, Thomas Jefferson University, 111 South 11th Street, Philadelphia, PA 19107, USA
* Corresponding author. Department of Anesthesiology, Thomas Jefferson University, 111 South 11th Street, Gibbon Building, Suite 8280, Philadelphia, PA 19107.
E-mail address: Jordan.Goldhammer@Jefferson.edu

Anesthesiology Clin 34 (2016) 659–668
http://dx.doi.org/10.1016/j.anclin.2016.06.003
1932-2275/16/© 2016 Elsevier Inc. All rights reserved.
anesthesiology.theclinics.com

SICKLE CELL ANEMIA

Sickle cell disease (SCD) results from a variety of inherited genetic mutations in the hemoglobin (Hgb) beta gene resulting in defective β-globin synthesis and culminating in attenuated oxygen transport. One particular Hgb beta gene mutation produces an altered β-globin molecule known as Hgb S (HbS). Two genotypes are expressed: (1) heterozygous (sickle cell trait [SCT]) and (2) homozygous (SCD).

Sickle Cell Disease

The clinical characteristics of SCD include anemia and recurrent vaso-occlusive crises that commonly affect the cardiac, pulmonary, renal, neurologic, and musculoskeletal systems. Within the natural history of SCD, a growing body of literature suggests that cardiovascular disease may play a role in disease progression and early mortality.[1] In a cohort study of 240 patients with SCD, cardiopulmonary compromise resulted in 39.5% of the recorded mortalities.[1] Causes of cardiovascular mortality include myocardial ischemia, malignant arrhythmia, heart failure, and pulmonary hypertension.

Chronic anemia of SCD results in an increased cardiac output and intravascular volume retention to maintain oxygen delivery. Increased intravascular volume results in left ventricular dilation and eccentric hypertrophy. Arrhythmias, including atrial fibrillation, supraventricular tachycardia, and ventricular fibrillation, frequently arise secondary to chronic volume overload and have been linked to cardiovascular mortality. Baseline QT prolongation has been reported in 38% of pediatric and young adult patients with SCD.[2] Left ventricular systolic function is typically preserved; however, myocardial hypertrophy and increased left ventricular mass lead to diastolic dysfunction and increased left ventricular filling pressure. Diastolic dysfunction has been associated with increased age, hypertension, and renal failure and has been identified as an independent risk factors for mortality in patients with SCD.[3,4]

Chronic hemolytic anemia results in release of free Hgb and other red blood cell intracellular enzymes that inhibit nitric oxide signaling pathways causing vasoconstriction.[3] Within the pulmonary vasculature, this mechanism is responsible for the development of primary pulmonary hypertension. Pulmonary hypertension, either secondary to volume overload and underlying diastolic heart failure, or as a primary pathology, is encountered in up to 60% of adult patients with SCD and contributes to early cardiovascular mortality.[5,6] Increased pulmonary pressures should be treated aggressively to reduce right ventricular afterload and mitigate right ventricular failure.

Myocardial infarction in the SCD population results from microvascular vessel occlusion and thus coronary angiography is typically normal.[7] Supportive care, including hydration, supplemental oxygen therapy, and blood transfusion, may be initiated; however, exchange transfusion seems to be the definitive therapy during severe coronary ischemia. Exchange transfusion to replace HbS with normal adult Hgb (HbA) results in reduced microvascular viscosity, inhibition of the inflammatory cascade, and restoration of the intrinsic nitric oxide pathway.[8]

Patients with SCD frequently present for anesthesia and surgery. An understanding of the pathophysiology of this disease is critical to provide optimal care. Perioperative transfusion has been shown to decrease both vaso-occlusive and cardiac complications in patients undergoing low-risk and medium-risk surgery.[9] A transfusion threshold of 10 g/dL is generally recommended; however, the need for exchange transfusion and reduced HbS level is less clear. Conservative transfusion (maintain Hgb of 10 g/dL), compared with aggressive transfusion (maintain Hgb ≥10 g/dL and exchange transfusion to decrease HbS <30%), results in 50% less blood administration and similar complication rates in low-risk to moderate-risk surgery.[10] Major cardiac surgery has been undertaken using both aggressive exchange transfusion and conservative transfusion protocols with similar complication rates.[11,12]

In patients with SCD and coexisting cardiac disease, a conservative transfusion strategy to a target Hgb of 10 g/dL should be undertaken. Although aggressive exchange transfusion may significantly reduce HbS content, the risk of blood product administration and volume overload must be reconciled in this population. Those with underlying pulmonary hypertension, diastolic dysfunction, or cardiomyopathy require titrated transfusion and volume administration to avoid exacerbation of right heart failure or malignant arrhythmias.

Sickle Cell Trait

SCT is a carrier state of the HbS mutation occurring in 1.6% of the US population.[13] Patients with SCT have a higher incidence of urologic disease, including hematuria, chronic kidney disease, and renal medullary carcinoma. A small percentage of these patients may display some vaso-occlusive phenomena; however, cardiovascular manifestations of SCD are absent and life expectancy is typically normal. Patients with SCT presenting for surgery and anesthesia should be managed according to their underlying comorbidities; no discrete management due to their status as an SCT carrier is indicated.

ANEMIA OF CHRONIC DISEASE

Anemia of chronic disease is typically a mild anemia with a normocytic, normochromic profile primarily due to reduced red blood cell production. Anemia of chronic disease (female Hgb <12 g/dL and male Hgb <13 g/dL) is associated with increased age, diabetes, renal insufficiency, chronic immune activation, and cardiac disease and is present in 10% of those with coronary disease and as high as 79% of patients with advanced heart failure.[14–16] In the general population, observational studies have shown the noninferiority of restrictive transfusion protocols (compared with more liberal targets) in the perioperative period; however, less robust clinical data exist for patients with perioperative anemia and advanced cardiac disease. One study evaluated the natural history of anemia, following a subset of anemic patients who refused blood transfusion in the perioperative period. In those patients with coexisting cardiac disease, the refusal of blood products was associated with an increased risk of death.[17] A randomized pilot trial of 110 anemic patients with acute coronary syndrome or stable angina undergoing cardiac catheterization revealed greater than twice the risk of myocardial infarction, unscheduled revascularization, or death within 30 days when treated with a restrictive (transfusion for symptomatic anemia or Hgb <8 g/dL) transfusion protocol.[18] Recent registry data, however, further obfuscate the decision whether or not to transfuse these patients; data have shown an increased risk of cardiovascular morbidity with as little as 1 unit of red blood cell transfusion during the perioperative period.[19] In support of restrictive transfusion practices, a post hoc analysis of a subset of 796 patients with known coronary disease from a large, randomized, controlled trial of hip fracture patients randomized to restrictive (Hgb <8 mg/dL or symptomatic anemia) or liberal (Hgb <10 mg/dL) transfusion found similar 30-day mortality rates between the 2 groups.[20,21] In addition, subgroup analysis of patients with cardiovascular disease from the Transfusion Requirements in Critical Care trial found no difference in 30-day, 60-day, ICU, or in-hospital mortality when randomized to restrictive (Hgb 7.0–9.0 g/dL) or liberal (Hgb 10.0–12.0 g/dL) transfusion.[22,23] Even in the setting of acute coronary syndrome liberal transfusion is not without risk, because a greater degree of complications related to heart failure has been observed in anemic patients.[24]

Although patients with ongoing ischemia may benefit from transfusion to restore myocardial oxygen delivery, the treatment of anemia in those patients with coronary artery disease (CAD) or severe heart failure should be approached in a methodical fashion based on underlying symptomatology, with a focus on end-organ perfusion and oxygenation. Physical examination (mental status and self-reported energy level), laboratory monitoring (arterial lactate and acid/base status), and physiologic monitoring (heart rate, blood pressure, cardiac index, and urine output) should all be used to optimize goal directed transfusion therapy in this complex patient population.

PLATELET ABNORMALITIES
Thrombocytosis

Essential thrombocytosis (ET) is a rare disorder affecting approximately 3/1,000,000 patients and is associated with both thrombosis and hemorrhage. Acute coronary thrombosis may occur in up to 9.4% of patients with ET.[25] Age, smoking, hypertension, hyperlipidemia, history of thrombotic events, duration of thrombocytosis, and platelet count greater than 1,500,000/μL are associated with increased thrombotic risk.[26,27] Patients with existing risk factors and a history of occlusive CAD requiring stents or open revascularization should be treated aggressively with a platelet-lowering regimen to decrease the likelihood of stent thrombosis or recurrent thrombotic occlusion. Hydroxyurea has been used in both ET and polycythemia vera and, when compared with control, decreases both platelet count and thrombotic events in those patients at high risk for thrombotic complications from thrombocytosis.[28,29] Strategies to decrease platelet count, generally below 600,000/μL, have been proved to reduce thrombosis.[27,28] Aspirin and hydroxyurea should, where feasible, be continued throughout the perioperative period in patients with ET. High-risk patients, especially those with a history of CAD, should be aggressively managed with hydroxyurea to a target platelet count less than 600,000/μL to decrease the incidence of thrombotic complications. If signs of acute coronary syndrome develop, emergent cardiac catheterization is indicated, because the inciting lesion should be assumed to be occlusive coronary thrombosis until proved otherwise.

Idiopathic Thrombotic Purpura

Idiopathic thrombocytopenic purpura (ITP) is an acquired deficiency of both platelet count and function. ITP may be classified as either primary (idiopathic) or secondary (typically due to infection such as hepatitis C, HIV, or other autoimmune syndromes, such as systemic lupus erythematosus). Thrombocytopenia in ITP is caused by antibodies to platelet antigens resulting in decreased platelet lifespan and impaired platelet production. Circulating platelets are often large and immature, increasing the risk of thrombotic events.[30] Although rare, coexisting ITP and CAD have been managed by either traditional coronary artery bypass or percutaneous intervention; however, both pose significant management dilemmas. Open revascularization is associated with increased bleeding risk due to thrombocytopenia, whereas stent implantation is complicated by the need for postintervention antiplatelet therapy. Intravenous immunoglobulin and steroid therapy, coupled with perioperative platelet transfusion, has been used with acceptable results; however, in those with ITP, both open revascularization and percutaneous intervention are associated with a moderate increase in bleeding.[31] A preponderance of percutaneous interventions in these patients have used bare metal stents in an effort to limit the duration of postintervention antiplatelet therapy.[31,32] A critical assessment of the balance of thrombosis prevention and bleeding risk must be achieved. Aspirin and clopidogrel have been used successfully; however, glycoprotein IIb/IIIa inhibitors are associated with uncontrolled bleeding and should be avoided.[33,34] Postintervention antiplatelet agents can be used until the platelet count falls below 20,000/μL or clinical bleeding occurs.

Thrombotic Thrombocytopenic Purpura

Thrombotic thrombocytopenic purpura (TTP) is a rare and often fatal disorder characterized by thrombocytopenia, hemolytic anemia, renal failure, and mental status changes. The incidence of TTP in the general population is approximately 3.7/1,000,000; however, after percutaneous coronary intervention, the incidence is much higher due to antiplatelet-induced TTP.[35] TTP has been reported in 1/4,814 patients treated with ticlopidine.[36] Clopidogrel has a safer side-effect profile; however, reports of TTP after administration exist.[37] Early diagnosis and treatment of antiplatelet-induced TTP are essential because mortality approaches 67% without prompt plasmapharesis.[36]

ANTICOAGULATION FOR CARDIAC DEVICES
Artificial Valves

Artificial heart valves may be implanted for acute or chronic valvular dysfunction, resulting in stenotic or regurgitant heart disease. Two main classes of devices are mechanical valves and bioprosthetic valves. Bioprosthetic valves may be either a cadaveric homograft or a xenograft composed of porcine or bovine pericardium mounted on a stent. Although the lifespan of bioprosthetic valves is generally reduced compared with mechanical valves, use of the tissue material precludes the need for anticoagulation unless special circumstances arise. In contrast, mechanical valves are composed of pyrolytic carbon and last an indefinite period of time. Because of the high rate of thrombosis, however, mechanical valves require aggressive long-term anticoagulation. According to American Heart Association/American College of Cardiology guidelines, patients with a mechanical valve in the mitral position should be anticoagulated to a target median international normalized ratio (INR) of 3.0.[38] Due to an accelerated transvalvular flow pattern, the target median INR of a valve in the aortic position in those without thrombotic risk factors (atrial fibrillation, left ventricular dysfunction, hypercoagulable state, and previous thrombotic event) is 2.5.[38] Although major guidelines differ in their specific recommendation, aspirin, in addition to warfarin, is generally recommended in those without increased bleeding risk.[38–40]

Anticoagulation therapy in preparation for noncardiac surgery must take into account both the bleeding risk of surgery and the thrombotic risk of abruptly discontinuing anticoagulation. In general, minor dental or cutaneous procedures may be accomplished without interruption of anticoagulation; however, if the surgical site is not amenable to local hemostasis or major surgery is planned, a preoperative INR less than 1.5 is desirable. Warfarin should be discontinued 5 to 6 days prior to surgical intervention and anticoagulant bridging with a heparin analog is indicated.

On some occasions, patients on chronic anticoagulation for mechanical heart valves may suffer from warfarin overdose. This is typically manifest by an elevated INR and frequently results from medication mismanagement or a change in absorption pharmacokinetics. If no significant bleeding occurs, warfarin can be held and oral vitamin K administered until target INR is reached. In those with severe bleeding, prothrombin complex concentrates or fresh frozen plasma may be used to expeditiously normalize the INR. Complications from severe bleeding generally outweigh the risk of valve thrombosis. Anticoagulation can be safely interrupted for 7 to 14 days even in those at high risk for thromboembolic events.[41]

Pregnant patients with mechanical heart valves pose multiple challenges. Parturients are hypercoagulable due to changes in blood viscosity, decreased fibrinolysis, and up-regulation of clotting factors. All pregnant patients with artificial heart valves should be deemed high risk because the percentage of pregnancies ending with both a live mother and child is approximately 81%.[42] Adequate anticoagulation to prevent mechanical valve thrombosis must be balanced against the risks of bleeding and teratogenicity of the anticoagulant. In a large registry series, 4.5% of such patients experienced mechanical valve thrombosis, with half of the events occurring in the first trimester.[42] Anticoagulation regimens in the first trimester remain a matter of debate. Warfarin has proven to be superior to heparin analogs for thrombosis prophylaxis; however, concerns for teratogenicity, miscarriage (<24 weeks), and late fetal death (>24 weeks) exist.[42] Multiple medication regimens have been studied, including warfarin, unfractionated heparin, and low-molecular-weight heparin. Current guidelines suggest either administration of low-dose (<5 mg/d) warfarin or discontinuation of warfarin in the first trimester.[38] If resumed, complete discontinuation of warfarin is indicated after 36 weeks in preparation for delivery. Anticoagulant coverage can be provided during warfarin-free periods or, alternatively, maintained for the duration of pregnancy with unfractionated or low-molecular-weight heparin. Regardless of the medication choice; pregnancy in this patient population is best managed by a multidisciplinary team and the risk/benefit of anticoagulant medications must be discussed with the patient.

Ventricular Assist Device

A left ventricular assist device (LVAD) can be used in 3 clinical scenarios:

1. Acute ventricular failure as a bridge to recovery
2. Chronic ventricular failure as a bridge to heart transplantation
3. Permanent implantation in those not suitable for heart transplantation

All LVADs fall into 1 of 2 physiologic categories based on how blood is circulated through the device: pulsatile or nonpulsatile. Nonpulsatile, or continuous, flow LVADs are smaller in size and have greater durability compared with pulsatile flow LVADs.[43]

Careful consideration of the anticoagulation status in patients with an LVAD is important for optimal management. Thrombus formation within the device, reported to occur between 2% and 12% at 24 months, can lead to embolic events or LVAD failure.[44] LVAD patients are anticoagulated with a regimen consisting of antiplatelet agents and warfarin. Target median INR varies between centers from 2.0 to 2.5.[43]

Major bleeding may occur in patients with an LVAD secondary to aggressive anticoagulation, hemolysis, and down-regulation of clotting factors. Although the etiology is not yet completely understood, many continuous-flow LVADs cause reduced levels of von Willebrand factor, which may further increase the risk of bleeding. The need to reverse or withhold anticoagulation depends on the severity and location of hemorrhage. Prothrombin complex concentrates or fresh frozen plasma can be administered to reverse warfarin. Anticoagulation therapy should immediately resume when the risk of thrombosis outweighs the risk of further bleeding.

The extended lifespan of new-generation LVADs, coupled with their use for destination therapy, has resulted in a large proportion of these patients presenting for elective, noncardiac surgery. In patients without additional indication for anticoagulation (atrial fibrillation or left ventricular thrombus) cessation of warfarin 5 to 6 days before surgery and continuation of aspirin has reduced the need for perioperative blood transfusion without an increase in thrombosis.[45] In patients at high risk for thrombosis, anticoagulation bridging with a heparin analog is indicated. Warfarin anticoagulation can be safely resumed in the postoperative period when bleeding risk has subsided.

HEART FAILURE WITH REDUCED EJECTION FRACTION

Heart failure is associated with significant morbidity and mortality from thromboembolic events leading to stroke, myocardial infarction, deep vein thrombosis, and pulmonary embolus. The pathophysiology of thromboembolism in heart failure is primarily related to blood stasis within the left ventricle, endothelial dysfunction, and increased platelet activation. The addition of anticoagulant and/or antithrombotic therapy in those with coexisting atrial fibrillation or previous thromboembolic event is recommended; however, anticoagulant therapy for patients in sinus rhythm with reduced ejection fraction is less clear. Multiple randomized controlled trials have compared the use of warfarin, aspirin, and clopidogrel in this patient population with conflicting results.[46–48] Aspirin has been associated with increased risk for hospitalization and gastrointestinal bleeding; however, this may be due to an as-yet undefined interaction with ACE inhibitors.[49] Baseline warfarin use has been associated with a reduction in all-cause mortality and acute coronary syndrome; however, the rate of major bleeding is increased compared with aspirin or clopidogrel.[49] Antiplatelet and antithrombotic use in patients with normal sinus rhythm and reduced ejection fraction should be dictated based on underlying comorbidities and heart failure pathology. Aspirin is a mainstay treatment of patients with underlying coronary disease and heart failure secondary to ischemic cardiomyopathy. Alternatively, warfarin can be used to decrease thrombosis risk and improve intermediate morbidity and mortality in those with reduced ejection fraction and normal cardiac rhythm; however, therapy should be reserved only for patients at low risk for bleeding complications.

SUMMARY

Patients with concomitant hematologic and cardiac issues represent challenges to everyone involved in their perioperative care. An understanding of the pertinent pathophysiology, the appropriate therapy, and the risks are essential. In the end, management decisions should be based on a thoughtful discussion with other involved providers and a balanced approach that explicitly addresses the risk and benefit of each intervention.

REFERENCES

1. Fitzhugh CD, Lauder N, Jonassaint JC, et al. Cardiopulmonary complications leading to premature deaths in adult patients with sickle cell disease. Am J Hematol 2010;85(1):36–40.
2. Liem RI, Young LT, Thompson AA. Prolonged QTc interval in children and young adults with sickle cell disease at steady state. Pediatr Blood Cancer 2009;52(7): 842–6.
3. Gladwin MT, Sachdev V. Cardiovascular abnormalities in sickle cell disease. J Am Coll Cardiol 2012;59(13):1123–33.
4. Sachdev V, Machado RF, Shizukuda Y, et al. Diastolic dysfunction is an independent risk factor for death in patients with sickle cell disease. J Am Coll Cardiol 2007;49(4):472–9.

5. Vichinsky EP. Pulmonary hypertension in sickle cell disease. N Engl J Med 2004; 350(9):857–9.

6. Voskaridou E, Christoulas D, Terpos E. Sickle-cell disease and the heart: Review of the current literature. Br J Haematol 2012;157(6):664–73.

7. Pavlu J, Ahmed RE, O'Regan DP, et al. Myocardial infarction in sickle-cell disease. Lancet 2007;369(9557):246.

8. Pannu R, Zhang J, Andraws R, et al. Acute myocardial infarction in sickle cell disease: a systematic review. Crit Pathw Cardiol 2008;7(2):133–8.

9. Howard J, Malfroy M, Llewelyn C, et al. The transfusion alternatives preoperatively in sickle cell disease (TAPS) study: a randomised, controlled, multicentre clinical trial. Lancet 2013;381(9870):930–8.

10. Vichinsky EP, Haberkern CM, Neumayr L, et al. A comparison of conservative and aggressive transfusion regimens in the perioperative management of sickle cell disease. the preoperative transfusion in sickle cell disease study group. N Engl J Med 1995;333(4):206–13.

11. Edwin F, Aniteye E, Tettey M, et al. Hypothermic cardiopulmonary bypass without exchange transfusion in sickle-cell patients: a matched-pair analysis. Interact Cardiovasc Thorac Surg 2014;19(5):771–6.

12. Yousafzai SM, Ugurlucan M, Al Radhwan OA, et al. Open heart surgery in patients with sickle cell hemoglobinopathy. Circulation 2010;121(1):14–9.

13. Ojodu J, Hulihan MM, Pope SN, et al, Centers for Disease Control and Prevention (CDC). Incidence of sickle cell trait–united states, 2010. MMWR Morb Mortal Wkly Rep 2014;63(49):1155–8.

14. Boyd CM, Leff B, Wolff JL, et al. Informing clinical practice guideline development and implementation: Prevalence of coexisting conditions among adults with coronary heart disease. J Am Geriatr Soc 2011;59(5):797–805.

15. Felker GM, Adams KF Jr, Gattis WA, et al. Anemia as a risk factor and therapeutic target in heart failure. J Am Coll Cardiol 2004;44(5):959–66.

16. Silverberg DS, Wexler D, Blum M, et al. The use of subcutaneous erythropoietin and intravenous iron for the treatment of the anemia of severe, resistant congestive heart failure improves cardiac and renal function and functional cardiac class, and markedly reduces hospitalizations. J Am Coll Cardiol 2000;35(7): 1737–44.

17. Carson JL, Duff A, Poses RM, et al. Effect of anaemia and cardiovascular disease on surgical mortality and morbidity. Lancet 1996;348(9034):1055–60.

18. Carson JL, Brooks MM, Abbott JD, et al. Liberal versus restrictive transfusion thresholds for patients with symptomatic coronary artery disease. Am Heart J 2013;165(6):964–71.e1.

19. Whitlock EL, Kim H, Auerbach AD. Harms associated with single unit perioperative transfusion: retrospective population based analysis. BMJ 2015;350:h3037.

20. Carson JL, Terrin ML, Noveck H, et al. Liberal or restrictive transfusion in high-risk patients after hip surgery. N Engl J Med 2011;365(26):2453–62.

21. Kansagara D, Dyer E, Englander H, et al. Treatment of anemia in patients with heart disease: a systematic review. Ann Intern Med 2013;159(11):746–57.

22. Hebert PC, Wells G, Blajchman MA, et al. A multicenter, randomized, controlled clinical trial of transfusion requirements in critical care. transfusion requirements in critical care investigators, canadian critical care trials group. N Engl J Med 1999;340(6):409–17.

23. Hebert PC, Yetisir E, Martin C, et al. Is a low transfusion threshold safe in critically ill patients with cardiovascular diseases? Crit Care Med 2001;29(2):227–34.

24. Cooper HA, Rao SV, Greenberg MD, et al. Conservative versus liberal red cell transfusion in acute myocardial infarction (the CRIT randomized pilot study). Am J Cardiol 2011;108(8):1108–11.

25. Rossi C, Randi ML, Zerbinati P, et al. Acute coronary disease in essential thrombocythemia and polycythemia vera. J Intern Med 1998;244(1):49–53.

26. Griesshammer M. Risk factors for thrombosis and bleeding and their influence on therapeutic decisions in patients with essential thrombocythemia. Semin Thromb Hemost 2006;32(4 Pt 2):372–80.

27. Cortelazzo S, Viero P, Finazzi G, et al. Incidence and risk factors for thrombotic complications in a historical cohort of 100 patients with essential thrombocythemia. J Clin Oncol 1990;8(3):556–62.

28. Cortelazzo S, Finazzi G, Ruggeri M, et al. Hydroxyurea for patients with essential thrombocythemia and a high risk of thrombosis. N Engl J Med 1995;332(17): 1132–6.

29. Squizzato A, Romualdi E, Passamonti F, et al. Antiplatelet drugs for polycythaemia vera and essential thrombocythaemia. Cochrane Database Syst Rev 2013;(4):CD006503.

30. Sarpatwari A, Bennett D, Logie JW, et al. Thromboembolic events among adult patients with primary immune thrombocytopenia in the United Kingdom general practice research database. Haematologica 2010;95(7):1167–75.

31. Russo A, Cannizzo M, Ghetti G, et al. Idiopathic thrombocytopenic purpura and coronary artery disease: comparison between coronary artery bypass grafting and percutaneous coronary intervention. Interact Cardiovasc Thorac Surg 2011;13(2):153–7.

32. Chan Wah Hak CM, Tan YO, Chan C. Coronary artery stenting in a patient with chronic immune thrombocytopenic purpura: A clinical conundrum. BMJ Case Rep 2012;2012. http://dx.doi.org/10.1136/bcr-02-2012-5802.

33. Mendez TC, Diaz O, Enriquez L, et al. Severe thrombocytopenia refractory to platelet transfusions, secondary to abciximab readministration, in a patient previously diagnosed with idiopathic thrombocytopenic purpura. A possible etiopathogenic link. Rev Esp Cardiol 2004;57(8):789–91.

34. Marques LG, Furukawa MK, Leitao TP, et al. Percutaneous transluminal coronary angioplasty in a patient with idiopathic thrombocytopenic purpura. Arq Bras Cardiol 2005;84(4):337–9.

35. Torok TJ, Holman RC, Chorba TL. Increasing mortality from thrombotic thrombocytopenic purpura in the united states–analysis of national mortality data, 1968-1991. Am J Hematol 1995;50(2):84–90.

36. Steinhubl SR, Tan WA, Foody JM, et al. Incidence and clinical course of thrombotic thrombocytopenic purpura due to ticlopidine following coronary stenting. EPISTENT investigators. evaluation of platelet IIb/IIIa inhibitor for stenting. JAMA 1999;281(9):806–10.

37. von Mach MA, Eich A, Weilemann LS, et al. Subacute coronary stent thrombosis in a patient developing clopidogrel associated thrombotic thrombocytopenic purpura. Heart 2005;91(2):e14.

38. Nishimura RA, Otto CM, Bonow RO, et al. 2014 AHA/ACC guideline for the management of patients with valvular heart disease: a report of the American College of Cardiology/American heart association task force on practice guidelines. Circulation 2014;129(23):e521–643.

39. Whitlock RP, Sun JC, Fremes SE, et al, American College of Chest Physicians. Antithrombotic and thrombolytic therapy for valvular disease: Antithrombotic therapy and prevention of thrombosis, 9th ed: American college of chest

physicians evidence-based clinical practice guidelines. Chest 2012;141(Suppl 2):e576S–600S.

40. Joint Task Force on the Management of Valvular Heart Disease of the European Society of Cardiology (ESC), European Association for Cardio-Thoracic Surgery (EACTS), Vahanian A, et al. Guidelines on the management of valvular heart disease (version 2012). Eur Heart J 2012;33(19):2451–96.

41. Phan TG, Koh M, Wijdicks EF. Safety of discontinuation of anticoagulation in patients with intracranial hemorrhage at high thromboembolic risk. Arch Neurol 2000;57(12):1710–3.

42. van Hagen IM, Roos-Hesselink JW, Ruys TP, et al. Pregnancy in women with a mechanical heart valve: Data of the european society of cardiology registry of pregnancy and cardiac disease (ROPAC). Circulation 2015;132(2):132–42.

43. Slaughter MS, Pagani FD, Rogers JG, et al. Clinical management of continuous-flow left ventricular assist devices in advanced heart failure. J Heart Lung Transplant 2010;29(4 Suppl):S1–39.

44. Baumann Kreuziger LM. Management of anticoagulation and antiplatelet therapy in patients with left ventricular assist devices. J Thromb Thrombolysis 2015;39(3): 337–44.

45. Morgan JA, Paone G, Nemeh HW, et al. Non-cardiac surgery in patients on long-term left ventricular assist device support. J Heart Lung Transplant 2012;31(7): 757–63.

46. Massie BM, Collins JF, Ammon SE, et al. Randomized trial of warfarin, aspirin, and clopidogrel in patients with chronic heart failure: The warfarin and antiplatelet therapy in chronic heart failure (WATCH) trial. Circulation 2009;119(12):1616–24.

47. Homma S, Thompson JL, Pullicino PM, et al. Warfarin and aspirin in patients with heart failure and sinus rhythm. N Engl J Med 2012;366(20):1859–69.

48. Cokkinos DV, Haralabopoulos GC, Kostis JB, et al, HELAS Investigators. Efficacy of antithrombotic therapy in chronic heart failure: The HELAS study. Eur J Heart Fail 2006;8(4):428–32.

49. Prom R, Usedom JE, Dull RB. Antithrombotics in heart failure with reduced ejection fraction and normal sinus rhythm: an evidence appraisal. Ann Pharmacother 2014;48(2):226–37.

Surgical Critical Care for the Trauma Patient with Cardiac Disease

 CrossMark

Michael M. Woll, MD[a], Linda L. Maerz, MD[b],*

KEYWORDS

- Geriatric trauma • Preexisting cardiac disease • Shock • Targeted resuscitation
- Myocardial ischemia • Cardiogenic shock • Blunt cardiac injury • Arrhythmias

KEY POINTS

- Effects of aging on cardiac performance include naturally occurring structural and functional changes of the aging heart as well as pathology associated with aging, including ischemic heart disease, arrhythmias, and valvular disease.
- Shock is defined by inadequate delivery of oxygen and nutrients required for normal cellular function. Differential diagnosis in the immediate postinjury period includes hemorrhagic shock, traumatic shock, and primary myocardial dysfunction.
- Targeted assessment of perfusion and resuscitation is essential in the management of any injured patient but is particularly important in the geriatric trauma patient with preexisting cardiac dysfunction.
- Management of cardiac dysfunction in the trauma patient includes an appreciation of the inherent effects of trauma on cardiac function as well as treatment of myocardial ischemia and infarction, cardiogenic shock, blunt cardiac injury, and arrhythmias.

INTRODUCTION

Evolution of Trauma Epidemiology in the United States: Geriatric Trauma and Preexisting Cardiac Disease

The elderly population is rapidly increasing in number. By 2040, more than 82 million Americans will be over age 65.[1] More Americans are living into their eighth and ninth decades and lead active lives, making them susceptible to injury. A minor injury in a young patient without cardiac disease can quickly overwhelm the cardiac reserve of an elderly patient, leading to significant physiologic derangement. The challenge to

Disclosure Statement: The authors have nothing to disclose.
[a] Section of General Surgery, Trauma & Surgical Critical Care, Department of Surgery, Yale School of Medicine, 330 Cedar Street, BB 310, PO Box 208062, New Haven, CT 06520-8062, USA; [b] Section of General Surgery, Trauma & Surgical Critical Care, Department of Surgery, Yale School of Medicine, 330 Cedar Street, BB 310, PO Box 208062, New Haven, CT 06520-8062, USA
* Corresponding author.
E-mail address: linda.maerz@yale.edu

Anesthesiology Clin 34 (2016) 669–680
http://dx.doi.org/10.1016/j.anclin.2016.06.004
1932-2275/16/© 2016 Elsevier Inc. All rights reserved.
anesthesiology.theclinics.com

all team members caring for the elderly is to rapidly identify underlying cardiac disease and intervene in a manner that limits the duration of myocardial oxygen supply–demand imbalance.

Effects of Aging on Cardiac Performance

Structural and functional changes of the aging heart

Aging produces many structural and functional changes in the heart. Myocytes decrease in number and are replaced with extracellular collagen matrix, resulting in decreased compliance of the ventricles. The number of sinoatrial (SA) node cells decreases, such that a 75-year-old man has only 10% of the SA nodal cells that he had at age 20. Therefore, conduction abnormalities and a prolonged PR interval are common. Stiffening of the aorta leads to uncoupling from the ventricle, increasing afterload and leading to myocardial hypertrophy and septal thickening. The net result is a stiff ventricle that fills more slowly, relying on atrial contraction in late diastole rather than passive early diastolic filling. A decrease in the average heart rate is compensatory, so that stroke volume is preserved at rest. In the absence of physiologic stress, these changes are imperceptible.[2]

Exercise tolerance significantly declines with aging. Maximum oxygen consumption decreases by 50% from age 20 to age 80. Structural changes play a role, but the transition to a hyposympathetic state accounts for much of this decline. In spite of an increase in circulating catecholamines, the cardiac response to adrenergic stimulation is blunted, because there are fewer adrenergic receptors in the aged heart. SERCA2 is an intracellular pump that facilitates the reuptake of calcium into the sarcoplasmic reticulum and is downregulated in the elderly. This results in prolongation of the cardiac action potential and compounds the diminished lusitropic state. Moreover, derangements in the myocyte–calcium interaction diminish intrinsic cardiac contractility.[3]

Pathology associated with aging: preexisting cardiac disease

Ischemic heart disease Although mortality from ischemic heart disease in the United States has decreased by 50% from its peak in 1963, it remains the leading cause of death in Americans.[4] Atherosclerosis creates fixed defects of the coronary arteries, limiting the ability to increase blood flow at times of increased myocardial demand, and creates an oxygen supply–demand imbalance, diminished cardiac reserve, and demand-related ischemia. Improved prevention and treatment of ischemic heart disease have dramatically reduced mortality, but survivors of ischemia are left with diminished cardiac reserve, a significant physiologic burden for those who sustain traumatic injuries.

Arrhythmias Atrial fibrillation, supraventricular tachycardia, and ventricular ectopic beats are more common in elderly patients. The incidence of atrial fibrillation is 10 times higher in those over age 65 compared with the general population. In the setting of decreased ventricular compliance and the increased importance of organized atrial contraction to maintain stroke volume, atrial fibrillation can cause significant degradation of cardiac output, which compounds the physiologic burden in the elderly trauma patient.

Valvular disease Nkomo and colleagues[5] reported an 8.5% incidence of valvular disease in patients aged 65 to 74 years and an 13.2% incidence in patients over age 75. This was associated with a 14% increase in mortality at 5 years compared with those without valvular disease. Mitral regurgitation (MR) and aortic regurgitation (AR) were more common than aortic stenosis (AS) in this study. However, AS is especially significant in the trauma population. Increased resistance to left ventricular ejection results in ventricular hypertrophy and decreased compliance. With increasing severity of AS, the ventricle becomes reliant on atrial contractility to sustain cardiac output. Therefore, even slight changes in preload can result in significant decompensation. Additionally, AS and associated syncope may be the antecedent precipitant of traumatic injuries in elderly patients and should be identified prior to operative interventions.[6]

Cardiovascular medications in the geriatric patient population
Calcium channel blockers (CCBs) and beta (β) blockers (BBs) are frequently prescribed agents for blood pressure or rate control in the geriatric population.[7] Both CCBs and BBs have significant negative inotropic and chronotropic effects, which significantly blunt the adrenergic response to trauma and prevent compensatory mechanisms from reestablishing homeostasis after injury. Additionally, these and other antiarrhythmic medications prevent tachycardia and, thereby, may delay diagnosis and intervention for traumatic hemorrhage.

MANAGEMENT GOALS
Identification of the Shock State and Relationship to Cardiac Dysfunction

Definition and phenotype of shock
Shock causes inadequate delivery of oxygen and nutrients required for normal cellular function.[8] Shock results from injury and the myriad host responses designed to redirect the physiology back toward homeostasis. With significant trauma, uncontrolled hemorrhage, or ongoing sepsis, inflammation is propagated. A systemic cascade of events results in ongoing physiologic derangement and organ dysfunction. As shock progresses, cellular function shifts to anaerobic metabolism, resulting in metabolic acidosis. Prolonged cellular acidosis results in decreased activity of cellular enzymes, alterations in gene expression, and interference with membrane ion exchange, resulting in cell swelling and further reduction in plasma volume. As the metabolic crisis and cellular swelling progress, lysosomal and cell membranes rupture, and cell death ensues.

Apropos to the trauma patient, with increasing grades of hemorrhage, adrenergic stimulation of the heart results in an increase in heart rate to maintain cardiac output. A normal adult heart can meet this demand by increasing the heart rate up to 170 to 190 beats per minute, depending on the premorbid level of conditioning.[9] Release of vasoactive peptides results in the shunting of blood away from splanchnic, renal, and musculocutaneous circulations to vital organs, such as the brain and heart. The physical manifestations of shock include mental status changes, diaphoresis, hypothermia, pallor, mottled extremities, and oliguria.

Immediate postinjury differential diagnosis of shock
Hemorrhagic shock Tissue hypoperfusion may be masked by the aforementioned mechanisms in the geriatric trauma patient. Multiple authors have demonstrated that traditional vital signs are insensitive markers for significant hypovolemia in geriatric patients.[10,11] The elderly have a lower maximum heart rate and decreased peripheral vascular compliance, rendering them hypertensive at baseline. A common pitfall in the evaluation of geriatric trauma patients is the mistaken impression that normal blood pressure and heart rate indicate normovolemia.[12] Therefore, a high index of suspicion is required to identify tissue hypoperfusion. At least initially, shock in the trauma patient is presumed to be hemorrhagic and prompts fluid and blood product administration while hemorrhage control is achieved.

Traumatic shock The systemic response to injury does not necessarily correlate with the degree of hemorrhage. For example, a small-volume blood loss associated with significant blunt trauma can elicit a profound systemic inflammatory response similar to the systemic inflammatory response syndrome (SIRS).[13] Some authors propose that release of cellular organelles into the circulation, especially after reperfusion, stimulates an intense immune response. Others cite microcirculatory dysfunction and gut ischemia resulting from redistribution of cardiac output, with resultant bacterial translocation and endotoxemia.[14–16]

Primary myocardial dysfunction Failure to respond to resuscitation in spite of hemorrhage control or the absence of significant injuries identifiable during the primary and secondary surveys should raise the possibility of concomitant cardiac pathology. Additionally, particularly in the geriatric population, a cardiac event may have triggered the trauma.

Response to hypovolemia in the geriatric patient
The altered response to hypovolemia in the geriatric patient deserves emphasis and specific comment. Catecholamine insensitivity, atherosclerosis, myocardial fibrosis, and conduction abnormalities attenuate the elderly patient's chronotropic response to hypovolemia. Additionally, baseline hypertension is more prevalent in elderly patients, rendering a normal systolic blood pressure misleading. Accordingly, a narrowed pulse pressure may be the first indicator of hypovolemic shock in the elderly patient.

Targeted Assessment of Perfusion and Resuscitation

Shock index versus traditional vital signs
As noted previously, traditional vital signs may be insensitive markers for significant hypovolemia in geriatric trauma patients. The utility of traditional vital signs has been questioned as being too insensitive to detect the early stages of hemorrhagic shock, given the wide range of normal. The shock index, defined as the systolic blood pressure divided by the heart rate, has been proposed as a measure of significant hemorrhage.[17] Shock index has been validated in several trials as being sensitive to hemorrhage requiring a massive transfusion in young patients, but is less so with patients older than 65 years of age.

End-organ perfusion
With loss of greater than 30% of the circulating blood volume, symptoms of decreased end-organ perfusion appear.[8] The brain and the kidneys are 2 organs that are readily amenable to assessment with respect to perfusion. Mental confusion may be difficult to distinguish from dementia in an elderly trauma patient; nonetheless, hemorrhagic shock must be ruled out in the elderly patient presenting with an abnormal mental status. Activation of the renin–angiotensin cascade results in afferent arteriolar constriction, decreased renal blood flow, and oliguria. Diminished end-organ perfusion portends cardiovascular collapse if the hemorrhage is not controlled and resuscitation not promptly initiated.

Central venous pressure
Early goal-directed therapy (EGDT) has been adopted into the Surviving Sepsis Campaign guidelines.[18] These guidelines prescribe volume resuscitation to achieve a central venous pressure (CVP) of 8 to 12 mm Hg, a mean arterial pressure of 65 to 90 mm Hg, and a central venous oxygen saturation of 70%. However, CVP

measurement as an endpoint of resuscitation has not been uniformly accepted and, in fact, has been challenged.[19]

Pulmonary artery catheter measurements

In the past, the pulmonary artery catheter (PAC) was a standard tool in the hemodynamic monitoring of critically ill patients. In recent years, inappropriate use and inaccurate interpretation of the data have been demonstrated to cause harm.[20–22] With declining use of the PAC, fewer clinicians have the expertise to use these devices and interpret the associated data. Therefore, the PAC has a limited role in the management of the trauma patient.

Central venous oxygen saturation

Matching oxygen supply to tissue demand is the goal of resuscitation. With decreased perfusion of the peripheral tissues, oxygen extraction increases, resulting in a lower venous oxygen saturation. Continuous measurement of the central venous oxygen saturation ($S_{cv}O_2$) offers the ability to gauge the adequacy of resuscitation and changes in perfusion status. Some authors have proposed a target of 70%, but trending the values to assess the impact of resuscitation and detect changes in perfusion is likely more useful than targeting an absolute percentage.[23]

Venous lactate and base deficit

In conditions of low oxygen tension, such as shock, cells shift to the anaerobic pathway of glycolysis in order to meet their metabolic needs, resulting in lactic acid production. In hemorrhagic shock, lactic acid is not cleared and leads to metabolic acidosis.[9] Venous lactate is an indicator of inadequate resuscitation and persistence of the oxygen debt. When measured serially, it offers another data set as a means to assess the dynamic adequacy of resuscitation.[24]

Ultrasonography

Bedside ultrasonography has become an increasingly important diagnostic and therapeutic tool for the management of trauma patients. Transthoracic ultrasound offers a real-time image of cardiac contractility and valvular function.[25] The inferior vena cava (IVC) collapsibility index, defined as the difference in IVC diameter measured ultrasonographically during inspiration and expiration divided by the maximal diameter, can identify hypovolemia.[26] A collapsibility index of greater than 12% in spontaneously breathing patients and 18% in mechanically ventilated patients is predictive of fluid responsiveness.[27]

Functional hemodynamic monitoring

Functional hemodynamic monitoring (FHM) is the process of assessing the dynamic response of a measured hemodynamic variable to a defined, reproducible, and readily reversible extrinsic stress.[28] A simple example is administration of a fluid challenge and observation of a physiologic response, such as change in mean arterial pressure.

Pulse pressure and stroke volume variation

Pulse pressure variation (PPV) is the difference in the pulse pressure between inspiration and expiration and is measured by tracking an arterial line tracing. Commercial devices provide algorithm-driven parameters to refine the displayed PPV. A PPV greater than 11% to 13% is predictive of volume responsiveness.[29] Devices to assess stroke volume variation (SVV) utilize ultrasound or an arterial line tracing to analyze the contour of the arterial pulse and calculate the stroke volume. An SVV of at least 14% is predictive of fluid responsiveness in surgical patients, burn patients, and patients with cardiac dysfunction.[30]

Management of Cardiac Dysfunction in the Trauma Patient

Inherent effects of trauma on cardiac function

Acidosis and hypothermia Hemorrhagic shock results in anaerobic glycolysis due to failure to deliver adequate oxygen to the tissues. Lactic acidosis progresses to systemic acidosis, which blunts the inotropic and chronotropic response of β-adrenergic receptors to stimulation by epinephrine and norepinephrine. Even mild acidosis impairs the function of slow calcium channels in cardiac myocytes, resulting in depressed contractility. This is exacerbated by hypothermia, which is common in trauma patients. Severe hypothermia (core body temperature <30° C) significantly increases the risk for arrhythmias. Furthermore, skin thickness decreases by 20% in the elderly, leading to impaired thermoregulatory capability.[8]

Systemic inflammatory response syndrome Trauma and shock induce a SIRS response that may be incommensurate with the degree of blood loss. This is likely due to destruction of the endothelial glycocalyx, resulting in activation of immune effector cells and microcirculatory dysfunction that persists beyond restoration of blood volume. Additionally, adrenergic stimulation activates cytokine production and stimulates the immune response, which consists of inflammatory and immunologic mediators that are part of the local response to injury and infection, but cause global derangement in tissues and organs when released into the systemic circulation.[1] Tumor necrosis factor-alpha (TNF-α), interleukin-6 (IL-6), and IL-8 levels are elevated in both septic and hemorrhagic shock. They are responsible for a peripheral vasodilation, cellular metabolic changes, and modulation of immune effector cells; additionally, they may lead to myocardial injury by direct cytotoxic effects.[31]

Myocardial ischemia and infarction

Cardiac troponin levels Type 1 myocardial infarction (MI) is spontaneous, caused by plaque rupture, and is the most common type of MI in the nonsurgical population. Type 2 MI is caused by demand ischemia and is the more common type encountered in trauma and postoperative populations.

Cardiac troponin (cTn) is released as a result of myocardial cell injury and is specific to the myocardium. Given the sensitivity of present assays, elevated cTn may exist in the setting of myocardial injury without infarction. Because of multiple confounding physiologic factors and masking of typical symptoms by pain due to distracting injuries, the diagnosis of MI in the trauma patient can be difficult and requires a high index of suspicion.

Significance of elevated troponin levels without myocardial infarction Elevated cTn levels indicate myocardial cell death, but do not necessarily diagnose MI. Multiple investigations in both medical and trauma intensive care units (ICUs) have demonstrated a significant increase in mortality in critically ill patients who have elevated cTn levels when compared to similarly matched cohorts in whom cTn levels remain normal.[31–34] When viewed as an indicator of myocardial cell damage resulting from oxygen supply–demand imbalance, even mildly elevated cTn levels should be addressed by improving myocardial oxygen delivery and decreasing demand.

Diagnosis of myocardial infarction Type 1 MI is caused by plaque rupture and is associated with ST-segment elevation (STEMI) on electrocardiogram (EKG) and elevated cTn levels. Type 2 MI is far more common in the trauma setting and results from prolonged oxygen supply–demand imbalance, which may manifest as ST segment depression on EKG. Tachycardia is the most important cause of oxygen supply–demand imbalance. In patients with significant coronary artery disease, an increase in the heart rate from a baseline of 50 to 60 beats per minute (bpm) to 80 to 90 bpm can lead to prolonged ischemia and MI.[35] Once hemorrhage has been controlled, if there is ongoing concern for hypoperfusion, a formal echocardiogram is indicated. Wall motion abnormalities in the setting of rising cTn levels suggest MI.

Treatment of acute myocardial infarction Treatment of acute myocardial infarction (AMI) in the trauma patient is often complicated by the competing risk of bleeding associated with acute injuries. Treatment is directed at restoration of blood flow to the infarcted region in order to salvage endangered myocardium in the penumbra of the infarct. Regardless of the type of MI, the immediate management is the same. Hypovolemia and hypothermia are corrected. Oxygenation is optimized with administration of supplemental oxygen or mechanical ventilation if indicated. Pain control is of utmost importance, particularly in the injured patient, in order to decrease adrenergic stimulation and myocardial oxygen consumption. Because of their negative inotropic effects, CCBs and BBs have a limited role in the acute setting; however, they improve survival when used for long-term therapy. Nitrates are administered if the systolic blood pressure is greater than 90 mm Hg. They exert a vasodilatory effect through the formation of nitric oxide (NO) and resultant vascular smooth muscle relaxation. These effects are dose dependent; venous effects predominate at low doses, and arterial tone is decreased at higher doses. Caution must be exercised in the trauma patient to ensure adequate volume status prior to administration of nitrates in order to avoid hypotension and resultant further compromise of coronary perfusion. The positive effects of nitrates on myocardial oxygen delivery are due to improved subendocardial perfusion.[9] Early administration of aspirin is a cornerstone of AMI therapy and must be weighed against the risk of bleeding. Judgment must be exercised in the presence of intracranial hemorrhage, thrombocytopenia, or ongoing hemorrhage. Each case must be individually assessed with respect to risk–benefit analysis of antiplatelet therapy.[36]

In any patient with AMI, options for anatomic revascularization include percutaneous coronary intervention (PCI) and coronary artery bypass grafting (CABG). Inherent in both of these procedures is the requirement for either antiplatelet therapy, systemic anticoagulation, or both. Systemic thrombolysis is another option when PCI is not readily available. All of these procedures obviously predispose to recurrent or ongoing hemorrhage in the trauma patient. At particularly significant risk are those patients who have suffered traumatic brain injury.[37] Decisions regarding utility of these procedures, anticoagulation, and antiplatelet therapy are made on a case-by-case basis in a multidisciplinary manner, weighing the benefits of augmented coronary perfusion against the risk of significant hemorrhage.

Cardiogenic shock
Pathogenesis and general principles of management Even when adequately resuscitated, those patients who lack sufficient cardiac reserve to meet the physiologic stress of the traumatic insult will require cardiac support. The most common cause of cardiogenic shock is systolic dysfunction resulting from left ventricular (LV) failure. Fixed coronary artery defects and loss of cardiac reserve result in decreased myocardial performance in the setting of demand ischemia. The resultant hypotension compromises coronary perfusion pressure. Compromised stroke volume and cardiac output ensue, further exacerbating myocardial ischemia and dysfunction. Diastolic dysfunction leads to elevated LV end-diastolic pressure and pulmonary congestion. Hypoxemia results in further exacerbation of the myocardial oxygen supply–demand imbalance.[38]

Treatment of cardiogenic shock begins with correction of hypovolemia, of particular importance in the severely injured trauma patient. In diastolic dysfunction, the heart is preload dependent, so filling pressures should be optimized and can be monitored with functional hemodynamic monitoring devices, transesophageal echocardiography (TEE), or transthoracic echocardiography (TTE). Oxygenation is optimized with mechanical ventilation if indicated. Of note, positive pressure ventilation can adversely affect preload by decreasing venous return. If hypotension persists in spite of these measures, pharmacologic support is required.

Pharmacologic agents Both vasopressors and inotropes play a role in the pharmacologic management of cardiogenic shock. Some of these agents have both vasopressor and inotropic effects, dependent on the dose employed.

At high doses, norepinephrine (NE) acts as a potent vasoconstrictor, exerting its effects through α- and β-adrenergic mechanisms. Thus, at high doses, it can increase afterload and thereby increase myocardial oxygen consumption. However, at lower doses, the β-adrenergic effects predominate, which increase both myocardial contractility and relaxation. Dopamine (DA) similarly increases both blood pressure and cardiac output through stimulation of α- and β-beta adrenergic receptors as well as DA1 and DA2 receptors. Its effects are dose dependent. At high doses (>10 μg/kg/min), α-adrenergic effects predominate, leading to vasoconstriction, tachycardia, and increased myocardial oxygen consumption. Accordingly, NE has demonstrated superior survival compared with DA in the treatment of cardiogenic shock.[39]

Dobutamine, a synthetic catecholamine, exerts specific inotropic effects through β_1-adrenergic receptors. It is a first-line agent in the treatment of cardiogenic shock in patients who have adequate preload and systolic blood pressure above 80 mm Hg. It improves cardiac contractility and output without increasing myocardial oxygen demand. However, use may be limited by the precipitation of tachyarrhythmias and hypotension. These effects can be offset by the concomitant administration of phenylephrine, a selective α_1 agonist. Epinephrine is a naturally occurring catecholamine that is a potent α- and β-adrenergic agonist. At low doses, β effects predominate and can be used for ventricular dysfunction refractory to dobutamine. However, epinephrine is limited by its propensity for renal artery constriction, arrhythmias, and metabolic derangements, including ketoacidosis and hyperglycemia.[1]

Amrinone and milrinone are phosphodiesterase III inhibitors that have positive inotropic effects and decrease afterload by decreasing vasomotor tone. They should be used with caution in patients who have borderline blood pressure, as they may precipitate hypotension. They have longer half-lives than dobutamine, which prevent them from being titrated to effect in a short timeframe.

Intra-aortic balloon pump counterpulsation Intra-aortic balloon pump (IABP) counterpulsation can serve as a bridge to intervention to correct anatomic etiologies of myocardial failure, such as valvular disease (other than aortic insufficiency) or critical coronary artery stenosis. This device reduces afterload by synchronizing balloon inflation to an EKG monitor. Use of the IABP alone has not demonstrated improved mortality. In patients at high risk for bleeding, such as acute trauma patients, its use is limited by the need for systemic anticoagulation. There are no prospective studies involving trauma patients, but there are case reports of success as a means to provide support and allow time for definitive interventions.[40]

Blunt cardiac injury
Blunt cardiac injury (BCI) usually results from motor vehicle crashes. BCI encompasses a wide range of diagnoses and is present in approximately 20% of blunt

trauma victims, but with severe thoracic trauma or multisystem trauma, the risk approaches 76%.[41] Injuries that should raise suspicion for BCI include sternal fracture, pulmonary contusion, scapular fracture, multiple rib fractures, and seat belt sign. The most common site of injury is the right ventricle, although multiple chambers can be involved. Manifestations of BCI include septal rupture, free wall rupture, coronary artery thrombosis, valvular dysfunction, cardiac failure, minor EKG/enzyme abnormalities, or complex arrhythmias.[42] However, the most common manifestation of BCI is occasional premature ventricular complexes.[1]

All patients presenting with chest trauma or a mechanism suggestive of chest trauma (ie, high-speed motor vehicle crash) should undergo EKG evaluation. However, a normal EKG does not rule out BCI and may miss 13% of significant BCI.[43] Therefore, cTn levels should be measured in patients who have suspicion of BCI due to mechanism or an abnormal EKG. Those patients with normal EKGs and normal cTn can be discharged from the emergency department if there are no other indications for admission.[43] Patients with an abnormal EKG or elevated cTn should be placed in a monitored setting for 24 to 48 hours.

Patients who are or become hypotensive should undergo echocardiography. Coronary artery thrombosis and dissection have been described in multiple case reports.[44] An abnormal EKG and abnormal wall motion noted on echocardiogram should prompt urgent cardiology consultation, as coronary lesions are often amenable to PCI with clot evacuation and stenting. Echocardiography may also demonstrate valvular pathology. The most common valvular injury is aortic insufficiency, most likely resulting from a sudden increase in aortic pressure against a closed aortic valve.[45]

Arrhythmias

General principles Acidosis and increased levels of circulating catecholamines inherent to the stress response of surgery and trauma predispose these patients to the development of arrhythmias. Approximately 12% to 40% of patients admitted to the ICU experience a dysrhythmia during their admission. Tachyarrhythmias comprise 90% of the arrhythmias encountered in the ICU. ST is the most common EKG abnormality, but is not considered a dysrhythmia. Rather, sinus tachycardia (ST) is a physiologic response to increased tissue demand for oxygen. Thus, predisposing factors such as fever, pain, and anemia should be identified and corrected to avoid increased myocardial oxygen demand and potential demand ischemia.

The first step in management of arrhythmias is to assess for stability. Unstable patients suffering from tachyarrhythmias may require immediate direct current (DC) cardioversion when mental status changes, oliguria, ischemia, congestive heart failure, or hypotension result from the arrhythmia. An EKG, cTn level, serum electrolytes, and chest radiograph should be obtained. Physiologic factors predisposing to dysrhythmias should be identified and corrected, including electrolyte derangements and conditions contributing to acidosis, including hypovolemia and hypoventilation.

Atrial fibrillation Atrial fibrillation is the most common supraventricular dysrhythmia observed in the ICU. It is commonly associated with left atrial distension caused by fluid shifts. In patients with underlying heart disease, such as MS or AS and hypertrophic cardiomyopathy, the loss of organized atrial contraction can result in cardiogenic shock or myocardial ischemia. The immediate goal of therapy is to control the heart rate to facilitate diastolic filling. If the patient is unstable, DC cardioversion should be performed. For stable patients, rate control with BBs, CCBs, digoxin, or amiodarone can be used. Although BBs tend to be more effective than CCBs and are considered first-line agents, both classes of medication should be used with caution in trauma patients because of the potential for hypotension, particularly if the degree of hypovolemia is underappreciated. In patients with an ejection fraction of less than 40%, amiodarone should be the first-line agent. Class III antiarrhythmic agents can be used as second-line drugs to convert patients to sinus rhythm. However, the Atrial Fibrillation Follow-up Investigation of Rhythm Management trial demonstrated no long-term benefit of conversion over rate control in high-risk, hemodynamically stable elderly patients.[46]

SUMMARY

Effects of aging on cardiac performance include naturally occurring structural and functional changes of the aging heart as well as pathology associated with aging, including ischemic heart disease, arrhythmias, and valvular disease. Shock causes inadequate delivery of oxygen and nutrients required for normal cellular function. Differential diagnosis in the immediate postinjury period includes hemorrhagic shock, traumatic shock, and primary myocardial dysfunction. Targeted assessment of perfusion and resuscitation are essential in the management of any injured patient, but are particularly important in the geriatric trauma patient with preexisting cardiac dysfunction. Management of cardiac dysfunction in the trauma patient includes an appreciation of the inherent effects of trauma on cardiac function as well as treatment of myocardial ischemia and infarction, cardiogenic shock, blunt cardiac injury, and arrhythmias.

REFERENCES

1. Yelon JA. The geriatric patient. In: Mattox KL, Moore EE, Feliciano DV, editors. Trauma. 7th edition. New York: McGraw-Hill Medical; 2013. p. 874–5.
2. Strait JB, Lakatta EG. Aging-associated cardiovascular changes and their relationship to heart failure. Heart Fail Clin 2012;8:143–64.
3. Fleg JL, Strait J. Age-associated changes in cardiovascular structure and function: a fertile milieu for future disease. Heart Fail Rev 2012;17:545–54.
4. Schoen FJ, Mitchell RN. The heart. In: Kumar V, Abbas AK, Aster JC, editors. Robbins and Cotran pathologic basis of disease. 9th edition. Philadelphia: Elsevier/Saunders; 2015. p. 523–78.
5. Nkomo VT, Gardin JM, Skelton TN, et al. Burden of valvular heart diseases: a population-based study. Lancet 2006;368:1005–11.
6. Loxdale SJ, Sneyd JR, Donovan A, et al. The role of routine pre-operative bedside echocardiography in detecting aortic stenosis in patients with a hip fracture. Anaesthesia 2012;67:51–4.
7. Chen N, Zhou M, Yang M, et al. Calcium channel blockers versus other classes of drugs for hypertension. Cochrane Database Syst Rev 2010;(8):CD003654.
8. American College of Surgeons Committee on Trauma. Shock. In: Advanced trauma life support student course manual. 9th edition. Chicago: American College of Surgeons; 2012. p. 62–8, 69–81.
9. Hall JE. Cardiac output, venous return, and their regulation. In: Hall JE, editor. Guyton and Hall textbook of medical physiology. 13th edition. Philadelphia: Elsevier; 2016. p. 245–58.
10. Salottolo KM, Mains CW, Offner PJ, et al. A retrospective analysis of geriatric trauma patients: venous lactate is a better predictor of mortality than traditional vital signs. Scand J Trauma Resusc Emerg Med 2013;21:7.

11. Zarzaur BL, Croce MA, Magnotti LJ, et al. Identifying life-threatening shock in the older injured patient: an analysis of the National Trauma Data Bank. J Trauma 2010;68:1134–8.
12. Demetriades D, Chan LS, Bhasin P, et al. Relative bradycardia in patients with traumatic hypotension. J Trauma 1998;45:534–9.
13. Magnotti LJ, Upperman JS, Xu DZ, et al. Gut-derived mesenteric lymph but not portal blood increases endothelial cell permeability and promotes lung injury after hemorrhagic shock. Ann Surg 1998;228:518–27.
14. Peitzman AB, Billiar TR, Harbrecht BG, et al. Hemorrhagic shock. Curr Probl Surg 1995;32:925–1002.
15. Gierer P, Hoffmann JN, Mahr F, et al. Sublethal trauma model with systemic endotoxemia for the study of microcirculatory disorders after the second hit. J Surg Res 2008;147:68–74.
16. Iba T, Miki T, Hashiguchi N, et al. Combination of antithrombin and recombinant thrombomodulin attenuates leukocyte–endothelial interaction and suppresses the increase of intrinsic damage-associated molecular patterns in endotoxemic rats. J Surg Res 2014;187:581–6.
17. Olaussen A, Peterson EL, Mitra B, et al. Massive transfusion prediction with inclusion of the pre-hospital Shock Index. Injury 2015;46:822–6.
18. Dellinger RP, Levy MM, Rhodes A, et al. Surviving sepsis campaign: international guidelines for management of severe sepsis and septic shock, 2012. Intensive Care Med 2013;39:165–228.
19. Marik PE, Baram M, Vahid B. Does central venous pressure predict fluid responsiveness? A systematic review of the literature and the tale of seven mares. Chest 2008;134:172–8.
20. Binanay C, Califf RM, Hasselblad V, et al. Evaluation study of congestive heart failure and pulmonary artery catheterization effectiveness: the ESCAPE trial. JAMA 2005;294:1625–33.
21. Connors AF Jr, Speroff T, Dawson NV, et al. The effectiveness of right heart catheterization in the initial care of critically ill patients. SUPPORT Investigators. JAMA 1996;276:889–97.
22. Wheeler AP, Bernard GR, Thompson BT, et al. Pulmonary-artery versus central venous catheter to guide treatment of acute lung injury. N Engl J Med 2006; 354:2213–24.
23. Reinhart K, Kuhn HJ, Hartog C, et al. Continuous central venous and pulmonary artery oxygen saturation monitoring in the critically ill. Intensive Care Med 2004; 30:1572–8.
24. Barbee RW, Reynolds PS, Ward KR. Assessing shock resuscitation strategies by oxygen debt repayment. Shock 2010;33:113–22.
25. Ferrada P, Vanguri P, Anand RJ, et al. A, B, C, D, echo: limited transthoracic echocardiogram is a useful tool to guide therapy for hypotension in the trauma bay—a pilot study. J Trauma Acute Care Surg 2013;74:220–3.
26. Huang SJ, McLean AS. Appreciating the strengths and weaknesses of transthoracic echocardiography in hemodynamic assessments. Cardiol Res Pract 2012; 2012:894308.
27. Wesson HK, Khan S, Ferrada P. Ultrasound as a tool for fluid status assessment in the trauma and critically ill patient. Int J Surg 2015. http://dx.doi.org/10.1016/j.ijsu.2015.9.063.
28. Pinsky MR. Functional haemodynamic monitoring. Curr Opin Crit Care 2014;20: 288–93.

29. Michard F, Teboul JL. Using heart-lung interactions to assess fluid responsiveness during mechanical ventilation. Crit Care 2000;4:282–9.

30. Reuter DA, Kirchner A, Felbinger TW, et al. Usefulness of left ventricular stroke volume variation to assess fluid responsiveness in patients with reduced cardiac function. Crit Care Med 2003;31:1399–404.

31. Korff S, Katus HA, Giannitsis E. Differential diagnosis of elevated troponins. Heart 2006;92:987–93.

32. Turley AJ, Gedney JA. Role of cardiac troponin as a prognosticator in critically ill patients. Crit Care 2005;9:E30.

33. Ammann P, Maggiorini M, Bertel O, et al. Troponin as a risk factor for mortality in critically ill patients without acute coronary syndromes. J Am Coll Cardiol 2003; 41:2004–9.

34. Ostermann M, Lo J, Toolan M, et al. A prospective study of the impact of serial troponin measurements on the diagnosis of myocardial infarction and hospital and six-month mortality in patients admitted to ICU with non-cardiac diagnoses. Crit Care 2014;18:R62.

35. Landesberg G, Beattie WS, Mosseri M, et al. Perioperative myocardial infarction. Circulation 2009;119:2936–44.

36. Lewis HD Jr, Davis JW, Archibald DG, et al. Protective effects of aspirin against acute myocardial infarction and death in men with unstable angina. Results of a Veterans Administration cooperative study. N Engl J Med 1983;309:396–403.

37. Rabin J, Harris DG, Crews GA, et al. Early aortic repair worsens concurrent traumatic brain injury. Ann Thorac Surg 2014;98:46–51.

38. Mega JL, Morrow DA. ST-elevation myocardial infarction. In: Mann DL, Zipes DP, Libby P, et al, editors. Braunwald's heart disease: a textbook of cardiovascular medicine. 10th edition. Philadelphia: Elsevier/Saunders; 2015. p. 1095–154.

39. De Backer D, Biston P, Devriendt J, et al. Comparison of dopamine and norepinephrine in the treatment of shock. N Engl J Med 2010;362:779–89.

40. Bates ER, Stomel RJ, Hochman JS, et al. The use of intra-aortic balloon counterpulsation as an adjunct to reperfusion therapy in cardiogenic shock. Int J Cardiol 1998;65(Suppl 1):S37–42.

41. Schultz JM, Trunkey DD. Blunt cardiac injury. Crit Care Clin 2004;20:57–70.

42. Mattox KL, Flint LM, Carrico CJ, et al. Blunt cardiac injury. J Trauma 1992;33: 649–50.

43. Velmahos GC, Karaiskakis M, Salim A, et al. Normal electrocardiography and serum troponin I levels preclude the presence of clinically significant blunt cardiac injury. J Trauma 2003;54:45–50.

44. Maron BJ, Doerer JJ, Haas TS, et al. Sudden deaths in young competitive athletes: analysis of 1866 deaths in the United States, 1980-2006. Circulation 2009;119:1085–92.

45. Marcolini EG, Keegan J. Blunt cardiac injury. Emerg Med Clin North Am 2015;33: 519–27.

46. Wyse DG, Waldo AL, DiMarco JP, et al. A comparison of rate control and rhythm control in patients with atrial fibrillation. N Engl J Med 2002;347:1825–33.

Surgical Critical Care for the Patient with Sepsis and Multiple Organ Dysfunction

 CrossMark

Gary J. Kaml, MD[a],*, Kimberly A. Davis, MD, MBA, FCCM[b]

KEYWORDS

- Multiple organ dysfunction syndrome • Sepsis • Septic shock • Surgical critical care
- Severe sepsis • Sepsis treatment

KEY POINTS

- Sepsis and multiple organ dysfunction syndrome (MODS) are common problems among surgical intensive care unit patients, and a significant source of cost, morbidity, and mortality.
- The concept of sepsis must incorporate both the infectious insult and the host's response to that insult.
- Early recognition of the symptoms, physiologic disturbances, and laboratory findings of sepsis, and prompt and aggressive interventions, are critical to the success of therapy.
- Treatment of the patient with MODS should focus on control and treatment of an infectious source, along with supportive therapy to maintain organ homeostasis.
- Despite advances in treatment, sepsis and MODS carry a significant mortality rate; early discussion helps to establish expectations and goals of care.

INTRODUCTION

Sepsis and multiple organ dysfunction syndrome (MODS) are clinical entities commonly seen in the critically ill surgical patients. Advances in medical therapies have resulted in a more elderly population, and have allowed critically ill and injured patients to survive their initial illness, only to develop sepsis thereafter. There are an estimated 1.1 million cases of sepsis in the United States annually, costing more than $24.3 billion.[1]

Disclosure Statement: The authors have nothing to disclose.
[a] Section of General Surgery, Trauma, and Surgical Critical Care, Department of Surgery, Yale School of Medicine, 330 Cedar Street, BB310, PO Box 208062, New Haven, CT 06520-8062, USA; [b] Department of Surgery, Quality and Performance Improvement, Yale-New Haven Hospital, Yale School of Medicine, 330 Cedar Street BB310, New Haven, CT 06520-8062, USA
* Corresponding author.
E-mail address: gary.kaml@yale.edu

Anesthesiology Clin 34 (2016) 681–696
http://dx.doi.org/10.1016/j.anclin.2016.06.005
1932-2275/16/© 2016 Elsevier Inc. All rights reserved.

The concept of sepsis as a discrete clinical entity was first outlined by Bone and co-workers[2] in 1989, and can be defined as the invasion of microorganisms and/or their toxins into the patient's bloodstream, in concert with the patient's response to that infection characterized by systemic inflammation. Sepsis is characterized by hemostatic dysregulation and endothelial dysfunction, resulting in compromise of both the circulatory system and intracellular homeostasis. The resultant cellular hypoxia and programmed cell death (apoptosis) are responsible for organ dysfunction and death.

INCIDENCE AND RISK FACTORS

Sepsis is common in the intensive care unit (ICU), and 10% to 15% of patients in the ICU develop septic shock, with a mortality rates of 50% to 60%.[3] Sepsis remains the number one cause of death in noncardiac ICUs, and surgical patients account for one-third of sepsis cases in the United States.[1,4] In surgical patients, sepsis and septic shock are 10 times more common than perioperative myocardial infarction and pulmonary embolism, with septic shock carrying the highest mortality.[5]

Common sources of sepsis in surgical patients include surgical wound and organ space infections, pneumonia, urinary tract infections, and catheter-associated bloodstream infections. Among hospital-acquired infections, nosocomial pneumonias are most common at 43%, followed by urinary tract infections at 25%. Catheter-associated bloodstream infections increased with the increased use of central lines, invasive monitoring, and parenteral nutrition since the 1970s but have declined over the past decade in response to standardization of catheter insertion bundles. Surgical site infections also continue to decline owing to improvements in perioperative antibiotics and sterile technique but still account for 10% of nosocomial infections.[6] Polymicrobial infections are more common in patients with organ space infections.

Advanced age and male gender are known risk factors for the development of sepsis. Chronic health issues such as obesity, alcohol use, immune status, physical conditioning, and medical comorbidities can contribute to the genesis and progression of sepsis. Finally, we are just beginning to understand that genetic factors may be an influence in sepsis development and patient survival.[7–10]

PATHOGENIC STIMULUS

Fundamental to the diagnosis of sepsis is the presence of infection. Although activation of the systemic inflammatory response syndrome (SIRS) is the final common pathway leading to MODS, signal pathways vary depending on the infecting organism. In gram-negative sepsis, the initiation of the host immune response is mediated primarily by lipopolysaccharide from the bacterial cell wall. Lipopolysaccharide binds to CD14 and Toll-like receptor-4 receptors to induce activation of a transcription factor known as nuclear factor kappa-B.[11,12] Nuclear factor kappa-B then activates gene promoters, which results in the transcription and expression of genes for cytokines and other proinflammatory mediators.[13] Gram-positive bacteria lack lipopolysaccharide, and are characterized by cell wall components (peptidoglycans and others), as well as specific bacterial toxins. The main pattern of recognition in gram-positive bacteremia is via lipoteichoic acid, a cell wall component found in all gram-positive bacteria that, along with other components of gram positive bacteria, interacts with the Toll-like receptor-2 receptor.[14] The resulting release of tumor necrosis factor (TNF)-α, interleukin (IL)-6, and IL-10 seem to be through a similar pathway of signal transduction.[13] The initiation of the host response and release of proinflammatory mediators in fungal and viral infections is less well-understood. The recognition of viruses is generally through endosomal Toll-like receptors.

IMMUNOLOGIC RESPONSE

Sepsis induces a host immune response that is complex and far-reaching. The primary mediators involved are TNF-α and IL-1β, which are released by CD4 T cells and macrophages early in the infectious process. Inflammation is then amplified when these cytokines induce the release of several secondary mediators, including IL-6, IL-8, platelet activating factor, and others (**Fig. 1**). The complement system also plays an important role in the proinflammatory response. C5a is a cleavage product of the complement cascade that appears early in the septic process, and stimulates macrophages to produce proinflammatory mediators. Later in the septic process, migration inhibitory factor and high-mobility group box protein-1 promote continued activation of T cells, macrophages, and phagocytic cells.

The host's inflammatory reaction is a necessary one, and is designed to allow the patient to overcome the infectious insult, as long as the process remains localized and well-balanced. However, when the host's response becomes unbalanced and systemic, SIRS occurs. The explanation as to why certain patients maintain a normal, balanced reaction to infectious challenge and others progress to SIRS is not well-understood. Some evidence points to genetic variations in certain cytokines, such as IL-6, TNF-α, and CD14.[7-10]

The normal inflammatory response to infection is a balance between proinflammatory and antiinflammatory processes. As is often found in many physiologic processes, proinflammatory mediators are countered by antiinflammatory mediators, such as IL-4 and IL-10. The actions of TNF-α and IL-1 are blunted by the release of soluble receptors and antagonists to these cytokines. T cells, neutrophils, and macrophages can become unresponsive to infectious stimuli in a process known as anergy.[15] The antiinflammatory response is furthered by the process of apoptosis, in which genetic programming results in the "suicide" of immune-effector cells via a release of proteases. The loss of CD4 and CD8 T cells, B cells, dendritic cells, and others is commonly seen in the enhanced apoptosis of sepsis.[16] The concept of the antiinflammatory response in sepsis has been labeled compensatory antiinflammatory response syndrome, and although some investigators propose that this antiinflammatory process may result in a blunted immune response and impair the ability of the patient to clear the infection,[17] the interplay of hyperinflammatory and antiinflammatory states remains uncertain.

The loss of hemostatic balance and dysfunction of the vascular endothelium are critical elements in the physiologic manifestations of sepsis. Increased levels of IL-6 promote the expression of tissue factor from mononuclear and endothelial cells, resulting in the induction of intravascular thrombin formation.[18] This process is known as disseminated intravascular coagulation (DIC), and is countered by the actions of antithrombin, as well as the thrombomodulin/protein C/protein S system. The consumption of these anticoagulant substances, as well as their reduced synthesis (both seen in sepsis), results in a procoagulant state.[19,20] The vascular endothelium responds to cytokine stimulation with an increased expression of inducible nitric oxide synthase,[21,22] resulting in a surge of nitric oxide and hypotension owing to overwhelming vasodilation. In a normal inflammatory response, endothelial cells express various adhesion molecules on their surface to stimulate the migration of leukocytes toward the site of infection. However, in a systemic inflammatory response, the widespread expression of these adhesion molecules causes leukocyte rolling and

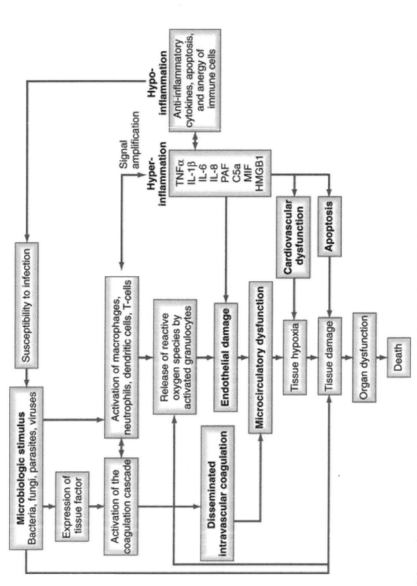

Fig. 1. Pathophysiology of sepsis. HMGB, high mobility group B; IL, interleukin; MIF, migration inhibitory factor; TNF, tumor necrosis factor. (*From* Reinhart K, Bloos F. The pathophysiology of sepsis and multiple organ dysfunction. In: Vincent JL, Abraham E, Moore FA, et al, editors. The textbook of critical care. 6th edition. Philadelphia: Elsevier Saunders; 2011. p. 984; with permission.)

adhesion along vascular surfaces. This process induces a respiratory burst, releasing cytotoxic substances. The subsequent endothelial damage produces the "leaky" capillaries and tissue edema so often seen in the septic patient.

Patients with septic shock have, by definition, dysfunction of the cardiovascular system. Endothelial damage results in massive fluid shift into the extravascular tissues, which is worsened by the third space loss of albumin, reducing plasma oncotic pressure. Endothelial injury also causes the release of nitric oxide and other vasodilatory compounds, resulting in collapse of vascular tone creates the characteristic profound arterial hypotension seen in septic shock. Nitric oxide also diminishes myocardial function by interfering with intracellular use of calcium by the myocytes and may also cause direct myocardial injury via peroxynitrate formation.[23] The end result is an impaired myocardial contractility, which is compensated by left ventricular diastolic dilation and increased left ventricular end-diastolic volume.[24,25] Finally, pathologic changes in the microvasculature impair peripheral oxygen delivery owing to leukocyte adherence and intravascular microthrombi formation, decreasing red blood cell flow. In sepsis, red blood cells exhibit an impaired ability to deform within the microvasculature, worsening the problem of impaired oxygen delivery. Ultimately, the hypovolemic state, loss of vascular tone, compromised cardiac function, and microcirculatory shunting result in profound impairment of oxygen delivery to peripheral tissues.

SYSTEMIC INFLAMMATORY RESPONSE SYNDROME AND THE SEPSIS SPECTRUM

Sepsis progresses on a continuum. Standard definitions of the sepsis spectrum exist, and range from SIRS through septic shock and multiple organ failure.[26] The diagnosis of SIRS is generally confirmed by the presence of 2 or more of the following criteria: temperature greater than 38°C or less than 35°C; heart rate greater than 90 beats/min; respiratory rate greater than 20 breaths/min, or $Paco_2$ less than 32 mm Hg, and a white blood cell count greater than 12,000/mm^3 or less than 4000/mm^3. SIRS in the presence of a culture-proven or clinically suspected infection is defined as sepsis. Severe sepsis and septic shock are associated with hypoperfusion and organ system dysfunction (**Box 1**). Clinically, septic shock presents with hypotension, oliguria, altered mental status, and decreased skin perfusion, often in association with a metabolic acidosis. MODS represents the final stage of this process, when the function of multiple organ systems is severely impaired.

QUANTIFYING ORGAN DYSFUNCTION

There are several published systems for the stratifying the severity of organ dysfunction in critically ill patients. These systems focus on the failure of individual organ systems, assigning a score to each system based on the abnormality of a measurable value. Scoring systems allow for comparison of outcomes related to differing therapeutic approaches and attempt to match patients for severity of illness. Disease-specific scoring systems promote standardized assessment, enabling uniformity of research. In addition, these scores allow a clinician to confirm the severity of the patient's illness. They support objective assessments of disease severity to ensure that a particular institution's mortality rate is similar to expected benchmarks. Finally, scores can be used to triage patients within an institution to ensure appropriate levels of care and monitoring.

These scoring systems use different methodologies. Some systems include preexisting comorbidities and therapies undertaken before admission to the surgical ICU (including care given in other ICUs). Other systems focus on direct measurements

---

Box 1
Features of severe sepsis

Severe sepsis definition = sepsis-induced tissue hypoperfusion or organ dysfunction (any of the following thought to be owing to the infection)

Sepsis-induced hypotension

Lactate above upper limits laboratory normal

Urine output <0.5 mL/kg/h for >2 hours despite adequate fluid resuscitation

Acute lung injury with Pao_2/Fio_2 <250 in the absence of pneumonia as infection source

Acute lung injury with Pao_2/Fio_2 <200 in the presence of pneumonia as infection source

Creatinine >2.0 mg/dL (176.8 μmol/L)

Bilirubin >2 mg/dL (34.2 μmol/L)

Platelet count <100,000 μL

Coagulopathy (international normalized ratio >1.5)

From Dellinger RP, Levy MM, Rhodes A, et al. Surviving sepsis campaign: International guidelines for management of severe sepsis and septic shock: 2012. Crit Care Med 2013;41:586; with permission.

---

of physiologic parameters and laboratory values. All tend to arrive at the final goal of determining hospital mortality. The ideal scoring system has good discrimination (the ability to correctly order patients in terms of their predicted mortality relative to each other), and good calibration (how well a system accurately predicts actual likelihood of mortality in a cohort). Some systems render a score upon admission to the ICU, whereas others produce sequential scores over an individual's stay in the ICU. Scores that can be obtained at the time of admission to the ICU include the Mortality Predictive Model, the Acute Physiology and Chronic Health Evaluation, and the Simplified Acute Physiology Score. Scoring systems that allow sequential determination include the Sequential Organ Failure Assessment, the Organ System Failure Score, and the Multiple Organ Dysfunction Score.

TREATMENT OF SEPSIS

The Surviving Sepsis guidelines were revised in 2012, and provide a framework for the management of the septic patient.[27] Briefly, blood cultures should be obtained before the initiation of antimicrobial therapy as long as the initiation of therapy is not delayed. Broad-spectrum antimicrobial therapy should be administered within 1 hour of diagnosis, and should have activity against all likely pathogens. Antifungal and antiviral therapies should be considered in patients with known immunocompromise or a history of organ transplantation.

After the initiation of antimicrobial therapy, attention should be diverted to obtaining source control. A specific anatomic diagnosis of infection should be identified or excluded as rapidly as possible, and intervention undertaken for source control within the first 12 hours after the diagnosis of sepsis. Whenever possible, the intervention with the least physiologic insult should be used, that is, percutaneous drainage rather that surgical drainage of an organ space infection. If an intravascular device is identified as a possible source of sepsis, said device should be removed as soon as feasible once alternate vascular access is established.

Surgical therapy comes with the risk of surgical complications. In addition to nonsurgical sources of sepsis (urinary tract infection, pneumonia, central line–associated infection), surgery patients have a substantial risk for surgical site infection, organ space infection, and *Clostridium difficile* colitis. Anastomotic leaks, retained foreign bodies, and wound and deep space infections can be a significant source of septic shock. Intraabdominal infection is the source of 69% of sepsis cases in surgical patients.[28]

C difficile infection should be suspected in any patient who has been in a hospital or other health care setting, or one who has been on antibiotic therapy. The white blood cell count is elevated, often strikingly high, and radiologic studies can reveal diffuse inflammation of the colon and ascites. Early surgical consultation and intervention is indicated for patients with end organ insufficiency or insipient failure.

DIAGNOSIS AND MANAGEMENT OF ORGAN DYSFUNCTION

Hypoperfusion associated with severe sepsis and septic shock can result in end-organ damage and dysfunction. MODS represents the final stage of this process, when the function of multiple organ systems is severely impaired.

Cardiovascular Derangements

Sepsis results in reduction of cardiac function and peripheral vascular resistance, as well as an increase in microvascular permeability. Patients manifest a hyperdynamic circulatory profile and volume loss into soft tissues. The end result is poor oxygen delivery at the level of the tissue, with microvascular shunting a result of the vasodilation, and edema resulting in decreased oxygen diffusion across membranes into cells. This shunting results in decreased oxygen extraction at the level of the tissue, and a high mixed venous oxygen saturation ($S_{mv}O_2$). Myocardial dysfunction in the setting of attempts at fluid resuscitation often takes the form of biventricular dilation, affecting the right ventricle more severely owing to the development of pulmonary hypertension related to acute lung injury.

The initial resuscitation phase embraces the concept of early goal-directed therapy, and should be completed within 6 hours of the identification of sepsis. Crystalloid resuscitation remains the standard of care and should be guided by measurements of central venous pressure. The Surviving Sepsis Campaign supports resuscitation to a goal central venous pressure of 8 to 12 mm Hg. Other markers for adequacy of resuscitation include a mean arterial pressure of greater than 65 mm Hg, a urine output of greater than 0.5 mL/kg/h, a central venous O_2 saturation of greater than 70%, resolution of the patient's metabolic acidosis, and normalization of lactate levels (**Box 2**).

Colloids and blood products are rarely indicated in the initial resuscitation of a septic patient. Specifically, hydroxyethyl starch containing fluids are contraindicated because their use is associated with increased mortality and need for renal replacement therapy (RRT).[29,30] Earlier studies found equipoise between patients resuscitated with crystalloid versus albumin, and, thus crystalloid has traditionally been the preferred agent for volume resuscitation owing to lower costs. However, the CRISTAL trial (Colloids Compared to Crystalloids in Fluid Resuscitation of Critically Ill Patients: A Multinational Randomised Controlled Trial) did support the use of albumin in the resuscitation of patients in hypovolemic shock, resulting in a lower fluid requirement and less vasopressor use.[31] Packed red blood cell transfusion is indicated if the patient has a hemoglobin level of less than 7.0 g/dL, but should be avoided if possible owing to the immunosuppressive effects of transfusion. Transfusion at higher hemoglobin

---

Box 2
Surviving sepsis care bundles for initial resuscitation

Surviving Sepsis Campaign Bundles

To be completed within 3 hours:
1. Measure lactate level
2. Obtain blood cultures before administration of antibiotics
3. Administer broad spectrum antibiotics
4. Administer 30 mL/kg crystalloid for hypotension or lactate $\geq$4 mmol/L

To be completed within 6 hours:
5. Apply vasopressors (for hypotension that does not respond to initial fluid resuscitation) to maintain a mean arterial pressure (MAP) of $\geq$65 mm Hg
6. In the event of persistent arterial hypotension despite volume resuscitation (septic shock) or initial lactate $\geq$4 mmol/L (36 mg/dL):
   a. Measure central venous pressure (CVP)[a]
   b. Measure central venous oxygen saturation (Scvo$_2$)[a]
7. Remeasure lactate if initial lactate was elevated[a]

[a] Targets for quantitative resuscitation included in the guidelines are CVP of $\geq$8 mm Hg, Scvo$_2$ of $\geq$70%, and normalization of lactate.
From Dellinger RP, Levy MM, Rhodes A, et al. Surviving sepsis campaign: International guidelines for management of severe sepsis and septic shock: 2012. Crit Care Med 2013;41:591; with permission.

---

levels has not shown significant differences in 90-day mortality, ischemic events, nor use of life support.[32]

If the patient remains hypotensive despite adequate volume loading, then vasopressor medications should be added to achieve the goal mean arterial pressure. The first-line agent is norepinephrine, with the addition of vasopressin or epinephrine if the first-line agent fails to meet blood pressure goals. These medications should be delivered through a central venous catheter, and patients receiving pressor therapy should have an arterial line placed. Inotropic support may be of utility in patients with demonstrated myocardial dysfunction not responsive to pressor therapy.

Respiratory Derangements

The spectrum of acute lung injury and acute respiratory distress syndrome (ARDS), characterized by tachypnea, hypoxia, and hypocapnia often requires mechanical ventilation. The Pao$_2$/Fio$_2$ ratio is a well-established and objective measure of the severity of this process, and a ratio of less than 300 mm Hg is the generally accepted threshold for the diagnosis for mild ARDS, 100 to 200 mm Hg for moderate ARDS, and less than 100 mm Hg for severe ARDS.[33] Another criterion for the diagnosis of ARDS includes fluffy bilateral infiltrates seen on chest radiography in the absence of congestive heart failure.

Treatment for acute respiratory failure is supportive. Care should be taken to avoid the deleterious effects of alveolar collapse, barotrauma, and volutrauma. Lower tidal volumes with higher respiratory rates may be beneficial.[34] Positive end-expiratory pressure should be used to prevent alveolar collapse and resultant atelectasis-induced trauma. In patients with refractory hypoxemia, prone positioning or the institution of airway pressure release ventilation may facilitate alveolar recruitment.

Although noninvasive positive-pressure ventilation can be beneficial in avoiding intubation in patients with exacerbations of chronic obstructive pulmonary disease, its use in patients with sepsis and acute lung injury/ARDS is limited. Patients should be placed on noninvasive positive-pressure ventilation only if the benefits are thought to outweigh the risks, and after careful consideration.

Gastrointestinal Derangements

Critically ill patients, especially those who require prolonged mechanical ventilation or have a coagulopathy, are at risk for stress gastritis and ulcer formation. These patients are effectively treated with either histamine receptor blockers or proton pump inhibitors. Intolerance of enteral feedings is also common and may reflect postoperative opioid use, surgical ileus, pulmonary or intraabdominal infection, or a combination of these factors. Hepatic failure can occur, either owing to ischemic hepatitis, ICU jaundice, or venous congestion in the setting of cardiac dysfunction. Ischemic hepatitis is characterized by dramatically elevated transaminase levels, an increased international normalized ratio, and hypoglycemia, and is treated by resuscitation. ICU jaundice is more common, and is marked by hyperbilirubinemia.

Patients with sepsis are catabolic, and require nutritional repletion. Enteral nutrition, delivered either orally or via a feeding tube, should be initiated within 48 hours of diagnosis. While the patient is in shock, the focus should be on the maintenance of gut integrity through the use of trophic tube feeds. Thereafter, feedings can be increased to goal rates. Parenteral nutrition should be reserved for those patients with an intolerance to enteral nutrition for more than 7 days, and for those patients with an absolute contraindication to enteral nutrition.[35]

Renal Derangements

Acute renal failure (ARF) is a common feature in MODS, and sepsis is the leading cause of ARF in the ICU.[36] ARF is the rapid loss of glomerular filtration rate over a period of hours or days, and is usually marked by a increasing plasma creatinine and blood urea nitrogen levels. Early dysfunction is usually the result of renal hypoperfusion during the shock state while late dysfunction can be owing to toxic injury and other factors. Causes of ARF in patients with MODS are either prerenal (hypovolemic) or renal (likely acute tubular necrosis). Postrenal causes are uncommon. Acute tubular necrosis is the result of hypoxic and/or oxidative injury result in an abnormal tubular integrity, where obstructing debris in the tubule and a "backing up" of ultrafiltrate through the tubule wall. One notable cause of ARF may be abdominal compartment syndrome, which often results from large volume crystalloid resuscitation and results in increased abdominal pressure compromising renal blood flow. Generally, an abdominal pressure of greater than 25 mm Hg or an abdominal perfusion pressure of less than 60 mm Hg should raise suspicion of abdominal compartment syndrome and prompt surgical evaluation for possible decompression.

Unfortunately, there is little one can do to mitigate the emergence of ARF beyond ensuring an adequate renal perfusion and avoidance of nephrotoxic substances. RRT is often required to manage this condition. Indications for RRT include metabolic acidosis, electrolyte abnormalities (hyperkalemia and/or hyperphosphatemia), or severe volume overload. Options for RRT include continuous and intermittent therapy. In patients with severe sepsis, the use of continuous RRT is favored because it mitigates ongoing hemodynamic instability.

Hematologic Derangements

Patients with MODS commonly have perturbations in hematologic function. Thrombocytopenia can be seen in up to 53% of ICU patients, and can be associated with poor prognosis.[37] Low platelet counts may be exacerbated by recent surgical intervention and acute blood loss. Sepsis may cause DIC, which is the result of aberrant activation of the clotting cascade, combined with the activation of fibrinolytic mechanisms. DIC results in the consumption of platelets and clotting factors, leading to depletion and simultaneous hemorrhage and thrombosis. DIC is characterized by thrombocytopenia concurrent with prolonged activated prothrombin and activated partial thromboplastin times, decreased fibrinogen, and increased fibrin degradation products.

Treatment of hematologic alterations is supportive. Packed red blood cell transfusion is indicated if the patient has a hemoglobin level of less than 7.0 g/dL, and should be undertaken to achieve a goal between 7.0 and 9.0. Platelet transfusion should be reserved for patients with levels of less than 10,000 mm^3 (in the absence of active bleeding), or of less than 20,000 mm^3 with a high risk of bleeding. A threshold level of less than 50,000 mm^3 can be used for patients with active bleeding, or the need for surgery or other invasive procedures. Cryoprecipitate should be administered to keep fibrinogen levels greater than 80 to 100 mg/dL. Finally, fresh frozen plasma can be transfused to maintain the prothrombin time and activated partial thromboplastin time at less than 1.5 times their normal range.

Endocrine Derangements

The 3 most common alterations in endocrine function in sepsis and MODS are insulin deficiency, adrenal deficiency, and vasopressin deficiency. Insulin deficiency manifests as hyperglycemia, which may impact immune function and wound healing. Maintaining glucose levels using insulin has been shown to decrease mortality, but recent definitive trial data have pointed away from tight glycemic control toward a more permissive glucose target. Functional adrenal deficiency may manifest as hypotension unresponsive to pressor therapy, but continues to be difficult to diagnose in critically ill patients. Several studies trialing exogenous steroid therapy in septic shock have shown benefit,[38–42] especially in the setting of fluid- and pressor-refractory shock. Finally, sepsis results in abnormally low levels of circulating vasopressin, and administration of intravenous vasopressin is indicated as a second-line agent to improve blood pressure or reduce norepinephrine dosage.[27]

PROGNOSTIC INDICATORS

The factors impacting prognosis and outcomes in sepsis are numerous, but can be divided into 3 main categories:

1. The site and type of infection,
2. The severity of the patient's response to the infectious insult, and
3. The timing and appropriateness of therapy.

Sepsis owing to community-acquired organisms carries a lower mortality rate than those events caused by nosocomial pathogens.[43,44] Bloodstream infections owing to methicillin-resistant Staphylococcus aureus, methicillin-sensitive S aureus, Candida, and non-Candida fungi, pseudomonas, and polymicrobial infections carry higher rates of mortality than other organisms.[44] The site of infection also impacts survival. Sepsis stemming from gastrointestinal, pulmonary, or unknown sites carries a higher risk of mortality, whereas urinary tract-related sepsis has a lower risk.[45]

Factors regulating a patient's response to infectious insult are even more numerous, and far less understood. Genetic factors may play a role in determining which patients maintain an appropriate and localized inflammatory response, while others manifest an uncontrolled, systemic one. One hypothesis for this variation centers on single nucleotide polymorphisms in the genes that code for certain cytokines. These minor mutations maintain the overall function of the cytokine, but have been implicated in increased rates of the development of sepsis and poorer outcomes in septic shock.[7–10]

The early evidence supporting the true impact of timely initiation of therapy for patients with sepsis has been challenged recently. Early fluid resuscitation has been shown to improve survival,[46] and the implementation of "sepsis bundles" and early goal-directed therapy to guide treatment has been demonstrated to reduce mortality in some studies,[47–50] but has been refuted in more recent literature.[51–53] The initiation of early appropriate antimicrobial therapy has been shown to improve mortality, including therapy started before ICU arrival,[54–56] although other studies have challenged this notion.[57,58]

OUTCOMES

The sepsis spectrum has a significant mortality rate. Overall mortality estimates range from 10% to 52%,[43,59,60] and generally increase with the severity of the septic process with SIRS, sepsis, severe sepsis, and septic shock patients experiencing mortality rates of 7%, 16%, 20%, and 46%.[61] The mortality related to the sepsis spectrum seems to be decreasing over recent years,[1,59,60,62] although this may be the result of changes in hospital coding and documentation practices.[1] The development and application of sepsis "bundles" has been proposed as the reason for this decline,[63,64] although the evidence for this is conflicting, perhaps owing to varying degrees of compliance.[64] The use of performance metrics to ensure bundle compliance resulted in a 25% reduction in relative risk of mortality.[65]

The effects of sepsis often do not end upon hospital discharge. Patients who survive sepsis to the point of hospital discharge have an increased risk of death, as well as subsequent episodes of sepsis and hospital readmission.[66–68] Although most deaths occur within 6 months, increased mortality is seen up to 2 years after discharge.[68,69] The common 90-day readmission diagnoses for patients surviving sepsis are heart failure, pneumonia, exacerbations of chronic obstructive pulmonary disease, and urinary tract infections.[70] Patients who survive sepsis to hospital discharge are commonly placed in short- or long-term care facilities, have increased health care use, and frequently experience a diminished quality of life.[68,71–73]

WITHDRAWAL OF SUPPORT AND END-OF-LIFE CARE

Despite the efforts of the best medical teams with the most advanced technology and treatments, many patients with sepsis and multiple organ dysfunction will progress to death. Physicians caring for critically ill patients have an obligation to inform patients and their families about the prognosis of their condition. Upon admission to the ICU and recognition of critical illness, all attempts should be made to discuss the patient's wishes regarding goals of care as soon as possible, and certainly within the first 72 hours. In the setting of known MODS, the clinician should present the likelihood of survival and meaningful recovery in layman's terms but using available data regarding probability of survival. In some cases, a time-limited period of aggressive management may be appropriate, with further discussions based on patient progress. Many hospitals now have interdisciplinary care teams to assist with end-of-life care issues, whose involvement has been shown to increase patient satisfaction and reduce ICU costs.[74]

SUMMARY

Sepsis and MODS continue to be a significant cause of morbidity and mortality in the ICU, using an enormous amount of resources and health care dollars. Sepsis involves the interplay of the infectious insult and the patient's inflammatory response thereto, both of which are necessary factors in the progression along the spectrum from sepsis to MODS. The inflammatory response is a complex process that is characterized by a procoagulant state, endothelial injury, cardiac dysfunction, vasodilation, hypovolemia owing to fluid shift, microcirculatory dysfunction, and hemodynamic collapse. MODS is present when this process results in the dysfunction or failure of more than one organ system, and sharply increases mortality rates. The current standards of therapy for sepsis have been established through the efforts of the Surviving Sepsis Campaign, which provides a framework for evidence-based care. Timely recognition of the signs and symptoms of early sepsis, aggressive volume resuscitation to established endpoints, and appropriate support with vasopressors and antimicrobial medications are the goals of early resuscitative efforts. Eradication of the infection by achieving source control and providing proper antibiotic therapy is critical to the resolution of the septic process. In patients who progress to MODS, the clinician must work to support and maintain the homeostasis of the failing organ systems. Mortality rates from septic shock and MODS are improving, but remain high, and physicians must embrace the reality that not all can be saved. An early and meaningful discussion with the patient and their family regarding expectations, prognosis, and goals of care can help to guide the clinician, allow for informed decision making, reduce excessively heroic and costly therapies, and permit the family to come to terms with the patient's critical illness.

REFERENCES

1. Lagu T, Rothberg MB, Shieh MS, et al. Hospitalizations, costs, and outcomes of severe sepsis in the united states 2003 to 2007. Crit Care Med 2012;40(3): 754–61.
2. Bone RC, Fisher CJ Jr, Clemmer TP, et al. Sepsis syndrome: a valid clinical entity. methylprednisolone severe sepsis study group. Crit Care Med 1989;17(5): 389–93.
3. Vincent JL, Sakr Y, Sprung CL, et al. Sepsis in European intensive care units: results of the SOAP study. Crit Care Med 2006;34(2):344–53.
4. Angus DC, Linde-Zwirble WT, Lidicker J, et al. Epidemiology of severe sepsis in the united states: analysis of incidence, outcome, and associated costs of care. Crit Care Med 2001;29(7):1303–10.
5. Moore LJ, Moore FA, Todd SR, et al. Sepsis in general surgery: the 2005-2007 national surgical quality improvement program perspective. Arch Surg 2010; 145(7):695–700.
6. Richards M, Thursky K, Buising K. Epidemiology, prevalence, and sites of infections in intensive care units. Semin Respir Crit Care Med 2003;24(1):3–22.
7. Gordon AC, Lagan AL, Aganna E, et al. TNF and TNFR polymorphisms in severe sepsis and septic shock: a prospective multicentre study. Genes Immun 2004; 5(8):631–40.
8. Heidecke CD, Hensler T, Weighardt H, et al. Selective defects of T lymphocyte function in patients with lethal intraabdominal infection. Am J Surg 1999;178(4): 288–92.
9. D'Avila LC, Albarus MH, Franco CR, et al. Effect of CD14 -260C>T polymorphism on the mortality of critically ill patients. Immunol Cell Biol 2006;84(4):342–8.

10. Sutherland AM, Walley KR, Manocha S, et al. The association of interleukin 6 haplotype clades with mortality in critically ill adults. Arch Intern Med 2005; 165(1):75–82.

11. Medzhitov R, Preston-Hurlburt P, Janeway CA Jr. A human homologue of the drosophila toll protein signals activation of adaptive immunity. Nature 1997; 388(6640):394–7.

12. Macdonald J, Galley HF, Webster NR. Oxidative stress and gene expression in sepsis. Br J Anaesth 2003;90(2):221–32.

13. Cohen J. The immunopathogenesis of sepsis. Nature 2002;420(6917):885–91.

14. Yoshimura A, Lien E, Ingalls RR, et al. Cutting edge: recognition of gram-positive bacterial cell wall components by the innate immune system occurs via toll-like receptor 2. J Immunol 1999;163(1):1–5.

15. Hotchkiss RS, Nicholson DW. Apoptosis and caspases regulate death and inflammation in sepsis. Nat Rev Immunol 2006;6(11):813–22.

16. Hotchkiss RS, Swanson PE, Freeman BD, et al. Apoptotic cell death in patients with sepsis, shock, and multiple organ dysfunction. Crit Care Med 1999;27(7): 1230–51.

17. Loisa P, Rinne T, Laine S, et al. Anti-inflammatory cytokine response and the development of multiple organ failure in severe sepsis. Acta Anaesthesiol Scand 2003;47(3):319–25.

18. Massignon D, Lepape A, Bienvenu J, et al. Coagulation/fibrinolysis balance in septic shock related to cytokines and clinical state. Haemostasis 1994;24(1): 36–48.

19. Fourrier F, Chopin C, Goudemand J, et al. Septic shock, multiple organ failure, and disseminated intravascular coagulation. compared patterns of antithrombin III, protein C, and protein S deficiencies. Chest 1992;101(3):816–23.

20. Weiler H. Regulation of inflammation by the protein C system. Crit Care Med 2010;38(2 Suppl):S18–25.

21. Taylor BS, Geller DA. Molecular regulation of the human inducible nitric oxide synthase (iNOS) gene. Shock 2000;13(6):413–24.

22. Reinhart K, Bayer O, Brunkhorst F, et al. Markers of endothelial damage in organ dysfunction and sepsis. Crit Care Med 2002;30(5 Suppl):S302–12.

23. Bloos FM, Morisaki HM, Neal AM, et al. Sepsis depresses the metabolic oxygen reserve of the coronary circulation in mature sheep. Am J Respir Crit Care Med 1996;153(5):1577–84.

24. Bouhemad B, Nicolas-Robin A, Arbelot C, et al. Acute left ventricular dilatation and shock-induced myocardial dysfunction. Crit Care Med 2009;37(2):441–7.

25. Ognibene FP, Parker MM, Natanson C, et al. Depressed left ventricular performance. response to volume infusion in patients with sepsis and septic shock. Chest 1988;93(5):903–10.

26. American college of chest physicians/society of critical care medicine consensus conference: definitions for sepsis and organ failure and guidelines for the use of innovative therapies in sepsis. Crit Care Med 1992;20(6):864–74.

27. Dellinger RP, Levy MM, Rhodes A, et al. Surviving sepsis campaign: international guidelines for management of severe sepsis and septic shock: 2012. Crit Care Med 2013;41(2):580–637.

28. Moore LJ, McKinley BA, Turner KL, et al. The epidemiology of sepsis in general surgery patients. J Trauma 2011;70(3):672–80.

29. Brunkhorst FM, Engel C, Bloos F, et al. Intensive insulin therapy and pentastarch resuscitation in severe sepsis. N Engl J Med 2008;358(2):125–39.

30. Perner A, Haase N, Guttormsen AB, et al. Hydroxyethyl starch 130/0.42 versus ringer's acetate in severe sepsis. N Engl J Med 2012;367(2):124–34.

31. Annane D, Siami S, Jaber S, et al. Effects of fluid resuscitation with colloids vs crystalloids on mortality in critically ill patients presenting with hypovolemic shock: The CRISTAL randomized trial. JAMA 2013;310(17):1809–17.

32. Holst LB, Haase N, Wetterslev J, et al. Lower versus higher hemoglobin threshold for transfusion in septic shock. N Engl J Med 2014;371(15):1381–91.

33. ARDS Definition Task Force, Ranieri VM, Rubenfeld GD, et al. Acute respiratory distress syndrome: the Berlin definition. JAMA 2012;307(23):2526–33.

34. Ventilation with lower tidal volumes as compared with traditional tidal volumes for acute lung injury and the acute respiratory distress syndrome. the acute respiratory distress syndrome network. N Engl J Med 2000;342(18):1301–8.

35. Taylor BE, McClave SA, Martindale RG, et al. Guidelines for the provision and assessment of nutrition support therapy in the adult critically ill patient: Society of Critical Care Medicine (SCCM) and American Society for Parenteral and Enteral Nutrition (A.S.P.E.N. Crit Care Med 2016;44(2):390–438.

36. Andrikos E, Tseke P, Balafa O, et al. Epidemiology of acute renal failure in ICUs: a multi-center prospective study. Blood Purif 2009;28(3):239–44.

37. Tsirigotis P, Chondropoulos S, Frantzeskaki F, et al. Thrombocytopenia in critically ill patients with severe sepsis/septic shock: prognostic value and association with a distinct serum cytokine profile. J Crit Care 2016;32:9–15.

38. Annane D, Sebille V, Charpentier C, et al. Effect of treatment with low doses of hydrocortisone and fludrocortisone on mortality in patients with septic shock. JAMA 2002;288(7):862–71.

39. Bollaert PE, Charpentier C, Levy B, et al. Reversal of late septic shock with supra-physiologic doses of hydrocortisone. Crit Care Med 1998;26(4):645–50.

40. Briegel J, Forst H, Haller M, et al. Stress doses of hydrocortisone reverse hyper-dynamic septic shock: a prospective, randomized, double-blind, single-center study. Crit Care Med 1999;27(4):723–32.

41. Marik PE, Pastores SM, Annane D, et al. Recommendations for the diagnosis and management of corticosteroid insufficiency in critically ill adult patients: consensus statements from an international task force by the American College of Critical Care Medicine. Crit Care Med 2008;36(6):1937–49.

42. Annane D, Bellissant E, Bollaert PE, et al. Corticosteroids for treating sepsis. Cochrane Database Syst Rev 2015;(12):CD002243.

43. Labelle A, Juang P, Reichley R, et al. The determinants of hospital mortality among patients with septic shock receiving appropriate initial antibiotic treatment*. Crit Care Med 2012;40(7):2016–21.

44. Shorr AF, Tabak YP, Killian AD, et al. Healthcare-associated bloodstream infection: a distinct entity? insights from a large U.S. database. Crit Care Med 2006;34(10):2588–95.

45. Knaus WA, Sun X, Nystrom O, et al. Evaluation of definitions for sepsis. Chest 1992;101(6):1656–62.

46. Jones AE, Brown MD, Trzeciak S, et al. The effect of a quantitative resuscitation strategy on mortality in patients with sepsis: a meta-analysis. Crit Care Med 2008;36(10):2734–9.

47. Apibunyopas Y. Mortality rate among patients with septic shock after implementation of 6-hour sepsis protocol in the emergency department of Thammasat University Hospital. J Med Assoc Thai 2014;97(Suppl 8):S182–93.

48. Micek ST, Roubinian N, Heuring T, et al. Before-after study of a standardized hospital order set for the management of septic shock. Crit Care Med 2006;34(11): 2707–13.

49. Rivers E, Nguyen B, Havstad S, et al. Early goal-directed therapy in the treatment of severe sepsis and septic shock. N Engl J Med 2001;345(19):1368–77.

50. Cannon CM, Holthaus CV, Zubrow MT, et al. The GENESIS project (GENeralized early sepsis intervention strategies): a multicenter quality improvement collaborative. J Intensive Care Med 2013;28(6):355–68.

51. ARISE Investigators, ANZICS Clinical Trials Group, Peake SL, et al. Goal-directed resuscitation for patients with early septic shock. N Engl J Med 2014;371(16): 1496–506.

52. ProCESS Investigators, Yealy DM, Kellum JA, et al. A randomized trial of protocol-based care for early septic shock. N Engl J Med 2014;370(18):1683–93.

53. Mouncey PR, Osborn TM, Power GS, et al. Trial of early, goal-directed resuscitation for septic shock. N Engl J Med 2015;372(14):1301–11.

54. Puskarich MA, Trzeciak S, Shapiro NI, et al. Association between timing of antibiotic administration and mortality from septic shock in patients treated with a quantitative resuscitation protocol. Crit Care Med 2011;39(9):2066–71.

55. Garnacho-Montero J, Gutierrez-Pizarraya A, Escoresca-Ortega A, et al. Adequate antibiotic therapy prior to ICU admission in patients with severe sepsis and septic shock reduces hospital mortality. Crit Care 2015;19:302.

56. Kumar A, Roberts D, Wood KE, et al. Duration of hypotension before initiation of effective antimicrobial therapy is the critical determinant of survival in human septic shock. Crit Care Med 2006;34(6):1589–96.

57. Ryoo SM, Kim WY, Sohn CH, et al. Prognostic value of timing of antibiotic administration in patients with septic shock treated with early quantitative resuscitation. Am J Med Sci 2015;349(4):328–33.

58. Sterling SA, Miller WR, Pryor J, et al. The impact of timing of antibiotics on outcomes in severe sepsis and septic shock: a systematic review and meta-analysis. Crit Care Med 2015;43(9):1907–15.

59. Martin GS, Mannino DM, Eaton S, et al. The epidemiology of sepsis in the United States from 1979 through 2000. N Engl J Med 2003;348(16):1546–54.

60. Stevenson EK, Rubenstein AR, Radin GT, et al. Two decades of mortality trends among patients with severe sepsis: a comparative meta-analysis*. Crit Care Med 2014;42(3):625–31.

61. Rangel-Frausto MS, Pittet D, Costigan M, et al. The natural history of the systemic inflammatory response syndrome (SIRS). A prospective study. JAMA 1995; 273(2):117–23.

62. Kaukonen KM, Bailey M, Suzuki S, et al. Mortality related to severe sepsis and septic shock among critically ill patients in Australia and New Zealand, 2000-2012. JAMA 2014;311(13):1308–16.

63. Miller RR 3rd, Dong L, Nelson NC, et al. Multicenter implementation of a severe sepsis and septic shock treatment bundle. Am J Respir Crit Care Med 2013; 188(1):77–82.

64. Rhodes A, Phillips G, Beale R, et al. The surviving sepsis campaign bundles and outcome: results from the international multicentre prevalence study on sepsis (the IMPreSS study). Intensive Care Med 2015;41(9):1620–8.

65. Levy MM, Rhodes A, Phillips GS, et al. Surviving sepsis campaign: association between performance metrics and outcomes in a 7.5-year study. Intensive Care Med 2014;40(11):1623–33.

66. Jones TK, Fuchs BD, Small DS, et al. Post-acute care use and hospital readmission after sepsis. Ann Am Thorac Soc 2015;12(6):904–13.

67. Nesseler N, Defontaine A, Launey Y, et al. Long-term mortality and quality of life after septic shock: a follow-up observational study. Intensive Care Med 2013; 39(5):881–8.

68. Winters BD, Eberlein M, Leung J, et al. Long-term mortality and quality of life in sepsis: a systematic review. Crit Care Med 2010;38(5):1276–83.

69. Sasse KC, Nauenberg E, Long A, et al. Long-term survival after intensive care unit admission with sepsis. Crit Care Med 1995;23(6):1040–7.

70. Prescott HC, Langa KM, Iwashyna TJ. Readmission diagnoses after hospitalization for severe sepsis and other acute medical conditions. JAMA 2015;313(10): 1055–7.

71. Perl TM, Dvorak L, Hwang T, et al. Long-term survival and function after suspected gram-negative sepsis. JAMA 1995;274(4):338–45.

72. Prescott HC, Langa KM, Liu V, et al. Increased 1-year healthcare use in survivors of severe sepsis. Am J Respir Crit Care Med 2014;190(1):62–9.

73. Wang T, Derhovanessian A, De Cruz S, et al. Subsequent infections in survivors of sepsis: Epidemiology and outcomes. J Intensive Care Med 2014;29(2):87–95.

74. Gade G, Venohr I, Conner D, et al. Impact of an inpatient palliative care team: a randomized control trial. J Palliat Med 2008;11(2):180–90.

Anesthesia for Patients with Concomitant Cardiac and Renal Dysfunction

Radwan Safa, MD, PhD, Nicholas Sadovnikoff, MD*

KEYWORDS

- Renal failure • Cardiovascular disease • Anesthesia • Anesthetic goals • Surgery

KEY POINTS

- Renal disease and cardiovascular disease (CVD) are commonly encountered in the same patient.
- The dynamic interactions between renal disease and CVD have an impact on perioperative management.
- Renal failure is an independent risk factor for CVD and the link between the two disease states remains to be fully elucidated.

INTRODUCTION

Cardiovascular and renal disease are important, interrelated causes of perioperative morbidity and mortality. In the perioperative setting, renal dysfunction is an important predictor of major adverse cardiac events as evidenced by its inclusion as 1 of only 6 risk factors used to determine perioperative cardiac risk.[1] In the United States, the prevalence of CVD in patients with chronic kidney disease (CKD) is 9 times higher than it is in the general population[2] and CVD contributes to more than half of deaths among patients with renal failure.[3] Because it is increasingly common to encounter patients perioperatively with varying degrees of renal and cardiovascular dysfunction, a comprehensive understanding of the complexities emerging from simultaneous impairment of these organ systems is needed. Anesthetic goals in these circumstances setting may be competing or concordant depending on the nature and degree of cardiovascular and renal impairment.

The pathophysiologic basis for the relationship between CKD and CVD has not been clearly elucidated. Traditional CVD risk factors (ie, age, male gender, hypertension, smoking, and so forth) do not explain the entirety of the increased incidence of CVD in CKD patients. Conversely, although CKD-related risk factors, such as abnormal

Department of Anesthesiology, Perioperative and Pain Medicine, Brigham & Women's Hospital, 75 Francis Street, Boston, MA 02215, USA
* Corresponding author.
E-mail address: nsadovnikoff@partners.org

Anesthesiology Clin 34 (2016) 697–710
http://dx.doi.org/10.1016/j.anclin.2016.06.006
1932-2275/16/© 2016 Elsevier Inc. All rights reserved.

calcium and phosphorus homeostasis, and hypertension, are associated with cardio-vascular pathology, reversal of these of risk factors does not decrease CVD related mortality. Taken together, these data suggest a missing link between CKD and CVD. Although several hypotheses have been proposed, it remains an area of ongoing research.[4,5]

ANESTHETIC GOALS IN PATIENTS WITH KIDNEY DISEASE

The renal system plays a vital role in the maintenance of homeostasis and is primarily responsible for maintenance of fluid and electrolyte balance and excretion of meta-bolic waste products. It also plays an important role in regulation of vascular tone, he-matopoiesis, and bone metabolism. Both renal dysfunction and the therapies used to manage it have wide-ranging physiologic consequences relevant to perioperative care (**Box 1**).

Metabolic acidosis is common in patients with renal failure and is primarily due to impaired renal excretion of organic acids. The early stage of acute kidney injury is characterized by a nonanion gap acidosis secondary to impaired generation of ammonia. As the initiation phase progresses to the maintenance phase, an anion gap acidosis is observed secondary to impaired excretion of fixed acids. In a sponta-neously breathing patient with impaired renal function and consequent metabolic acidosis, respiratory function may be inadequate to normalize for the pH, and patients should be carefully monitored for signs of progression to respiratory failure.

Various electrolyte abnormalities can be expected in the setting of renal failure, including elevated potassium, magnesium, and phosphate, and decreased calcium and sodium. Because of impaired potassium handling, special consideration must be paid to blood product administration. In patients with elevated baseline potassium levels, the increase in serum potassium concentration associated with rapid transfu-sion of packed red blood cells is less well tolerated. Electrolyte abnormalities contribute to the high arrhythmia burden in patients with renal dysfunction. The great-est contributor to mortality in end-stage renal disease (ESRD) is sudden cardiac death, accounting for 25% of all-cause mortality in this population.[6] Arrhythmias in ESRD pa-tients are associated with poor prognosis. In diabetic patients with ESRD, the absence of sinus rhythm is associated with a 75% increase in cardiac death or myocardial infarction (MI).[7] Therefore, close monitoring with active prevention and treatment of ar-rhythmias becomes an important management priority.

Box 1
Systems review in patients with renal failure

- Electrolyte abnormalities
- Acid-base abnormalities
- Anemia
- Hypotension/blood pressure lability
- Impaired drug clearance
- Volume status
- Effects of renal replacement therapy
- Uremia
- Platelet dysfunction
- Difficult intravenous access

A combination of chronic anemia, impaired platelet function, and a diminished ability to replace red blood cells makes renal failure patients more vulnerable to intraoperative blood loss and its deleterious consequences. Since the introduction of recombinant erythropoietin for the treatment of ESRD-related anemia in 1989, much work has been directed toward determining the appropriate degree of hemoglobin (Hgb) correction. Multiple clinical benefits have been associated with correcting hematocrit to greater than 30% in patients with ESRD, including improved quality of life, exercise capacity, and cardiac function.[8,9] Although increasing hematocrit to greater than 30% was associated with important benefits, other data suggest that when higher hematocrit levels are targeted, the risks outweigh the benefits.[10] Besarab and colleagues[10] tested the hypothesis that morbidity and mortality would be reduced in ESRD patients with New York Heart Association classification heart disease stages I–III when hematocrit was increased to 42% compared with a control group with hematocrit sustained at 30%. The study was terminated early due to a trend toward increased risk of death in the higher hematocrit group, dampening the enthusiasm for targeting hematocrits in excess of 30%.

The impairment of glomerular filtration and tubular function in renal dysfunction has an impact on the elimination of numerous drugs. Water-soluble drugs are usually excreted unchanged whereas lipid-soluble drugs are converted to water-soluble metabolites, then excreted in the urine. The amount of drug and metabolite accumulation depends on the characteristics of the drug and the severity of renal failure. Relevant drug classes influenced by renal disease include certain hypnotics, nondepolarizing neuromuscular blocking agents, β-blockers, opioids, and antibiotics (**Table 1**). In addition to a direct effect on drug clearance, renal dysfunction indirectly alters drug pharmacokinetics via changes in protein binding. The protein binding of acidic drugs is decreased in serum from patients with renal failure. This decreased binding is thought to be due to retention of compounds that displace drugs from their binding site on albumin.

ANESTHETIC GOALS IN PATIENTS WITH CARDIOVASCULAR DISEASE

Cardiovascular complications, including perioperative MI (PMI), new or decompensated congestive heart failure (CHF), arrhythmia. and thromboembolism, are the

Table 1
Impact of renal failure on the pharmacokinetics of various medication classes

Drug Class	Pharmacokinetics Affected by Renal Failure	Pharmacokinetics Minimally Affected by Renal Failure
Benzodiazepines	Midazolam	Lorazepam
Hypnotics	Ketamine	Propofol Barbiturates Etomidate
Opioids	Morphine Hydromorphone Codeine Meperidine Methadone	Fentanyl Sufentanil Remifentanil
NMBs	Rocuronium Vecuronium Pancuronium	Atracurium Cisatracurium Mivacurium

Abbreviation: NMBs, neuromuscular blocking agents.

most common causes of postoperative morbidity and mortality.[1,11] With an aging population and advances in medical therapy, an increasing number of high-risk cardiovascular patients undergo surgery, and perioperative cardiovascular complications may become more common. Patients with preexisting cardiac disease are at highest risk of developing these complications. This section focuses on the anesthetic management of patients with coronary artery disease (CAD) as well as those with compromised systolic or diastolic function.

Coronary Artery Disease and Perioperative Myocardial Infarction

PMI is a feared complication with an early mortality rate ranging between 3.5% and 25%.[12] The pathophysiology of PMI is divided between 2 general mechanisms: acute coronary syndrome (ACS) and supply demand imbalance. ACS is caused by thrombosis secondary to rupture of a vulnerable atheromatous plaque whereas demand ischemia is caused by supply-demand imbalance in the absence of acute thrombosis. Although intraplaque inflammation is known to play a prominent role in the plaque instability associated with ACS, other perioperative stressors are thought to contribute. Hypertension and tachycardia have been shown promote plaque instability via shear stress and increased blood velocity.[13] Hence, good hemodynamic control during anesthetic induction and intraoperatively is essential. Tachycardia and hypertension also contribute significantly to demand ischemia, which is common in the postoperative period accounting for greater than 90% of postoperative ischemic events.[14,15]

Preoperative care of CVD patients presenting for noncardiac surgery is guided by stratification. Numerous risk indices and predictors of PMI have been published over the years, including the Revised Cardiac Risk Index[1] and the American College of Surgeons National Surgical Quality Improvement Program risk calculator (http://www.surgicalriskcalculator.com). The level of risk predicted by these indices informs further decisions regarding preoperative work up. If a patient has poor functional status and is deemed high risk for an adverse cardiovascular event, provocative testing (ie, stress testing) can be undertaken. In the event that reversible ischemia is observed, an important decision arises: whether to delay surgery to pursue revascularization via either percutaneous intervention (PCI) or coronary artery bypass grafting (CABG).

There are only weak data and no prospective studies in support of preoperative cardiac testing. The most widely cited study retrospectively reviewed the perioperative courses of 502 patients undergoing vascular surgery and found that those who had moderate to severe reversible ischemia on thallium scanning and underwent revascularization had lower mortality than those who did not.[16] Several prospective trials have assessed the utility of preoperative revascularization and preoperative cardiac testing. Coronary Artery Revascularization Prophylaxis (CARP) trial randomized 510 patients at increased risk for perioperative cardiac complications and clinically significant CAD to undergo either revascularization or no revascularization before elective major vascular surgery and found no difference in long-term mortality. A follow-up study randomized 510 patients with clinically significant CAD to revascularization or no revascularization before elective major vascular surgery and showed no difference in long term mortality.[17]

Patients with unstable angina or recent MI who undergo surgery are at very high risk for an adverse perioperative cardiac event. Current guidelines recommend delaying elective noncardiac surgery for 4 to 6 weeks after MI.[18] Likewise, patients who have undergone recent percutaneous coronary intervention are at increased risk of adverse perioperative cardiac events. These risks are primarily related to the premature discontinuation of antiplatelet therapy. The recommended waiting period for elective, noncardiac surgery after PCI is 6 months to 1 year. In those patients who require urgent or emergent surgery within 6 months of PCI, the risks of surgical bleeding must be weighed against the risks of premature interruption of antiplatelet agents.

Among the most important intraoperative anesthetic goals in patients with CVD are the prevention, detection, and treatment of myocardial ischemia. Ischemia represents an imbalance of oxygen supply and demand. Myocardial oxygen consumption depends on preload (ie, left ventricular distension increases wall stress) after load and heart rate. Myocardial ischemia is prevented and treated by optimizing these factors to the greatest extent possible. A low to normal heart rate allows adequate diastolic time for myocardial perfusion and minimizes oxygen consumption. Additionally, maintaining a normal to high BP, normal left ventricular end diastolic volume, normal arterial oxygen content, and normothermia help optimize myocardial supply-demand balance.

Heart Failure

Heart failure (HF) is a general term that refers to any structural or functional change in the heart that impairs the ventricles' ability to fill or eject blood. Although CAD is a more recognized risk factor for perioperative morbidity and mortality after major surgery, chronic stable HF is associated with a higher 30-day mortality and hospital readmission rate compared with CAD.[19,20] Assessment and maintenance of volume status are particularly important in HF patients. Impairment of either systolic or diastolic function predisposes patients to the development of elevated left ventricular filling pressures and pulmonary edema with minimal increases in intravascular volume. The detrimental impact of hypovolemia on forward flow is also magnified in this population; therefore, maintenance of euvolemia is particularly important.

Preexisting HF should be evaluated and treated to the greatest extent permitted by the urgency of surgery. Careful history and physical examination should be used to elucidate the cause of HF and evaluate for signs of inadequate treatment. A resting 12-lead electrocardiogram is recommended in all patients with HF except those undergoing low-risk surgery.[18] With respect to laboratory studies, obtaining a basic metabolic panel is appropriate because many patients are treated with loop diuretics and may present with electrolyte and acid-base abnormalities. In patients with chronic stable HF, routine preoperative radiographs and echocardiogram are not recommended.[18] Patients with signs or symptoms of new or worsening HF benefit from preoperative assessment of left ventricular function. A determination of the type of HF (systolic vs diastolic) has important implications for the anesthetic plan. In the setting of systolic dysfunction, inotropes may be favored over fluid administration to ensure end-organ perfusion and agents causing myocardial depression may be minimized. If diastolic dysfunction is identified, maintaining adequate preload intraoperatively becomes more important.

If at the time of presentation for nonemergent surgery, patients who are symptomatic or have signs of decompensated HF should have the procedure postponed, and their clinical status should be optimized. Treatment goals include optimizing volume status and end-organ perfusion, restoring normal oxygenation, and improving symptoms associated with pulmonary vascular congestion and/or low cardiac output. Medical management comprises several medication classes that may include diuretics, β-blockers, angiotensin-converting enzyme (ACE) inhibitors/angiotensin receptor blockers (ARBs), digoxin, and mineralocorticoid receptor antagonists. Because of their effects on the myocardium and vascular tone, CHF medications can magnify the hemodynamic swings associated with anesthesia and surgery. These medications should carefully reviewed preoperatively. In general, ACE inhibitors and ARBs may be continued if the patient is not hypotensive. Alternatively, the morning dose of ACE inhibitor/ARB may be held to decrease the risk of perioperative hypotension.[21] Chronically administered β-blockers should be continued. Patients not taking β-blockers, however, should not be started on these medications in the immediate perioperative period.[11] Aldosterone antagonists may be continued, although there is no evidence that they are useful in the perioperative period. Patients taking these should have potassium levels checked prior to surgery.

CONCOMITANT RENAL AND CARDIOVASCULAR DYSFUNCTION

It is now well known that CKD is a strong and independent risk factor for CVD.[22,23] In the United States, the prevalence of CVD in CKD is 63% whereas this rate is only 5.8% in people without CKD.[6] Patients with concomitant renal disease and CVD present a unique set of perioperative management goals, some of which are overlapping and some of which are concordant (**Table 2**).

Cardiorenal Syndrome

The cardiovascular and renal systems are closely interrelated with acute or chronic disruptions in one organ, often causing disruption in the other. They share common neurohormonal and biochemical feedback pathways and each organ has the ability to initiate disease in the other. Disease in one organ system rarely occurs in isolation. The term, *cardiorenal syndrome*, is used to describe the bidirectional relationship between HF and kidney disease and is defined explicitly as "a condition in which therapy to relieve congestive symptoms of HF is limited by a decline in renal function as manifested by a reduction in GFR [glomerular filtration rate]" (http://www.nhlbi.nih.gov/meetings/workshops/cardiorenal-hf-hd.htm).

Several different mechanisms are thought to contribute to the pathophysiology of cardiorenal syndrome. Reduced renal perfusion induced by low cardiac output was thought to play a central role, although this theory is not always applicable. Multiple studies have failed to demonstrate a relationship between cardiac output and worsening kidney function.[24,25] Compensatory neurohormonal activation in the setting of impaired left ventricular function serves to maintain systemic perfusion but ultimately contributes to worsening renal function. Activation of the renin-angiotensin-aldosterone system is thought to be particularly important in the progression of kidney

---

Table 2
Perioperative management considerations in patients with concomitant renal and cardiovascular disease

Phase of Care	Considerations
Preoperative	• Allow adequate time for venous and arterial access • Careful titration of anxiolytic medications
Intraoperative	• Avoid tachycardia and large hemodynamic swings • Neuraxial techniques associated with improved outcomes • Etomidate or propofol preferred for induction • Volatile agents preferred for maintenance • Goal-directed fluid therapy may improve outcomes • Careful titration of long-acting opioids
Postoperative	• Avoid NSAIDs • High risk of pulmonary edema • High risk of respiratory depression • High risk of cardiac events

disease. Angiotensin II has been shown to induce proteinuria and blockade of the angiotensin II receptor protects against renal fibrosis and inflammation.[26] ARB is protective against the progression of renal disease in several different populations.[27,28]

Preoperative Assessment

Preoperative assessment of patients with concomitant renal disease and CVD includes a history, physical examination, and appropriate studies. The history should focus on elucidating a patient's baseline disease and functional status as well as details of recent exacerbations. Medications regularly taken and those to be taken on the day of surgery should be clarified. Determination of preoperative fluid status is important particularly in patients with renal disease and systolic or diastolic dysfunction. Fluid status can vary widely depending on multiple factors, including dialysis schedule, diuretic use, and the degree of cardiac dysfunction. Although more objective assessments of fluid status are available in intubated patients (eg, pulse pressure variation), determination of fluid status in a spontaneously breathing patient is limited primarily to the bedside clinical examination. Conflicting goals, which must be balanced, include maintenance of adequate intravascular volume and minimizing hypotension while also minimizing volume overload and consequent pulmonary edema. For patients with some degree of preserved renal function, perioperative under-resuscitation represents a potential additional renal insult that may move patients further along the spectrum of renal failure.

Because of the substantially increased incidence of coronary disease in renal failure, signs and symptoms of cardiac ischemia should be thoroughly investigated. In the event that cardiac ischemia is discovered preoperatively, the decision to delay surgery and undertake revascularization must be weighed. Revascularization can be accomplished by either PCI or CABG. Despite that CVD is the leading cause of death in patients with CKD, most major randomized clinical trials assessing the use of coronary revascularization procedures exclude patients with renal insufficiency. In ESRD patients with CAD, the decision to pursue medical versus percutaneous or surgical management is guided primarily by observational studies. Multiple small retrospective studies have demonstrated higher long-term survival rates in ESRD patients who undergo CABG compared with percutaneous transluminal coronary angioplasty (PTCA).[29] In their study, Dewey and colleagues[30] demonstrated improved in hospital mortality in ESRD patients undergoing off-pump CABG, which avoids cardiopulmonary bypass, but also found significantly improved long-term survival with conventional on-pump CABG, where cardiopulmonary bypass is used. If a decision is made preoperatively to pursue coronary revascularization, patients with ESRD likely benefit more from conventional CABG than from off-pump CABG or PTCA.

Renal dysfunction, CAD, and CHF are each independently associated with increased arrhythmia burden; therefore, the risk of arrhythmias in patients with concomitant renal disease and CVD is cumulatively increased. The increased incidence of arrhythmias in patients with concomitant renal disease and CVD is multifactorial. Electrolyte abnormalities play an important role by altering the membrane potentials of myocardial cells, and chronic uremia can lead to cardiac autonomic neuropathy. Changes in myocardial structure and oxygenation significantly decrease the arrhythmia threshold. In addition to a standard chemistry panel, preoperative laboratory tests should, therefore, include calcium and magnesium.

Regional and Neuraxial

The risks and benefits of regional, neuraxial, and general anesthesia must be weighed in each clinical scenario (**Table 3**). Some considerations are broadly applicable, however, in patients with concomitant cardiovascular and renal disease. Regional or

Table 3
Advantages and disadvantages of neuraxial techniques in patients with renal failure

Advantages	Disadvantages
Minimize systemic medications	Hypotension
Minimize postoperative opioids	Tachycardia
Blockade of cardioaccelerator fibers with thoracic epidural	Altered pharmacokinetics of local anesthetics
Reduced cardiovascular complications[a]	Altered pharmacokinetics of anxiolytics
Reduced renal failure	Use limited by coagulopathy

[a] Reduced pulmonary embolism, deep vein thrombosis, and MI.

neuraxial techniques typically minimize the amount of systemic anesthetic medications administered over the course of the surgery, many of which of have cardiovascular depressant effects and are renally metabolized or eliminated, exerting prolonged activity in renal failure patients. In addition, regional and neuraxial anesthesia provide good intraoperative and postoperative analgesia, minimizing postoperative opioid requirements and the associated risk of respiratory depression. When large thoracic or abdominal procedures are anticipated, neuraxial anesthesia in the form of thoracic epidural blockade has the added benefit of blocking cardiac accelerator sympathetic fibers, thereby minimizing the increases in heart rate or contractility that can result from surgical stress. Multiple studies suggest improved cardiovascular and renal outcomes when neuraxial techniques are used, including reduced rates of MI, deep vein thrombosis, pulmonary embolism, transfusion requirements, and renal failure.[31–33] suggesting that these techniques should be offered when appropriate.

Coagulation abnormalities, including both hypercoagulabilty and hypocoagulabilty, are common in ESRD and CVD patients and may limit the utilization of regional techniques. In ESRD, coagulopathy is due to complex interactions of uremic toxins, the coagulation cascade, fibrinolytic system, and the endothelium.[34] The chronic inflammation associated with renal failure contributes to coagulopathy as well.[35] CAD is not directly associated with hypocoagulability; however, patients with CAD are commonly prescribed aspirin. Although aspirin therapy in and of itself is not a contraindication to neuraxial anesthesia (American Society of Regional Anesthesia and Pain Medicine guidelines), care should be taken when underlying coagulopathy is present.

There are several potential disadvantages to the use of regional techniques in patients with renal disease and CVD. A primary concern is myocardial ischemia induced by hypotension, tachycardia, or the combination of both. Hypotension associated with sympathectomy often induced by neuraxial techniques should be aggressively managed with a short-acting vasopressor, such as phenylephrine. Although judicious fluids are appropriate, large boluses may be problematic, particularly in patients with ESRD and CHF. Adequate analgesia and sedation are important in patients with CAD to minimize tachycardia-induced ischemia. The pharmacokinetics of local anesthetics and benzodiazepines are altered, however, in renal failure, making titration difficult. Poor drug clearance and decreased protein binding in renal disease prolong the duration of action of midazolam.[36] Likewise, the pharmacokinetics of local anesthetic may be altered in patients with renal failure secondary to decreased bicarbonate and decreased protein binding. Peripheral nerve blocks may, therefore, have prolonged onset and decreased duration of action. Because appropriate levels of sedation and analgesia may be difficult to achieve in the setting of advanced renal failure, the risk of tachycardia-induced ischemia should be weighed against the potential benefits of regional techniques.

Intraoperative Management

Vascular access may be more difficult in patients with renal disease and CVD, in particular venous access in ESRD patients. Those on hemodialysis have either a dialysis catheter or an arteriovenous fistula. Venipuncture at current or future fistula sites should be avoided, and hemodialysis catheters should not be used for access other than dialysis for reasons of sterility. Central venous cannulation may prove difficult, particularly if vessels have been previously accessed, and catheters should not be placed on the same side as an existing hemodialysis catheter. Furthermore, in patients for whom a dialysis fistula is planned, access should not be obtained in the larger veins of the extremity to be used; communication with the nephrologist or vascular surgeon regarding venous anatomy to be protected is recommended. Typically, patients with CAD most commonly also have peripheral vascular disease, and arterial access may prove difficult in this population. Arterial cannulation should likewise be limited to an extremity without a fistula. Adequate time should be allotted preoperatively in anticipation of difficult vascular access.

The goals of induction are to induce unconsciousness while minimizing hemodynamic changes that lead to myocardial oxygen imbalance. A standard approach is to use a hypnotic to induce unconsciousness, an opiate or lidocaine to blunt the sympathetic response to intubation, and a neuromuscular blocker to facilitate intubation. Etomidate is a frequently used induction agent because it has minimal effect on systemic vascular resistance and contractility and does not require dose adjustment in renal failure. Propofol is a reasonable alternative because metabolism is exclusively hepatic; however, propofol markedly decreases blood pressure through a combination of decreased systemic vascular resistance, increased venous capacitance, and direct depression of myocardial contractility. Induction doses should be reduced and boluses administered slowly. An α_1-receptor can be administered prophylactically to minimize hypotension. Fentanyl and remifentanil are the opiates of choice for attenuating the sympathetic response to intubation because they have pharmacokinetics independent of renal function and no active metabolites. Fentanyl has little direct affect myocardial contractility or vascular tone. An induction using high-dose fentanyl improves hemodynamic stability by minimizing requirements for other more vasoactive agents, such as propofol. Although ketamine is a useful induction agent because it preserves respiratory drive and is not affected by renal failure, it should be used cautiously in patients with CVD secondary to its sympathomimetic properties.

The choice of neuromuscular blocker depends on the need for rapid-sequence induction (RSI). If RSI is required, succinylcholine or high-dose rocuronium can be used. Succinylcholine does not cause an exaggerated hyperkalemic response in patients with renal failure more than for other patients and can be used safely provided there are no preoperative ECG changes and the serum potassium level is less than 5.5 mEQ/L.[37] Continuous succinylcholine infusions should be avoided because its major metabolite succinylmonocholine is active and is renally excreted. In cases of standard induction, cisatracurium is a reasonable choice because its pharmacokinetics are not affected by renal dysfunction. Laudanosine is a renally cleared byproduct produced by the Hoffmann degradation of cisatracurium and has been shown to be neurotoxic in animal studies. The significance of this finding is unclear because there is little evidence that laudanosine accumulation and related toxicity will likely ever be seen with the doses of cisatracurium used in clinical practice.[38]

Although surgery-specific or patient-specific factors may necessitate total intravenous anesthesia, a volatile agent is ideal for the maintenance of general anesthesia. Several studies have demonstrated that brief ischemic episodes protect myocardial cells against subsequent prolonged ischemic attack, a mechanism termed, *ischemic preconditioning*.[39,40] Volatile agents have been shown to mimic ischemic preconditioning and can theoretically lessen the risk of ischemia in patients with CVD undergoing surgery.[41] Another advantage of volatile agents is that they are minimally metabolized, and their pharmacokinetics and pharmacodynamics are, therefore, independent of renal function. There has been some concern about the accumulation of compound A, a renally toxic metabolite of sevoflurane. This concern was based on data from animal studies; however, no clinically significant association with renal injury has ever been demonstrated in humans.[42] Likewise, metabolism of isoflurane and sevoflurane results in the production of fluoride ions, which are nephrotoxic; however, clinically significant fluoride accumulation is not encountered in practice.[43]

Maintaining appropriate intravascular volume is important in patients with renal disease and CVD, in particular those with abnormal systolic or diastolic function. Hypervolemia is poorly tolerated in this population, making them especially susceptible to pulmonary edema. Static physiologic parameters, such as blood pressure, heart rate, urine output, and central venous and pulmonary artery occlusion pressure, are commonly used to guide fluid therapy. Central venous and pulmonary artery occlusion pressure have been shown to correlate poorly with cardiac preload and do not accurately predict impending pulmonary edema.[44,45] Heart rate, blood pressure, and urine output also may be normal despite mild hypovolemia. Dynamic indices, such as stroke volume and pulse pressure variation, can better predict fluid responsiveness and may be useful in fragile populations. Fixed-volume algorithms for intraoperative fluid administration should be avoided because of their tendency to cause fluid overload.[46,47] Goal-directed fluid therapy, in which fluids are administered to achieve a certain stroke volume or cardiac output, is associated with improved clinical outcomes, such as shorter hospital length of stay and decreased postoperative morbidity.[48,49] Because of their limited ability to tolerate hypervolemia, patients with concomitant renal and cardiac dysfunction require a more targeted approach to intraoperative fluid therapy. The use of dynamic indices of intravascular volume as well as goal-directed fluid therapy may improve outcomes in this population.

Optimum transfusion practice should minimize transfusions and maximize clinical outcomes. Much data have been generated supporting conservative transfusion thresholds.[50] Anemia is common in the setting of chronic renal disease and transfusion thresholds may require modification when concomitant CVD is present. Multiple societies have published transfusion guidelines with the general consensus that transfusion is not indicated for Hgb greater than 10 g/dL.[51–54] The lower threshold is more variable ranging from 6 g/dL to 8 g/dL. Although helpful as a general guideline, isolated Hgb measurements should not be the primary trigger to transfuse. Many factors must be considered, including symptoms, clinical status, and comorbidities. For asymptomatic patients with underlying CAD, multiple studies support a transfusion threshold of 8 g/dL (Transfusion Requirements in Critical Care [TRICC] and Functional Outcomes in Cardiovascular Patients Undergoing Surgical Repairs of Hip Fracture [FOCUS]) with a higher threshold of 10 associated with greater mortality. Symptomatic patients, patients who are actively bleeding, and patients with ACSs may benefit from higher transfusion thresholds in the range of 10 g/dL.[55,56]

Postoperative

A majority of cardiovascular events occur in the postoperative period. Therefore, particular attention should be paid to myocardial oxygen supply-demand balance during that phase of care. Stimuli for tachycardia, such as pain, hypovolemia, hypoxia, and arrhythmia, should be prevented and aggressively managed when they occur.

Likewise, increased afterload can tip the supply-demand balance toward ischemia. Pain is one of the most common causes of postoperative tachycardia and hypertension. Nonsteroidal anti-inflammatory drugs (NSAIDs) carry a black box warning due to an increased risk of thrombotic events, stroke, and MI in patients with CAD. They are contraindicated for the treatment of postoperative pain in the setting of CABG. Additionally, NSAIDs decrease renal blood flow and glomerular filtration rate through inhibition of renally active prostaglandins and should be avoided in patients with compromised renal function. Opiates continue to be the mainstay of postoperative pain control. In general, long-acting opiates, such as morphine and hydromorphone, should be used judiciously in patients with renal dysfunction because both drugs have active metabolites, which are renally cleared, increasing the risk of respiratory depression. Short-acting opiates, such as fentanyl and sufentanil, may be preferred because they have no active metabolites.

SUMMARY

Cardiovascular and renal disease are significant independent risk factors for perioperative morbidity and mortality. When encountered in the same patient, the dynamic interaction between these disease processes leads to both competing and concordant anesthetic goals. Disruption of homeostasis in the setting of renal failure introduces several risk factors for cardiac morbidity and mortality. Altered volume and electrolyte regulation potentiates the risk of pulmonary edema, CHF exacerbation, and arrhythmias in patients with underlying cardiomyopathy. Chronic anemia decreases oxygen carrying capacity, thereby increasing the risk of myocardial ischemia. Finally, altered drug clearance modifies the pharmacokinetics of various drugs used in the perioperative period and mandates particular attention to choice of drug and modification of dosing when needed. The dynamic interactions between the renal and cardiovascular systems play an important role in the maintenance of health as well as the pathophysiology of disease. These interactions and their implications must be recognized to most effectively identify and address patients' perioperative risks in planning their perioperative management.

REFERENCES

1. Lee TH, Marcantonio ER, Mangione CM, et al. Derivation and prospective validation of a simple index for prediction of cardiac risk of major noncardiac surgery. Circulation 1999;100(10):1043–9.
2. Gaita D, Mihaescu A, Schiller A. Of heart and kidney: a complicated love story. Eur J Prev Cardiol 2014;21(7):840–6.
3. Tonelli M, Wiebe N, Culleton B, et al. Chronic kidney disease and mortality risk: a systematic review. J Am Soc Nephrol 2006;17(7):2034–47 [Review].
4. Raggi P, Boulay A, Chasan-Taber S. Cardiac calcification in adult hemodialysis patients: a link between end-stage renal disease and cardiovascular disease? J Am Coll Cardiol 2002;39(4):695–701.
5. Arici M, Walls J. End-stage renal disease, atherosclerosis, and cardiovascular mortality: is C-reactive protein the missing link? Kidney Int 2001;59(2):407–14 [Review].
6. US Renal Data System. USRDS 2008 Annual Data Report: Atlas of End-Stage Renal Disease in the United States. Bethesda (MD): National Institutes of Health, National Institute of Diabetes and Digestive and Kidney Diseases; 2008.
7. Krane V, Heinrich F, Meesmann M, et al. Electrocardiography and outcome in patients with diabetes mellitus on maintenance hemodialysis. Clin J Am Soc Nephrol 2009;4(2):394–400.

8. Xia H, Ebben J, Ma JZ, et al. Hematocrit levels and hospitalization risks in hemo-dialysis patients. J Am Soc Nephrol 1999;10(6):1309–16.

9. Collins AJ, Ma JZ, Xia A, et al. Trends in anemia treatment with erythropoietin us-age and patient outcomes. Am J Kidney Dis 1998;32(6 Suppl 4):S133–41.

10. Besarab A, Bolton WK, Browne JK, et al. The effects of normal as compared with low hematocrit values in patients with cardiac disease who are receiving hemo-dialysis and epoetin. N Engl J Med 1998;339(9):584–90.

11. POISE Study Group, Devereaux PJ, Yang H, Yusuf S, et al. Effects of extended-release metoprolol succinate in patients undergoing non-cardiac surgery (POISE trial): a randomised controlled trial. Lancet 2008;371(9627):1839–47.

12. Landesberg G, Beattie WS, Mosseri M, et al. Perioperative myocardial infarction. Circulation 2009;119(22):2936–44 [Review].

13. Slager CJ, Wentzel JJ, FJH Gijsen, et al. The role of shear stress in the destabi-lization of vulnerable plaques and related therapeutic implications. Nat Clin Pract Cardiovasc Med 2005;2(9):456–64.

14. Landesberg G, Mosseri M, Zahger D, et al. Myocardial infarction after vascular surgery: the role of prolonged stress-induced, ST depression-type ischemia. J Am Coll Cardiol 2001;37(7):1839–45.

15. Landesberg G, Shatz V, Akopnik I, et al. Association of cardiac troponin, CK-MB, and postoperative myocardial ischemia with long-term survival after major vascular surgery. J Am Coll Cardiol 2003;42(9):1547–54.

16. Landesberg G, Mosseri M, Wolf YG, et al. Preoperative thallium scanning, selec-tive coronary revascularization, and long-term survival after major vascular sur-gery. Circulation 2003;108(2):177–83.

17. McFalls EO, Ward HB, Moritz TE, et al. Coronary-artery revascularization before elective major vascular surgery. N Engl J Med 2004;351(27):2795–804.

18. Fleisher LA, Fleischmann KE, Auerbach AD, et al. 2014 ACC/AHA guideline on perioperative cardiovascular evaluation and management of patients undergoing noncardiac surgery: executive summary: a report of the American College of Car-diology/American Heart Association Task Force on practice guidelines. Devel-oped in collaboration with the American College of Surgeons, American Society of Anesthesiologists, American Society of Echocardiography, American Society of Nuclear Cardiology, Heart Rhythm Society, Society for Cardiovascular Angiography and Interventions, Society of Cardiovascular Anesthesiologists, and Society of Vascular Medicine Endorsed by the Society of Hospital Medicine. J Nucl Cardiol 2015;22(1):162–215.

19. Hammill BG, Curtis LH, Bennett-Guerrero E, et al. Impact of heart failure on pa-tients undergoing major noncardiac surgery. Anesthesiology 2008;108:559.

20. Van Diepen S, Bakal JA, McAlister FA, et al. Mortality and readmission of patients with heart failure, atrial fibrillation, or coronary artery disease undergoing noncar-diac surgery: an analysis of 38 047 patients. Circulation 2011;124:289.

21. Fleisher LA, Eagle KA. Clinical practice. Lowering cardiac risk in noncardiac sur-gery. N Engl J Med 2001;345(23):1677–82.

22. Mann JF, Gerstein HC, Pogue J, et al. Cardiovascular risk in patients with early renal insufficiency: implications for the use of ACE inhibitors. Am J Cardiovasc Drugs 2002;2(3):157–62 [Review].

23. Shlipak MG, Simon JA, Grady D, et al. Renal insufficiency and cardiovascular events in postmenopausal women with coronary heart disease. J Am Coll Cardiol 2001;38(3):705–11.

24. De Silva R, Nikitin NP, Witte KK, et al. Incidence of renal dysfunction over 6 months in patients with chronic heart failure due to left ventricular systolic dysfunction: contributing factors and relationship to prognosis. Eur Heart J 2006;27:569.

25. Jessup M, Abraham WT, Casey DE, et al. 2009 focused update: ACCF/AHA Guidelines for the Diagnosis and Management of Heart Failure in Adults: a report of the American College of Cardiology Foundation/American Heart Association Task Force on Practice Guidelines: developed in collaboration with the International Society for Heart and Lung Transplantation. Circulation 2009;119:1977.

26. Ruiz-Ortega M, Rupérez M, Esteban V, et al. Angiotensin II: a key factor in the inflammatory and fibrotic response in kidney diseases. Nephrol Dial Transplant 2006;21(1):16–20 [Review].

27. Kiernan MS, Wentworth D, Francis G, et al. Predicting adverse events during angiotensin receptor blockertreatment in heart failure: results from the HEAAL trial. Eur J Heart Fail 2012;14:1401.

28. Vardeny O, Wu DH, Desai A, et al. Influence of baseline and worsening renal function on efficacy ofspironolactone in patients With severe heart failure: insights from RALES (Randomized Aldactone Evaluation Study). J Am Coll Cardiol 2012; 60:2082.

29. Ashrith G, Elayda MA, Wilson JM. Revascularization options in patients with chronic kidney disease. Tex Heart Inst J 2010;37(1):9–18.

30. Dewey TM, Herbert MA, Prince SL, et al. Does coronary artery bypass graft surgery improve survival among patients with end-stage renal disease? Ann Thorac Surg 2006;81(2):591–8.

31. Rodgers A, Walker N, Schug S, et al. Reduction of postoperative mortality and morbidity with epidural or spinal anaesthesia: results from overview of randomized trials. BMJ 2000;321:1493 [Review].

32. Guay J, Choi P, Suresh S, et al. Neuraxial blockade for the prevention of postoperative mortality and major morbidity: an overview of Cochrane systematic reviews. Cochrane Database Syst Rev 2014;(1):CD010108; [Review].

33. Barbosa FT, Jucá MJ, Castro AA, et al. Neuraxial anaesthesia for lower-limb revascularization. Cochrane Database Syst Rev 2013;(7):CD007083; [Review].

34. Jalal DI, Chonchol M, Targher G. Disorders of hemostasis associated with chronic kidney disease. Semin Thromb Hemost 2010;36:34–40.

35. Mezzano D, Pais EO, Aranda E, et al. Inflammation, not hyperhomocysteinemia, is related to oxidative stress and hemostatic and endothelial dysfunction in uremia. Kidney Int 2001;60:1844–50.

36. Spina SP, Ensom MH. Clinical pharmacokinetic monitoring of midazolam in critically ill patients. Pharmacotherapy 2007;27:389.

37. Thapa S, Brull SJ. Succinylcholine-induced hyperkalemia in patients with renal failure: an old question revisited. Anesth Analg 2000;91(1):237–41.

38. Fodale V, Santamaria LB. Laudanosine, an atracurium and cisatracurium metabolite. Eur J Anaesthesiol 2002;19(7):466–73.

39. Murry CE, Jennings RB, Reimer KA. Preconditioning with ischemia: a delay of lethal cell injury in ischemic myocardium. Circulation 1986;74(5):1124–36.

40. Przyklenk K, Bauer B, Ovize M, et al. Regional ischemic'preconditioning'protects remote virgin myocardium from subsequent sustained coronary occlusion. Circulation 1993;87(3):893–9.

41. Kunst G, Klein AA. Peri-operative anaesthetic myocardial preconditioning and protection - cellular mechanisms and clinical relevance in cardiac anaesthesia. Anaesthesia 2015;70(4):467–82 [Review].

42. Conzen PF, Kharasch ED, Czerner SF, et al. Lowflow sevoflurane compared with lowflow Isoflurane anesthesia in patients with stable renal insufficiency. Anesthesiology 2002;97:578.

43. Reichle FM, Conzen PF. Halogenated inhalational anaesthetics. Best Pract Res Clin Anaesthesiol 2003;17(1):29–46 [Review].

44. Marik PE, Baram M, Vahid B. Does central venous pressure predict fluid responsiveness? A systematic review of the literature and the tale of seven mares. Chest 2008;134(1):172–8 [Review].

45. Magder S. Fluid status and fluid responsiveness. Curr Opin Crit Care 2010;16(4): 289–96 [Review].

46. Holte K, Sharrock NE, Kehlet H. Pathophysiology and clinical implications of perioperative fluid excess. Br J Anaesth 2002;89(4):622–32.

47. Lobo DN, Macafee DA, Allison SP. How perioperative fluid balance influences postoperative outcomes. Best Pract Res Clin Anaesthesiol 2006;20(3):439–55 [Review].

48. Corcoran T, Rhodes JE, Clarke S, et al. Perioperative fluid management strategies in major surgery: a stratified meta-analysis. Anesth Analg 2012;114(3): 640–51 [Meta analysis].

49. Giglio MT, Marucci M, Testini M, et al. Goal-directed haemodynamic therapy and gastrointestinal complications in major surgery: a meta-analysis of randomized controlled trials. Br J Anaesth 2009;103(5):637–46.

50. Carson JL. Transfusion thresholds and other strategies for guiding allogeneic red blood cell transfusion. Cochrane Database Syst Rev 2012;(4):CD002042; [Review].

51. Practice Guidelines for blood component therapy: a report by the American Society of AnesthesiologistsTask Force on Blood Component Therapy. Anesthesiology 1996;84:732.

52. Hamm CW, Bassand JP, Agewall S, et al. ESC Guidelines for the management of acute coronary syndromes in patients presenting without persistent ST-segment elevation: The Task Force for the management of acute coronary syndromes (ACS) in patients presenting without persistent ST-segment elevation of the European Society of Cardiology (ESC). Eur Heart J 2011;32(23):2999–3054.

53. Ferraris VA, Brown JR, Despotis GJ, et al, Society of Thoracic Surgeons Blood Conservation Guideline Task Force. 2011 update to the Society of Thoracic Surgeons and the Society of Cardiovascular Anesthesiologists blood conservation clinical practice guidelines. Ann Thorac Surg 2011;91:944.

54. Napolitano LM, Kurek S, Luchette FA, et al. Clinical practice guideline: red blood cell transfusion in adult trauma and critical care. Crit Care Med 2009;37(12): 3124–57.

55. Carson JL, Brooks MM, Abbott JD, et al. Liberal versus restrictive transfusion thresholds for patients withsymptomatic coronary artery disease. Am Heart J 2013;165:964.

56. Kansagara D, Dyer E, Englander H, et al. Treatment of anemia in patients with heart disease: a systematic review. Ann Intern Med 2013;159:746 [Review].

Anesthesia for Patients with Anemia

Aryeh Shander, MD*, Gregg P. Lobel, MD, Mazyar Javidroozi, MD, PhD

KEYWORDS

• Anemia • Transfusion • Surgery • Iron • Patient blood management

KEY POINTS

- Anemia is common in perioperative settings and it is associated with worse clinical outcomes, including various complications and increased risk of morbidity and mortality.
- Factors contributing to anemia in surgical settings include nutritional deficiencies (including iron deficiency), inflammation, chronic underlying disorders, and surgical blood loss.
- Hospital-acquired anemia is increasingly recognized as an important contributor to worse outcomes in surgical patients, and it can persist long beyond the discharge.
- Allogeneic blood transfusion should not be considered as the default and first-line treatment of anemia given the associated risks and negative impact on the outcomes of patients and availability of other options.
- Patient blood management provides a multimodality framework for preventing and managing anemia in perioperative settings, with the ultimate goal of improving the outcomes of patients.

INTRODUCTION

As a simple and purportedly mundane diagnosis, anemia imposes a heavy burden on humankind. It is estimated that 1 out of every 3 to 4 people is anemic according to the criteria set by the World Health Organization (WHO; hemoglobin level <12 g/dL in adult nonpregnant women and <13 g/dL in adult men).[1–3] Kassebaum and colleagues[4] estimated that anemia had a global prevalence of 33% in 2010, and it caused 68.36 million years lived with disability, accounting for 8.8% of the total disability from all conditions.

Financial Support: None.

Conflicts of Interest: A. Shander has been a consultant or speaker with honorarium for, or has received research support from, Masimo, Gauss, and Vifor; he is a founding member of the Society for the Advancement of Blood Management (SABM). M. Javidroozi has been a consultant and contractor for SABM and Gauss Surgical. G.P. Lobel declares no relevant conflicts of interest.

Department of Anesthesiology and Critical Care Medicine, Englewood Hospital and Medical Center, TeamHealth Research Institute, 350 Engle Street, Englewood, NJ 07631, USA

* Corresponding author.

E-mail address: aryeh.shander@ehmchealth.org

Anemia is commonly found incidentally in patients across the spectrum of care, including those undergoing surgery. For surgical patients, many present to the operating room with anemia, whereas many patients develop new-onset (hospital-acquired) anemia following surgery and during hospital stay. Some patients leave the hospital with anemia, which persists for months.[5–8]

The omnipresent nature of anemia and the assumption that a quick and easy treatment is always available (blood transfusion) might lead some to think it is a simple and even acceptable condition. In reality, this notion lacks validity because anemia is not just a simple laboratory diagnosis and certainly not a so-called innocent bystander.[9] Development and progression of anemia is often a multifactorial process involving different causes. Inflammation (as commonly encountered in many chronic conditions) and iron deficiency (absolute or functional) are often among the key factors,[10,11] and, as shown by the function of hepcidin (and its counterpart, erythroferrone), they often go hand in hand.[12,13] Other factors, such as other nutritional deficiencies (zinc, folate, and B_{12}), blunted hematopoiesis, shortened survival of red blood cells, and blood loss, also commonly contribute to the development and exacerbation of anemia.[14]

Anemia has repeatedly been shown to be an independent predictor of worse outcomes across patient populations.[15] The role anemia can play in worsening outcomes is perhaps best exemplified in cardiorenal anemia syndrome: patients with chronic conditions such as heart failure and renal disease are at increased risk of development of anemia, whereas anemia works to exacerbate the underlying chronic conditions in a pernicious loop, leading to worse patient outcomes, including increased mortality.[16]

Anemia in the context of surgical patients is similarly troublesome. Acute blood loss in the surgical theater is a visible contributor to anemia, whereas diagnostic blood loss in the perioperative setting and during the hospital stay might be a less obvious but similarly important contributor.[17] Regardless of the cause, anemia takes its toll on surgical patients, because the independent link between anemia and worse outcomes has also been reported across various surgical populations.[14] In addition, anemia is a known risk factor for allogeneic blood transfusions, and transfusions are also independently linked with worse clinical outcomes.[15] Whenever faced with newly discovered anemia in the preoperative setting, clinicians should become alerted to potential underlying causes (eg, malignancy or chronic kidney disease) and consider referring the patients for additional investigation before surgery.[18]

Given all this, surgery and anesthesia in anemic patients requires a higher level of vigilance, to ensure proper diagnosis and management. Also important are the preventive measures, which can prove highly effective in this context. It is important for clinicians to screen for and recognize anemia as an important modifiable risk factor in their patients and take proper steps to address it.

DEFINITION OF ANEMIA AND ITS CONTROVERSIES

The WHO criteria define anemia based on hemoglobin concentrations.[3] This definition is rooted in the observed distribution of hemoglobin values across the populations (with stratifications for gender, age, and so forth). Values that are a few standard deviations more than or beyond the observed mean are considered abnormal. Although this practice is widely accepted and applied to various naturally occurring physiologic parameters, this approach has the potential pitfall of considering something to be normal based solely on its high prevalence. In the case of anemia, because the hemoglobin level is usually lower in women compared with men, the population-derived hemoglobin threshold to define anemia is also lower. As such, a woman with hemoglobin level of 12.5 g/dL is considered nonanemic, whereas a man with the same hemoglobin level is considered anemic.[19]

The population-derived definition of anemia should not be taken as justification for accepting lower levels of hemoglobin in women. Because of generally lower blood volume, women can be more susceptible to negative consequences of surgical blood loss.[20] In a surgical procedure with 600 mL of blood loss, the procedure would cause a 75-kg male patient to lose about 15% of his estimated blood volume, but the same amount of blood loss would cost a female 55-kg patient 21% of her estimated blood volume. Assuming the lower normal limits of preoperative hemoglobin level (13 g/dL for male and 12 g/dL for female patients) and blood loss occurring rapidly with no immediate volume replacement (ie, stable hemoglobin concentration during blood loss), the postbleeding, post–volume resuscitation hemoglobin levels of the male and female patients are 11 and 9.5 g/dL, respectively. It is therefore not surprising that, according to some studies, female gender is among the risk factors for allogeneic blood transfusion.[21–23]

Reliance on hemoglobin concentration (or hematocrit) for making a diagnosis of anemia (and making important treatment decisions such as ordering blood transfusion) has a few other potential pitfalls. Commonly used methods to measure hemoglobin level have an inherent margin of error, which can be as much as 1 g/dL.[24] In the example provided earlier, the hemoglobin concentration of the female patient before the bleeding might have been 11 g/dL not 12 g/dL as reported by the laboratory test, which brings her final hemoglobin level down to 8.7 g/dL following the blood loss and volume replacement.

As seen in this hypothetical example, when the blood loss happens quickly, hemoglobin concentration may not be reflective of the blood loss until volume replacement and hemodilution and volume redistribution occur. Hemoglobin concentrations can vary substantially over a short period of time as a result of changes in intravascular volume. As commonly seen in surgical cases under anesthesia, anesthetic agents may reduce blood pressure (eg, because of venodilation and cardiac depression). This reduced blood pressure can lead to infusion of intravenous fluids, which can result in hemodilution and further reduced hemoglobin concentration.

The issues surrounding the use of hemoglobin concentration or hematocrit levels are often not considered by clinicians when relying on them to make an important diagnosis (anemia) and make important clinical decisions for their patients (ordering blood or other treatments). Clinicians therefore should be reminded that the goal is not to treat a number but to treat a patient and the whole clinical picture, and the changes occurring over time, should be considered alongside laboratory test results.

The search for other alternatives to hemoglobin levels has been underway. A promising option is the red cell mass (RCM). The total blood volume is made up of the fraction taken by the blood cells (mainly red blood cells; RCM) and the remaining part, which is the plasma. As discussed earlier, hemoglobin and hematocrit levels are concentrations that should be considered in the context of total blood volume, whereas RCM indicates the total blood cell reserve of the patient that is available for oxygen delivery regardless of the plasma volume.[25] RCM has been used clinically for years (eg, in the assessment of polycythemia vera), but its measurement is cumbersome and not widely available. Other approaches, such as noninvasive continuous monitoring of hemoglobin level, have also become available and can prove useful in this context, but their accuracy and placement in clinical decision making are still being debated.[23,26,27]

RECENT FINDINGS ON PREVALENCE AND SIGNIFICANCE OF ANEMIA IN THE PERIOPERATIVE SETTING

Several studies have investigated the prevalence of anemia in the perioperative setting, and almost all have reported increased prevalence compared with the general population. There is variation in the observed/reported prevalence of anemia (most often according to the WHO criteria) across populations and studies, as indicated by the few recent examples cited here:

- Lasocki and colleagues[28] studied the data from more than 1500 patients who underwent major elective knee, hip, or spine surgery at 17 hospitals across 6 European countries. Preoperative anemia was detected in 14.1% of patients, whereas 85.8% of the patients were anemic in the postoperative period. Patients who had preoperative anemia had a mean hemoglobin reduction of 1.9 g/dL in the postoperative period, whereas patients who were not anemic at baseline experienced an astonishing 3-g/dL reduction in their hemoglobin levels in the postoperative period. Anemia was associated with increase rate of postoperative complications.
- Among more than 13,500 patients undergoing total joint arthroplasty in a single center, Viola and colleagues[29] detected preoperative anemia in 19% of the patients. Anemia was independently associated with increased risk of complications, particularly cardiac and genitourinary complications.
- In a nationwide study of more than 3 million total joint arthroplasty surgeries in the United States, Menendez and colleagues[30] identified anemia among the risk factors of in-hospital, postoperative myocardial infarction (odds ratio [OR] 1.4; 95% confidence interval [CI], 1.3–1.5).
- Uchida and colleagues[31] studied 337 patients admitted for percutaneous coronary intervention (PCI), and detected anemia at admission in 17.5% of the cases. Anemia at admission was an independent significant risk factor for adverse outcomes and worse prognosis during the median follow-up period of 4.5 years.
- Landes and colleagues[32] studied the predictors of long-term outcome in more than 11,000 patients who underwent PCI and reported that previous history of anemia was independently associated with mortality or myocardial infarction. The long-lasting negative impact of anemia at admission on worse outcomes is supported by other recent studies.[33]
- DeLarochellière and colleagues[34] reported anemia in 64.4% of 438 patients before undergoing transcatheter aortic valve replacement in a single-center study. At a 6-month follow-up visit, 62% of patients were still anemic. Anemia was independently associated with worsening of Duke Activity Status Index score and poor performance in the 6-minute walk test and other functional and quality-of-life measures The cause of anemia was considered to be potentially treatable (primarily iron deficiency) in 9 out of 10 anemic patients.[34]
- Shacham and colleagues[35] studied 1248 patients admitted with ST segment elevation myocardial infarction who underwent PCI, and reported that anemia at admission was independently associated with the increased risk of acute kidney injury.
- In a study of more than 2300 patients undergoing nonemergent isolated coronary artery bypass grafting surgery, Spiegelstein and colleagues[36] reported that lower preoperative hematocrit levels were independently associated with increased risk of perioperative major morbidity.
- Seicean and colleagues[37] investigated 668 patients undergoing open surgery for intracranial aneurysms (60% ruptured), and concluded that preoperative anemia

was independently associated with preoperative complications (OR, 1.9; 95% CI, 1.1–3.1), need for reoperation (OR, 2.1; 95% CI, 1.1–4.5) and longer hospital stay (OR, 2.5; 95% CI, 1.4–4.5).

- In a multicenter study of 684 patients undergoing radical cystectomy for transitional cell carcinoma of bladder, Gierth and colleagues[38] reported anemia in 39.3% of the patients. Anemia was an independent predictor of cancer recurrence, cancer mortality, and all-cause mortality.

The long list of the studies reporting on the high prevalence of anemia in surgical populations and the negative impact on clinical outcomes keeps growing. It is therefore appropriate to consider a recent meta-analysis on the association between preoperative anemia and outcomes in surgical patients by Fowler and colleagues.[39] They studied the results from 24 eligible observational studies involving approximately 950,000 surgical patients (excluding pediatric and obstetric populations as well as trauma, burn, and transplant surgeries). Across the studies, 39.1% of the patients had preoperative anemia. Presence of anemia was associated with increased risk of mortality (in-hospital or 30-day mortality: OR, 2.90; 95% CI, 2.30–3.68; $P<.001$), acute kidney injury (OR, 3.75; 95% CI, 2.95–4.76; $P<.001$), and infection (OR, 1.93; 95% CI, 1.17–3.18; $P = .01$). In the subgroup analysis of patients undergoing cardiac surgery, presence of anemia was linked with increased risk of stroke (OR, 1.28; 95% CI, 1.06–1.55; $P = .009$). Overall, anemic patients were at increased risk of receiving allogeneic blood transfusions during their course of care (OR, 5.04; 95% CI, 4.12–6.17; $P<.001$).[39]

Presence of anemia should alert clinicians to the increased risk of surgery-related complications, and anemia should be among the factors considered in preoperative risk assessment of patients. In a study among 4500 adult patients undergoing cardiac surgery, adding preoperative anemia to the European System for Cardiac Operative Risk Evaluation (EuroSCORE) II significantly improved the model's power to predict the probability of mortality: mortality increased from 3.4% in nonanemic patients to 7.7% in those with mild anemia (hemoglobin level, 11–12.9 g/dL in men and 11–11.9 g/dL in women) and 15.7% in those with moderate to severe anemia (hemoglobin level <11 g/dL).[40]

WHY IS ANEMIA HARMFUL?

Understanding the mechanism of injury of anemia and compensatory measures is important in selecting more effective management strategies. The perils of anemia are primarily considered in the context of its negative impact on oxygen carrying capacity of blood. Each gram of hemoglobin can bind as much as 1.39 mL of oxygen under ideal physiologic conditions, although the actual number is slightly less because of presence of other conformations of the hemoglobin molecule.[41,42] Reduced hemoglobin concentration in anemia reduces the capacity of blood to deliver oxygen throughout the body. Various safety and compensatory mechanisms are in place to mitigate the impact of anemia and to maintain the oxygen delivery to tissues despite the reduction. A few examples include:

- The effective hematocrit at microcirculation can stay almost unchanged in the face of substantial changes in systemic hematocrit level, because of the specific dynamics of blood cells in plasma as they travel through narrow capillaries (the Fahraeus effect).[43]
- Oxygen sensors throughout the body react to the reduced oxygen delivery and activate compensatory mechanisms at the subcellular level (eg, the hypoxia-inducible factor signaling pathway).[44]

- Another type of sensor in the renal cortex responds by increasing the release of erythropoietin to promote erythropoiesis.[45]
- Although the availability of oxygen in the alveoli is usually not a limiting factor, respiratory rate and ventilation are increased and ventilation-perfusion matching is improved through nitric oxide (NO)–mediated mechanisms.[46]
- Hypoxia is detected by the chemoreceptors of the aortic and carotid bodies,[47–49] which activate the sympathetic nervous system and increase cardiac output via positive inotropic and chronotropic changes, increasing contractility of heart muscle and pulse rate.
- To further increase the cardiac output, venous return and preload are increased, whereas afterload is reduced by systemic vasodilatation and decreased vascular resistance (mediated by increased NO activity, hypoxia-induced vasodilatation, increased recruitment of microvasculature, and the reduced viscosity of diluted blood).[50]
- The oxygen dissociation curve of hemoglobin is shifted to the right following increased accumulation of 2,3-diphosphoglycerate (2,3-DPG), reduced pH, and other NO-mediated signaling events, which facilitates release of oxygen and increases hemoglobin oxygen extraction ratio at tissue sites.[51–53]

Although these and other mechanisms are highly effective in mitigating the negative consequences of anemia, they all have limits that are reached sooner or later as hemoglobin level keeps decreasing. Once the limit is reached, oxygen delivery is no longer adequate to meet the needs of the cells, resulting in anaerobic metabolism, ischemia, injury, and death.[54]

The critical hemoglobin level below which tissue oxygen consumption is compromised is expected to occur only in extremely severe anemia.[55] Nonetheless, the harmful effects of anemia can still occur at much higher hemoglobin levels, and even in mild anemia.[56–58] There are several possible explanations:

- One possible cause is iron deficiency. In a patient with mild iron deficiency anemia, the iron deficiency is expected to be severe and iron storages are already depleted. Iron is a multifunctional element involved in multiple pathways, and iron deficiency is independently associated with worse outcomes even in the absence of anemia.[59,60]
- Reduced blood viscosity during anemia can undermine the rheologic characteristics of blood and its ability to sustain the microcirculation, although the effective hematocrit is expected to remain unchanged across a wide spectrum of hemoglobin levels.[61]
- Other conditions that can lead to anemia (eg, chronic illness and inflammation) can also affect the clinical outcomes of the patients. As discussed for cardiorenal anemia syndrome, the association between anemia and chronic diseases is often synergistic.[62]
- The harm may be attributed to the treatments given in response to anemia, namely allogeneic blood transfusions, which are known to be independently associated with worse clinical outcomes.[15,63,64]

It is important to recognize that patients often have a combination of these and other factors. Anemia, iron deficiency, chronic diseases, inflammation, allogeneic blood transfusions, and other conditions work together to affect the outcome. This view may also explain a recurring theme in the studies that evaluate each of these factors and try to assess their independent roles in worsening the outcomes. For example, studies of transfusion often debate whether transfusion is an independent risk factor for the worse outcomes or a marker of the underlying disorders. The same debate has been made over the role of anemia as an independent contributor to the worsening of the outcomes versus a marker of underlying comorbidities.[15,39] Both sides of these debates are likely to be valid to some extents, but it is important to remember that they are not mutually exclusive, and each factor can act as an independent risk factor while also being a marker of another underlying process.

In addition, it is important to remember that there can be significant variations in the susceptibility of individuals (and different organs) to the effects of anemia.[65] Some patients (eg, critically ill) may have higher oxygen consumption needs at the cellular level and a higher critical hemoglobin level.[54] Others, such as those with cardiac disease (although still debated), might be at risk because of a reduced margin in their compensatory mechanisms. As mentioned earlier, adjustment of hemoglobin oxygen extraction ratio is one of the strategies used during adaptation to anemia, but the extraction ratio is normally not the same in different tissues. For example, cardiac muscle has a much higher oxygen extraction ratio under normal physiologic conditions (particularly in the left ventricle), which leaves it with less room to increase in case of anemia. In patients with ischemic heart disease, this safety margin is further reduced, leaving them with less potential for compensation, although the dilutional effect of anemia may increase perfusion.[66] Another organ with increased susceptibility to hypoxia is the kidney, and some studies have supported the increased risk of renal failure associated with perioperative anemia.[67]

MANAGEMENT OF ANEMIA IN THE PERIOPERATIVE SETTING
Allogeneic Blood Transfusion

For years, blood transfusion has been, and continues to be, the default treatment of anemic surgical patients. Its seemingly innocuous nature, perceived availability, assumed low cost, ease of ordering, and the ability to observe the treatment effect immediately in terms of increased hemoglobin level have all contributed to its widespread use. Allogeneic blood transfusion has become the most commonly performed procedure in the hospitals in the United States.[68]

Every reason listed earlier for giving blood transfusions can be challenged and refuted. The evidence for the harmful effects of allogeneic blood transfusion is overwhelming. Several studies have shown that the patients who are transfused often have worse outcomes, including increased risk of mortality, morbidities (including stroke, renal injury, atrial fibrillation, thromboembolic events, infections, respiratory failure, and prolonged need for ventilatory support), and prolonged hospital stay.[15,69] The proposed reasons for harmful effects of blood are many, but one key consideration is that allogeneic blood transfusion is a live tissue transplant. The interaction of this foreign tissue with the body can produce numerous complex immunologic and inflammatory reactions. Furthermore, the tissue in this case (blood) has typically undergone various processing and prolonged storage ex vivo, which could further influence its effects on the body.[15]

Blood availability depends on a sophisticated chain of supply that can be broken at any of the numerous links: donor recruitment, processing, storage, and distribution. For instance, an aging population may lead to a situation in which fewer potential donors are available to meet the higher potential needs of more chronically ill elders.[70] Placing more restrictions on the permitted storage duration of blood (should studies support the harmful effects of prolonged storage of blood) can have a similar effect on the available blood supply.[71]

Studies have shown that the real cost of blood transfusion can be several times higher than the nominal fee of purchase that hospitals pay. Every step involved in recruiting donors to procuring blood, processing it, distributing it to the hospitals and transfusion centers, local storage, transfusion, and management of complications can be very costly.[72]

In addition, even though transfusion of blood leads to increased hemoglobin level, this does not necessarily translate into increased oxygen delivery. It takes some time for the transfused red blood cells to restore their depleted stores of 2,3-DPG. The impact of other aspects of storage lesions remains to be better understood. Also, many of the transfused red blood cells are already well beyond their prime time and are likely to be removed from the circulation soon, given the average 120-day lifespan of normal red blood cells in the body.[73]

Allogeneic blood transfusion is an effective treatment when used appropriately, and most of the issues arise when transfusions are used with little or no valid clinical justification, and when other less-risky alternatives are not explored and exploited.[69] Several randomized controlled trials have shown that more restrictive transfusion strategies are safe and effective in various patient population compared with more liberal use of blood. In a recent Cochrane meta-analysis by Brunskill and colleagues,[74] data from 2722 patients undergoing surgery for hip fracture from 6 trials comparing liberal transfusion strategies (usually target hemoglobin threshold of 10 g/dL) versus restrictive transfusion strategies (8 g/dL hemoglobin threshold) were pooled and analyzed. Despite a large number of patients having a history of cardiovascular disease, there was no significant difference in postoperative mortality between the liberal and restrictive transfusion strategies, a finding that casts doubt on the justification of liberal use of transfusion in these high-risk patients. These findings are supported by other recent trials in surgical populations, including those with higher baseline risk.[75,76] Note that transfusion practice trials have almost invariably focused on the use of allogeneic blood (at various triggers) for treatment of anemia, while ignoring the anemia per se and all other modalities available to treat it. Not reaching the preset transfusion trigger does not mean that the patient's anemia did not need proper attention.

Current guidelines should be followed for the use of allogeneic blood transfusions in surgical patients under anesthesia.[77] **Table 1** summarizes several available guidelines for this setting.[78–83] More importantly, clinicians should never lose sight of the other management strategies that can often be used successfully to reduce the need of patients for transfusion while maintaining and improving their outcomes.

Patient Blood Management

Patient blood management (PBM) is defined as "the timely application of evidence-based medical and surgical concepts designed to maintain hemoglobin concentration, optimize hemostasis and minimize blood loss in an effort to improve patient outcome."[84] The concept of PBM is rooted in earlier efforts to reduce the use of allogeneic blood components (blood conservation) or their complete avoidance when blood transfusion was not an option, as was the case for patients who refused transfusion (bloodless medicine and surgery).[85] The concept highlights a shift from a product-centered approach (focusing on avoidance of transfusion) to a patient-centered approach (focusing on improving the outcomes of patients).[85] The key strategies of PBM include[86,87]:

- Managing anemia
- Optimizing coagulation and hemostasis

Table 1
Transfusion guidelines for surgical patients

Guidelines	American Society of Anesthesiology (2006)[78]	Society of Thoracic Surgeons (2007)[79]	Italian Society of Transfusion Medicine and Immunohaematology (2011)[80-82]	American Association of Blood Banks (2012)[83]
Target population	General surgery	Cardiac surgery	General surgery	General hospitalized
When is blood transfusion usually indicated?	Hemoglobin <6 g/dL	• Hemoglobin <6 g/dL • Hemoglobin <7 g/dL in postoperative period • Possibly higher hemoglobin levels when risk of end-organ ischemia exists	• Hemoglobin <6 g/dL • Hemoglobin 6–8 g/dL in presence of risk factors • Hemoglobin 6–10 g/dL if symptoms of hypoxia are present	• Hemoglobin ≤7 g/dL in critically ill patients • Hemoglobin ≤8 g/dL in surgical patients, or patients with preexisting cardiovascular disease • When symptoms of hypoxia are present in context of anemia
When is blood transfusion rarely indicated?	Hemoglobin >10 g/dL	Hemoglobin >10 g/dL	Hemoglobin >10 g/dL	—
Gray areas	Hemoglobin 6–10 g/dL	—	—	Patients with acute coronary syndrome
Other factors to consider in making the decision	Ischemia, extent/rate of bleeding, volume status, risk factors for hypoxia complications	Age, severity of illness, cardiac function, ischemia, extent/rate of blood loss, mixed venous oxygen saturation	Rate of blood loss, risk factors, symptoms of hypoxia/ischemia	Symptoms of hypoxia (chest pain, orthostatic hypotension, unresponsive tachycardia, heart failure)

- Use of interdisciplinary blood conservation modalities
- Patient-centered decision making

Given the earlier discussion on the risks of anemia, management of anemia plays a central role in PBM. It is important to remember that anemia often does not occur overnight but it is the result of a long and convoluted chain of events that is acutely exacerbated by the surgical insult. For surgical patients, particularly when scheduled to undergo an elective surgical procedure, the focus of clinicians should be directed at the following:

- Detection and proper management of preexisting anemia
- Prevention of new-onset (hospital-acquired) anemia (or exacerbation of existing anemia)

As an example, an algorithm for detection, diagnosis, and management of anemia in surgical patients is provided in **Fig. 1**.[14,88] An elective procedure offers a great opportunity for screening for anemia and optimization of hemoglobin level before the surgery as long as anemia is detected early enough; preferably as early as 4 weeks ahead of the scheduled surgery.[88] Whenever possible, an elective procedure should be postponed until anemia is properly diagnosed and treated.[89]

Iron
Intravenous iron and erythropoiesis-stimulating agents (ESAs) are among the key tools available to clinicians for treatment of anemia. Munoz and colleagues[90] studied the short-term use of intravenous iron (iron sucrose, 100–200 mg up to 3 times perioperatively, or ferric carboxymaltose, 600 mg on the first postoperative morning) with or without ESA in the preoperative period among more than 2500 patients undergoing elective lower limb arthroplasty or hip fracture surgery.[90] Use of intravenous iron was associated with reduced allogeneic blood transfusion rate, reduced 30-day mortality, and shorter length of stay.

In a meta-analysis of 72 randomized controlled studies involving more than 10,000 patients comparing intravenous iron with oral iron or no iron for treatment of anemia, intravenous iron was associated with increased hemoglobin level (mean difference of 0.65 g/dL) and reduced risk of transfusion (relative risk [RR], 0.74; 95% CI, 0.62–0.88) but also increased risk of infection (RR, 1.33; 95% CI, 1.10–1.64) compared with oral or no iron.[91] The treatment was more effective when intravenous iron was used in combination with ESAs.[91] The increased risk of infection has been a concern with intravenous iron, although the association is not supported by several other studies.[92,93] Intravenous iron seems to be a safe and effective treatment of anemia in the perioperative setting.

Erythropoiesis-stimulating agents
In a meta-analysis of 26 trials involving 3560 patients, preoperative use of ESAs was associated with reduced transfusion in patients undergoing knee or hip surgery (RR, 0.48; 95% CI, 0.38–0.60). ESA therapy was associated with higher hemoglobin level (mean of 0.72; 95% CI, 0.47–0.96 g/dL) compared with the control group.[94] Thrombotic events are among the most serious complications of ESA therapy, but use of ESAs was not found to be associated with increased risk of thromboembolic events in this meta-analysis.[94]

It has been suggested that this risk is lower in surgical patients, who are typically treated for shorter periods of time with lower doses of ESAs in conjunction with anticoagulants, and do not carry the higher baseline risk for thromboembolic events typically seen in other populations treated with ESAs (eg, patients with chronic renal failure or malignancy).[95]

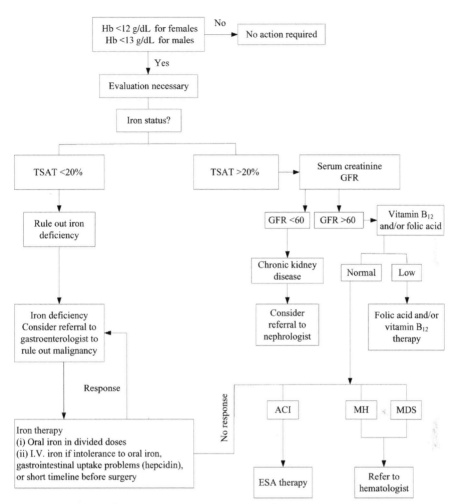

Fig. 1. An algorithm for detection and management of anemia in the perioperative setting. ACI, anemia of inflammation; ESA, erythropoiesis-stimulating agent; GFR, glomerular filtration rate; Hb, hemoglobin concentration; MDS, myelodysplastic syndrome; MH, malignant hematology; TSAT, transferrin saturation. (*Modified from* Shander A, Goodnough LT, Javidroozi M, et al. Iron deficiency anemia–bridging the knowledge and practice gap. Transfus Med Rev 2014;28:160; with permission.)

Hence, short-term treatment with ESAs, combined with intravenous iron during the preoperative period, seems to be safe and effective in treating anemia and reducing transfusions. It is estimated that, for every 3 to 6 patients treated, 1 episode of transfusion is avoided in this setting.[96]

Optimization of hemostasis

Patients going into the operating room (and coming out of it) should have a functioning clotting profile. Steps that clinicians can take include detailed history taking and risk assessment before surgery, adjustment of medications that could negatively affect coagulation, close monitoring of the coagulation system during the surgery, and appropriate use of topical and systemic hemostatic agents as needed.[97]

Antifibrinolytic agents, particularly tranexamic acid (TXA), have been widely studied in this context. A meta-analysis of 46 randomized controlled trials involving almost 3000 patients undergoing major orthopedic surgeries has indicated that TXA can significantly reduce total blood loss (by a mean of 408 mL; 95% CI, 311–506 mL), intraoperative blood loss (by a mean of 126 mL; 95% CI, 69–183 mL), postoperative blood loss (by a mean of 215 mL; 95% CI, 154–275 mL), volume of transfused blood (by 205 mL; 95% CI, 109–301 mL), and transfusion rate (RR, 0.51; 95% CI, 0.46–0.56), without any increase in the risk of thromboembolic events.[98]

Topical use of TXA has also been shown to be effective in reducing surgical bleeding. A meta-analysis of 29 trials on 2612 patients has indicated that topical use of TXA was associated with 29% less blood loss (95% CI, 28%–31%) and 55% lower transfusion rate (95% CI, 46%–55%) compared with no TXA or placebo.[99]

Other topical hemostatics can also help greatly with reducing surgical blood loss. For example, topical fibrin sealant has been shown to significantly reduce blood loss (by an average of 402 mL; 95% CI, 205–599 mL), and transfusion rate (RR, 0.62; 95% CI, 0.45–0.86) compared with control in a meta-analysis of 8 studies involving 558 patients undergoing total knee arthroplasty.[100] Topical use of hemostatic agents has the advantage of limiting the systemic exposure and the related potential adverse events. Tools such as electrocautery and argon beam can also aid effective hemostasis.

Autologous transfusion techniques

Any blood shed during the surgery should be retrieved, washed/filtered, and reinfused to the patient. Blood cell recovery systems are commercially available and they have been previously shown to reduce allogeneic transfusion rate by more than one-third (95% CI, 30%–45%), resulting in an average saving of 0.68 (95% CI, 0.49–0.88) units of red blood cells per patient, without negatively affecting clinical outcomes.[101]

Other autologous transfusion techniques include preoperative autologous donation and acute normovolemic hemodilution, in which a part of the patient's blood is removed and set aside before the surgery to be used in case of significant bleeding. These techniques require more planning and careful selection of the patients because their success depends on occurrence of significant blood loss, otherwise the harvested blood is at risk of being wasted.[102] Given the required logistics, issues of storage, possibility of making matters worse by causing iatrogenic anemia, and availability of other options such as blood cell recovery, preoperative autologous donation is often discouraged.[103]

Supportive care

Anemic patients require closer watch and additional supportive care during the surgery and in the postoperative period. Tachycardia increases the workload of the heart and its oxygen needs and it must be avoided as much as possible. Hypovolemia is often the cause. Hypothermia can negatively affect coagulation and it should be avoided unless clinically indicated for other purposes (eg, cardioplegia). Hyperthermia can also be harmful because the underlying increased metabolism means increased oxygen consumption and demand.[104]

Supplemental oxygen therapy is another effective supportive care for anemic patients undergoing surgery. Anemic patients have limited hemoglobin oxygen carrying capacity, but the amount of oxygen that can be carried dissolved in the plasma can marginally increase oxygen delivery to the tissues. Although too small to be considered under normal conditions, the amount of plasma-dissolved oxygen can increase to clinically significant quantities as the partial pressure of oxygen is increased in the alveoli.[89]

In addition, clinicians should remain vigilant with regard to any uncontrolled bleeding in the postoperative period. Patients should be immediately evaluated for suspected sources of bleeding, and returned to the operating room for exploration of possible causes immediately if needed.[89]

Managing hospital-acquired anemia

The negative contribution of hospital-acquired anemia (HAA) on patient outcomes is becoming increasingly recognized. Anemia can occur (or worsen) following the surgery and during the hospital stay. In a study of more than 188,000 hospital admissions, 74% of the patients developed HAA, and almost one-third of the cases were severe anemia.[105] HAA (even when mild) was associated with increased length of stay and hospital charges, whereas the risk of mortality was increased, particularly in more severe cases.[105] Preexisting anemia can also continue to get worse during the hospital stay, and this exacerbation of anemia is associated with a 2-fold increased risk of death, longer length of stay, and higher costs of hospital stay.[7]

Excessive diagnostic blood draws are among the factors contributing to HAA.[17] It has been estimated that a patient with initial hemoglobin level of 11 g/dL will reach a hemoglobin level of 7 g/dL within 9 to 14 days if subjected to a daily blood loss of about 43 mL as a result of diagnostic phlebotomies.[106] Efforts should be made to limit the volume and frequency of blood draws (and avoid the unnecessary ones) during the perioperative period. Standing orders and tests that are not likely to affect the management of the patients should be avoided.

New Frontiers

PBM is rapidly evolving as the safety and efficacy of existing treatments become better defined and new diagnostic and treatment modalities become available. There seems to be a substantial (but untapped) potential for intravenous iron (particularly the newer formulation) in the prevention and treatment of anemia in surgical patients, and it is hoped that more studies will lay out the groundwork for more routine use of these agents.[14]

Given its central role in regulating iron metabolism, hepcidin has generated substantial interest, both as a diagnostic parameter and as a therapeutic target.[107] The concept of anemia of inflammation is a recurring theme in the literature on anemia, but there is limited practical implication in the clinical arena. The hepcidin-erythroferrone axis is likely to be one of the main missing links between the concept and clinical practice, allowing clinicians to make the diagnosis of anemia of inflammation and provide targeted treatments.

The hemostatic management in surgery is also rapidly evolving. New diagnostic tools such as point-of-care monitoring and more specific tests can provide clinicians with a more accurate assessment of the status of the coagulation system.[108] In conjunction with the availability of more specific treatment options (eg, individual factors and concentrates as opposed to fresh frozen plasma), goal-directed and targeted management of coagulation deficiencies and coagulopathies is becoming a possibility.[109] As previously mentioned, technologies for noninvasive monitoring of hemoglobin and other important parameters are available, and it is expected that their roles as part of clinical management of patients will become better defined.[27]

Another field that once was heralded with much enthusiasm is artificial oxygen carriers and so-called artificial blood. In theory, these products can resolve many of the risks and issues surrounding the use of allogeneic blood. However, despite proof of concept and documented effectiveness as oxygen carriers, mounting safety concerns have prevented the clinical use of these products.[110,111]

SUMMARY

PBM is being recognized as the new standard of care by various entities, including WHO and the Joint Commission, and quality initiatives such as the Choosing Wisely campaign.[112–115] As PBM strategies become more widely adopted, reports of their impact on clinical practices and outcomes are emerging.

Implementing a PBM protocol for all patients undergoing major orthopedic surgery at a single center in France was associated with reduction in the number of severely anemic patients and reduced transfusion rates.[116] Loftus and colleagues[117] recently reported their successful experience with PBM in patients undergoing prosthetic joint arthroplasty, achieving reductions in transfusion rates and improved outcomes (fewer complications and readmissions and shorter hospital stays). Similar results have been observed by Gross and colleagues[118] in patients undergoing cardiac surgery. Also, following the observed failure of introducing transfusion guidelines alone in improving transfusion practices, Mehra and colleagues[119] achieved reduction in transfusions and costs with implementing a PBM program.

As a modifiable risk factor of worse outcomes, anemia in the perioperative setting should no longer be ignored. The first and foremost step is recognizing the problem and its impact. Once anemia is diagnosed, clinicians can use a host of readily available strategies, collectively known as PBM, to effectively manage anemia and only resort to transfusion therapy when appropriate. Other strategies are effective in preventing emergence of anemia and its exacerbation. In particular, HAA requires special attention given its high prevalence and lasting negative impact on the outcomes. In the current health milieu, proper management of anemia and other ailments can no longer be done during the brief time before or during the surgery but must be implemented throughout the course of care in surgical patients, paving the way to improved outcomes, including better quality of life.

REFERENCES

1. de Benoist B, McLean E, Egli I, et al, editors. Worldwide prevalence of anaemia 1993-2005: WHO global database on anaemia. Geneva (Switzerland): World Health Organization; 2008.
2. WHO. The global prevalence of anaemia in 2011. Geneva (Switzerland): World Health Organization; 2015.
3. WHO. Haemoglobin concentrations for the diagnosis of anaemia and assessment of severity. Vitamin and Mineral Nutrition Information System. 2011. Geneva (Switzerland): World Health Organization; 2014.
4. Kassebaum NJ, Jasrasaria R, Naghavi M, et al. A systematic analysis of global anemia burden from 1990 to 2010. Blood 2014;123:615–24.
5. Bateman AP, McArdle F, Walsh TS. Time course of anemia during six months follow up following intensive care discharge and factors associated with impaired recovery of erythropoiesis. Crit Care Med 2009;37:1906–12.
6. Salisbury AC, Kosiborod M, Amin AP, et al. Recovery from hospital-acquired anemia after acute myocardial infarction and effect on outcomes. Am J Cardiol 2011;108:949–54.
7. Koch CG, Li L, Sun Z, et al. From bad to worse: anemia on admission and hospital-acquired anemia. J Patient Saf 2014. [Epub ahead of print].

8. Koch CG, Li L, Sun Z, et al. Magnitude of anemia at discharge increases 30-day hospital readmissions. J Patient Saf 2014. [Epub ahead of print].

9. Nissenson AR, Goodnough LT, Dubois RW. Anemia: not just an innocent bystander? Arch Intern Med 2003;163:1400–4.

10. Joosten E, Lioen P. Iron deficiency anemia and anemia of chronic disease in geriatric hospitalized patients: how frequent are comorbidities as an additional explanation for the anemia? Geriatr Gerontol Int 2015;15:931–5.

11. Przybylowski P, Wasilewski G, Golabek K, et al. Absolute and functional iron deficiency is a common finding in patients with heart failure and after heart transplantation. Transplant Proc 2016;48:173–6.

12. Ganz T, Nemeth E. Hepcidin and iron homeostasis. Biochim Biophys Acta 2012; 1823:1434–43.

13. Kautz L, Jung G, Nemeth E, et al. Erythroferrone contributes to recovery from anemia of inflammation. Blood 2014;124:2569–74.

14. Shander A, Goodnough LT, Javidroozi M, et al. Iron deficiency anemia–bridging the knowledge and practice gap. Transfus Med Rev 2014;28:156–66.

15. Shander A, Javidroozi M, Ozawa S, et al. What is really dangerous: anaemia or transfusion? Br J Anaesth 2011;107(Suppl 1):i41–59.

16. von Haehling S, Anker SD. Cardio-renal anemia syndrome. Contrib Nephrol 2011;171:266–73.

17. Salisbury AC, Reid KJ, Alexander KP, et al. Diagnostic blood loss from phlebotomy and hospital-acquired anemia during acute myocardial infarction. Arch Intern Med 2011;171:1646–53.

18. Dahlerup JF, Eivindson M, Jacobsen BA, et al. Diagnosis and treatment of unexplained anemia with iron deficiency without overt bleeding. Dan Med J 2015;62: C5072.

19. Beutler E, Waalen J. The definition of anemia: what is the lower limit of normal of the blood hemoglobin concentration? Blood 2006;107:1747–50.

20. Munoz M, Gomez-Ramirez S, Kozek-Langeneker S, et al. 'Fit to fly': overcoming barriers to preoperative haemoglobin optimization in surgical patients. Br J Anaesth 2015;115:15–24.

21. Gombotz H, Rehak PH, Shander A, et al. Blood use in elective surgery: the Austrian benchmark study. Transfusion 2007;47:1468–80.

22. Gombotz H, Rehak PH, Shander A, et al. The second Austrian benchmark study for blood use in elective surgery: results and practice change. Transfusion 2014; 54(10 Pt 2):2646–57.

23. Rosencher N, Kerkkamp HE, Macheras G, et al. Orthopedic Surgery Transfusion Hemoglobin European Overview (OSTHEO) study: blood management in elective knee and hip arthroplasty in Europe. Transfusion 2003;43:459–69.

24. Giraud B, Frasca D, Debaene B, et al. Comparison of haemoglobin measurement methods in the operating theatre. Br J Anaesth 2013;111:946–54.

25. Jacob M, Annaheim S, Boutellier U, et al. Haematocrit is invalid for estimating red cell volume: a prospective study in male volunteers. Blood Transfus 2012; 10:471–9.

26. Suehiro K, Joosten A, Alexander B, et al. Continuous noninvasive hemoglobin monitoring: ready for prime time? Curr Opin Crit Care 2015;21:265–70.

27. Barker SJ, Shander A, Ramsay MA. Continuous noninvasive hemoglobin monitoring: a measured response to a critical review. Anesth Analg 2016;122: 565–72.

28. Lasocki S, Krauspe R, von HC, et al. PREPARE: the prevalence of perioperative anaemia and need for patient blood management in elective orthopaedic surgery: a multicentre, observational study. Eur J Anaesthesiol 2015;32:160–7.

29. Viola J, Gomez MM, Restrepo C, et al. Preoperative anemia increases postoperative complications and mortality following total joint arthroplasty. J Arthroplasty 2015;30:846–8.

30. Menendez ME, Memtsoudis SG, Opperer M, et al. A nationwide analysis of risk factors for in-hospital myocardial infarction after total joint arthroplasty. Int Orthop 2015;39:777–86.

31. Uchida Y, Ichimiya S, Ishii H, et al. Impact of admission anemia on coronary microcirculation and clinical outcomes in patients with ST-segment elevation myocardial infarction undergoing primary percutaneous coronary intervention. Int Heart J 2015;56:381–8.

32. Landes U, Kornowski R, Assali A, et al. Predictors of long term outcomes in 11,441 consecutive patients following percutaneous coronary interventions. Am J Cardiol 2015;115:855–9.

33. Zhang E, Li Z, Che J, et al. Anemia and inflammation in ST-segment elevation myocardial infarction. Am J Med Sci 2015;349:493–8.

34. DeLarochellière H, Urena M, Amat-Santos IJ, et al. Effect on outcomes and exercise performance of anemia in patients with aortic stenosis who underwent transcatheter aortic valve replacement. Am J Cardiol 2015;115:472–9.

35. Shacham Y, Gal-Oz A, Leshem-Rubinow E, et al. Association of admission hemoglobin levels and acute kidney injury among myocardial infarction patients treated with primary percutaneous intervention. Can J Cardiol 2015;31:50–5.

36. Spiegelstein D, Holmes SD, Pritchard G, et al. Preoperative hematocrit as a predictor of perioperative morbidities following nonemergent coronary artery bypass surgery. J Cardiovasc Surg 2015;30:20–6.

37. Seicean A, Seicean S, Alan N, et al. Preoperative anemia and perioperative outcomes in patients who undergo elective spine surgery. Spine (Phila Pa 1976) 2013;38:1331–41.

38. Gierth M, Mayr R, Aziz A, et al. Preoperative anemia is associated with adverse outcome in patients with urothelial carcinoma of the bladder following radical cystectomy. J Cancer Res Clin Oncol 2015;141:1819–26.

39. Fowler AJ, Ahmad T, Phull MK, et al. Meta-analysis of the association between preoperative anaemia and mortality after surgery. Br J Surg 2015;102:1314–24.

40. Scrascia G, Guida P, Caparrotti SM, et al. Incremental value of anemia in cardiac surgical risk prediction with the European System for Cardiac Operative Risk Evaluation (EuroSCORE) II model. Ann Thorac Surg 2014;98:869–75.

41. Otto JM, Montgomery HE, Richards T. Haemoglobin concentration and mass as determinants of exercise performance and of surgical outcome. Extrem Physiol Med 2013;2:33.

42. McLellan SA, Walsh TS. Oxygen delivery and haemoglobin. Contin Educ Anaesth Crit Care Pain 2004;4:123–6.

43. Chapler CK, Cain SM. The physiologic reserve in oxygen carrying capacity: studies in experimental hemodilution. Can J Physiol Pharmacol 1986;64:7–12.

44. Greer SN, Metcalf JL, Wang Y, et al. The updated biology of hypoxia-inducible factor. EMBO J 2012;31:2448–60.

45. Johannes T, Mik EG, Nohe B, et al. Acute decrease in renal microvascular P_{O_2} during acute normovolemic hemodilution. Am J Physiol Renal Physiol 2007;292: F796–803.

46. Deem S, Hedges RG, McKinney S, et al. Mechanisms of improvement in pulmonary gas exchange during isovolemic hemodilution. J Appl Physiol (1985) 1999; 87:132–41.
47. Halperin ML, Cheema-Dhadli S, Lin SH, et al. Properties permitting the renal cortex to be the oxygen sensor for the release of erythropoietin: clinical implications. Clin J Am Soc Nephrol 2006;1:1049–53.
48. Milsom WK, Burleson ML. Peripheral arterial chemoreceptors and the evolution of the carotid body. Respir Physiolo Neurobiol 2007;157:4–11.
49. Evans RG, Ince C, Joles JA, et al. Haemodynamic influences on kidney oxygenation: clinical implications of integrative physiology. Clin Exp Pharmacol Physiol 2013;40:106–22.
50. Metivier F, Marchais SJ, Guerin AP, et al. Pathophysiology of anaemia: focus on the heart and blood vessels. Nephrol Dial Transplant 2000;15(Suppl 3):14–8.
51. Li M, Bertout JA, Ratcliffe SJ, et al. Acute anemia elicits cognitive dysfunction and evidence of cerebral cellular hypoxia in older rats with systemic hypertension. Anesthesiology 2010;113:845–58.
52. McLaren AT, Mazer CD, Zhang H, et al. A potential role for inducible nitric oxide synthase in the cerebral response to acute hemodilution. Can J Anaesth 2009; 56:502–9.
53. El Hasnaoui-Saadani R, Pichon A, Marchant D, et al. Cerebral adaptations to chronic anemia in a model of erythropoietin-deficient mice exposed to hypoxia. Am J Physiol Regul Integr Comp Physiol 2009;296:R801–11.
54. Madjdpour C, Spahn DR, Weiskopf RB. Anemia and perioperative red blood cell transfusion: a matter of tolerance. Crit Care Med 2006;34:S102–8.
55. Shander A, Javidroozi M, Naqvi S, et al. An update on mortality and morbidity in patients with very low postoperative hemoglobin levels who decline blood transfusion (CME). Transfusion 2014;54:2688–95.
56. Aleksova A, Barbati G, Merlo M, et al. Deleterious impact of mild anemia on survival of young adult patients (age 45 ± 14 years) with idiopathic dilated cardiomyopathy: data from the Trieste Cardiomyopathies Registry. Heart Lung 2011; 40:454–61.
57. Lucca U, Tettamanti M, Mosconi P, et al. Association of mild anemia with cognitive, functional, mood and quality of life outcomes in the elderly: the "Health and Anemia" study. PLoS One 2008;3:e1920.
58. Riva E, Tettamanti M, Mosconi P, et al. Association of mild anemia with hospitalization and mortality in the elderly: the Health and Anemia population-based study. Haematologica 2009;94:22–8.
59. Klip IT, Comin-Colet J, Voors AA, et al. Iron deficiency in chronic heart failure: an international pooled analysis. Am Heart J 2013;165:575–82.
60. Pratt JJ, Khan KS. Non-anaemic iron deficiency - a disease looking for recognition of diagnosis: a systematic review. Eur J Haematol 2016;96(6):618–28.
61. Cabrales P, Martini J, Intaglietta M, et al. Blood viscosity maintains microvascular conditions during normovolemic anemia independent of blood oxygen-carrying capacity. Am J Physiol Heart Circ Physiol 2006;291:H581–90.
62. Lu KJ, Kearney LG, Hare DL, et al. Cardiorenal anemia syndrome as a prognosticator for death in heart failure. Am J Cardiol 2013;111:1187–91.
63. Marik PE. The hazards of blood transfusion. Br J Hosp Med (Lond) 2009;70: 12–5.
64. Shander A. Emerging risks and outcomes of blood transfusion in surgery. Semin Hematol 2004;41:117–24.

65. Lauscher P, Kertscho H, Schmidt O, et al. Determination of organ-specific anemia tolerance. Crit Care Med 2013;41:1037–45.

66. Duncker DJ, Bache RJ. Regulation of coronary blood flow during exercise. Physiol Rev 2008;88:1009–86.

67. Choi YJ, Kim SO, Sim JH, et al. Postoperative anemia is associated with acute kidney injury in patients undergoing total hip replacement arthroplasty: a retrospective study. Anesth Analg 2016;122(6):1923–8.

68. Pfuntner A, Wier LM, Stocks C. Most frequent procedures performed in U.S. Hospitals, 2011. Rockville (MD): Agency for Healthcare Research and Quality. Healthcare Cost and Utilization Project (HCUP); 2013.

69. Shander A, Fink A, Javidroozi M, et al. Appropriateness of allogeneic red blood cell transfusion: the international consensus conference on transfusion outcomes. Transfus Med Rev 2011;25:232–46.

70. Greinacher A, Fendrich K, Brzenska R, et al. Implications of demographics on future blood supply: a population-based cross-sectional study. Transfusion 2011;51:702–9.

71. McQuilten ZK, Mercer G, Phillips L, et al. A dynamic mathematical model of red blood cell clinical demand to assess the impact of prolonged blood shortages and transfusion restriction policies. Transfusion 2014;54:2705–15.

72. Shander A, Hofmann A, Ozawa S, et al. Activity-based costs of blood transfusions in surgical patients at four hospitals. Transfusion 2010;50:753–65.

73. Middelburg RA, van de Watering LM, Briet E, et al. Storage time of red blood cells and mortality of transfusion recipients. Transfus Med Rev 2013;27:36–43.

74. Brunskill SJ, Millette SL, Shokoohi A, et al. Red blood cell transfusion for people undergoing hip fracture surgery. Cochrane Database Syst Rev 2015;(4):CD009699.

75. Carson JL, Sieber F, Cook DR, et al. Liberal versus restrictive blood transfusion strategy: 3-year survival and cause of death results from the FOCUS randomised controlled trial. Lancet 2015;385:1183–9.

76. Murphy GJ, Pike K, Rogers CA, et al. Liberal or restrictive transfusion after cardiac surgery. N Engl J Med 2015;372:997–1008.

77. Shander A, Gross I, Hill S, et al. A new perspective on best transfusion practices. Blood Transfus 2013;11:193–202.

78. American Society of Anesthesiologists Task Force on Perioperative Blood Transfusion and Adjuvant Therapies. Practice guidelines for perioperative blood transfusion and adjuvant therapies: an updated report by the American Society of Anesthesiologists Task Force on Perioperative Blood Transfusion and Adjuvant Therapies. Anesthesiology 2006;105:198–208.

79. Ferraris VA, Ferraris SP, Saha SP, et al. Perioperative blood transfusion and blood conservation in cardiac surgery: the Society of Thoracic Surgeons and The Society of Cardiovascular Anesthesiologists clinical practice guideline. Ann Thorac Surg 2007;83:S27–86.

80. Liumbruno GM, Bennardello F, Lattanzio A, et al. Recommendations for the transfusion management of patients in the peri-operative period. I. The pre-operative period. Blood Transfus 2011;9:19–40.

81. Liumbruno GM, Bennardello F, Lattanzio A, et al. Recommendations for the transfusion management of patients in the peri-operative period. II. The intra-operative period. Blood Transfus 2011;9:189–217.

82. Liumbruno GM, Bennardello F, Lattanzio A, et al. Recommendations for the transfusion management of patients in the peri-operative period. III. The post-operative period. Blood Transfus 2011;9:320–35.

83. Carson JL, Grossman BJ, Kleinman S, et al. Red blood cell transfusion: a clinical practice guideline from the AABB*. Ann Intern Med 2012;157:49–58.
84. What is patient blood management? From the Society for the Advancement of Blood Management (SABM). Available at: http://www.sabm.org/. Accessed July 21, 2016.
85. Shander A, Javidroozi M, Perelman S, et al. From bloodless surgery to patient blood management. Mt Sinai J Med 2012;79:56–65.
86. Shander A, Hofmann A, Isbister J, et al. Patient blood management–the new frontier. Best Pract Res Clin Anaesthesiol 2013;27:5–10.
87. Shander A, Isbister J, Gombotz H. Patient blood management: the global view. Transfusion 2016;56(Suppl 1):S94–102.
88. Goodnough LT, Maniatis A, Earnshaw P, et al. Detection, evaluation, and management of preoperative anaemia in the elective orthopaedic surgical patient: NATA guidelines. Br J Anaesth 2011;106:13–22.
89. Shander A. Preoperative anemia and its management. Transfus Apher Sci 2014; 50:13–5.
90. Munoz M, Gomez-Ramirez S, Cuenca J, et al. Very-short-term perioperative intravenous iron administration and postoperative outcome in major orthopedic surgery: a pooled analysis of observational data from 2547 patients. Transfusion 2014;54:289–99.
91. Litton E, Xiao J, Ho KM. Safety and efficacy of intravenous iron therapy in reducing requirement for allogeneic blood transfusion: systematic review and meta-analysis of randomised clinical trials. BMJ 2013;347:f4822.
92. Susantitaphong P, Alqahtani F, Jaber BL. Efficacy and safety of intravenous iron therapy for functional iron deficiency anemia in hemodialysis patients: a meta-analysis. Am J Nephrol 2014;39:130–41.
93. Auerbach M, Adamson J, Bircher A, et al. On the safety of intravenous iron, evidence trumps conjecture. Haematologica 2015;100:e214–5.
94. Alsaleh K, Alotaibi GS, Almodaimegh HS, et al. The use of preoperative erythropoiesis-stimulating agents (ESAs) in patients who underwent knee or hip arthroplasty: a meta-analysis of randomized clinical trials. J Arthroplasty 2013;28:1463–72.
95. Tran DH, Wong GT, Chee YE, et al. Effectiveness and safety of erythropoiesis-stimulating agent use in the perioperative period. Expert Opin Biol Ther 2014; 14:51–61.
96. Lin DM, Lin ES, Tran MH. Efficacy and safety of erythropoietin and intravenous iron in perioperative blood management: a systematic review. Transfus Med Rev 2013;27:221–34.
97. Kozek-Langenecker SA. Coagulation and transfusion in the postoperative bleeding patient. Curr Opin Crit Care 2014;20:460–6.
98. Huang F, Wu D, Ma G, et al. The use of tranexamic acid to reduce blood loss and transfusion in major orthopedic surgery: a meta-analysis. J Surg Res 2014;186:318–27.
99. Ker K, Beecher D, Roberts I. Topical application of tranexamic acid for the reduction of bleeding. Cochrane Database Syst Rev 2013;(7):CD010562.
100. Liu J, Cao JG, Wang L, et al. Effect of fibrin sealant on blood loss following total knee arthroplasty: a systematic review and meta-analysis. Int J Surg 2014;12: 95–102.
101. Carless PA, Henry DA, Moxey AJ, et al. Cell salvage for minimising perioperative allogeneic blood transfusion. Cochrane Database Syst Rev 2010;(4):CD001888.

102. Frankel TL, Fischer M, Grant F, et al. Selecting patients for acute normovolemic hemodilution during hepatic resection: a prospective randomized evaluation of nomogram-based allocation. J Am Coll Surg 2013;217:210–20.
103. Shander A, Javidroozi M. Blood conservation strategies and the management of perioperative anaemia. Curr Opin Anaesthesiol 2015;28:356–63.
104. Shander A, Javidroozi M. Strategies to reduce the use of blood products: a US perspective. Curr Opin Anaesthesiol 2012;25:50–8.
105. Koch CG, Li L, Sun Z, et al. Hospital-acquired anemia: Prevalence, outcomes, and healthcare implications. J Hosp Med 2013;8:506–12.
106. Lyon AW, Chin AC, Slotsve GA, et al. Simulation of repetitive diagnostic blood loss and onset of iatrogenic anemia in critical care patients with a mathematical model. Comput Biol Med 2013;43:84–90.
107. Weiss G. Anemia of chronic disorders: new diagnostic tools and new treatment strategies. Semin Hematol 2015;52:313–20.
108. Johansson PI, Solbeck S, Genet G, et al. Coagulopathy and hemostatic monitoring in cardiac surgery: an update. Scand Cardiovasc J 2012;46:194–202.
109. Spahn DR. From plasma transfusion to individualized, goal-directed coagulation factor administration. J Cardiothorac Vasc Anesth 2013;27:S16–9.
110. Natanson C, Kern SJ, Lurie P, et al. Cell-free hemoglobin-based blood substitutes and risk of myocardial infarction and death: a meta-analysis. JAMA 2008;299:2304–12.
111. Baumler H, Xiong Y, Liu ZZ, et al. Novel hemoglobin particles–promising new-generation hemoglobin-based oxygen carriers. Artif Organs 2014;38:708–14.
112. WHA63.12-Availability, safety and quality of blood products. WHA resolution; Sixty-third World Health Assembly. Geneva (Switzerland): World Health Organization; 2010.
113. Implementation guide for The Joint Commission patient blood management performance measures. Chicago (IL): The Joint Commission; 2011.
114. Global Forum for Blood Safety: patient blood management - concept paper. Geneva (Switzerland): World Health Organization; 2011.
115. Murphy MF. The Choosing Wisely campaign to reduce harmful medical overuse: its close association with patient blood management initiatives. Transfus Med 2015;25:287–92.
116. Rineau E, Chaudet A, Chassier C, et al. Implementing a blood management protocol during the entire perioperative period allows a reduction in transfusion rate in major orthopedic surgery: a before-after study. Transfusion 2016;56:673–81.
117. Loftus TJ, Spratling L, Stone BA, et al. A patient blood management program in prosthetic joint arthroplasty decreases blood use and improves outcomes. J Arthroplasty 2016;31:11–4.
118. Gross I, Seifert B, Hofmann A, et al. Patient blood management in cardiac surgery results in fewer transfusions and better outcome. Transfusion 2015;55(5): 1075–81.
119. Mehra T, Seifert B, Bravo-Reiter S, et al. Implementation of a patient blood management monitoring and feedback program significantly reduces transfusions and costs. Transfusion 2015;55:2807–15.

Anesthesia Patients with Concomitant Cardiac and Hepatic Dysfunction

 CrossMark

Julianne Ahdout, MD[a],*, Michael Nurok, MBChB, PhD[b]

KEYWORDS

- Anesthesia • Liver dysfunction • Cardiac dysfunction • Perioperative management

KEY POINTS

- Patients with concomitant cardiac and hepatic dysfunction pose additional challenges and carry increased perioperative risk.
- Cirrhosis is associated with a wide range of cardiovascular abnormalities, including hyperdynamic circulation, cirrhotic cardiomyopathy, and pulmonary vascular abnormalities.
- Cirrhotic cardiomyopathy is characterized by increased cardiac output and compromised ventricular response to stress.
- Coronary artery disease has a significant unfavorable impact on mortality and morbidity in cirrhotic patients, especially following major surgery such as liver transplant.
- Cardiac studies done preoperatively should include electrocardiography and also echocardiography if risk factors for left ventricular dysfunction, cardiomyopathy, valvular lesions, or pulmonary vascular disorder are present.

INTRODUCTION

Hepatocardiac diseases can be categorized into heart diseases affecting the liver, liver diseases affecting the heart, and conditions affecting the heart and the liver at the same time. An estimated 1 in 700 patients scheduled to undergo elective surgery has abnormal liver enzyme levels. In addition, some investigators have estimated that as many as 10% of patients with advanced liver disease undergo surgery in the last 2 years of their lives.[1] Patients with hepatic dysfunction carry a particularly high risk for morbidity and mortality in the perioperative period caused by both the stress of surgery and the effects of general anesthesia.[2] Cardiac dysfunction increases the risks of

Disclosure: The authors have nothing to disclose.
[a] Department of Anesthesiology, Cedars-Sinai Medical Center, 8700 Beverly Boulevard, North Tower, Room 4209, Los Angeles, CA 90048, USA; [b] Cardiac Surgery Intensive Care Unit, Cedars-Sinai Medical Center, 127 South San Vicente Boulevard, Suite A3106, Los Angeles, CA 90048, USA
* Corresponding author.
E-mail address: Julianne.ahdout@cshs.org

Anesthesiology Clin 34 (2016) 731–745
http://dx.doi.org/10.1016/j.anclin.2016.06.008

anesthesia and surgery for patients who experience it. Namely, patients with coronary artery disease are at higher than average risk of perioperative cardiac complications.[3] Thus, patients with concomitant cardiac and hepatic dysfunction pose additional challenges and carry more risks perioperatively. Identifying and assessing surgical risk in any patient is a crucial task for anesthesiologists, but especially for patients with a growing list of chronic comorbidities. It is important for anesthesiologists to understand not only hepatic dysfunction and cardiac dysfunction independently but also the complex interaction between coexisting cardiac and hepatic dysfunction and the unique challenges that entails.

PATHOGENESIS AND PHYSIOLOGY

Clinically, anesthesiologists divide patients with liver disease into 2 major groups:

1. Patients with parenchymal liver disease (eg, acute and chronic viral hepatitis, liver cirrhosis)
2. Patients with cholestasis

Liver Cirrhosis and the Cardiovascular System

Cirrhosis is associated with a wide range of cardiovascular abnormalities, including hyperdynamic circulation, cirrhotic cardiomyopathy, and pulmonary vascular abnormalities. The pathogenic mechanisms of these cardiovascular changes are multifactorial and include neurohumoral and vascular dysregulations. Accumulating evidence suggests that cirrhosis-related cardiovascular abnormalities play a major role in the pathogenesis of multiple life-threatening complications, including hepatorenal syndrome, ascites, spontaneous bacterial peritonitis, gastroesophageal varices, and hepatopulmonary syndrome.[4]

Patients with cirrhosis from any cause have an enhanced activity of the sympathetic nervous system and hyperdynamic circulation showing increased cardiac output and reduced systemic vascular resistance (**Fig. 1**). These changes may induce myocardial remodeling and left ventricular hypertrophy, resulting in systolic and diastolic functional abnormalities and cardiomyopathy.[5]

Hyperdynamic State

Parenchymal liver disease is associated with a hyperdynamic circulatory state manifested by:

1. Increased heart rate
2. Increased cardiac output and circulatory blood volume
3. Reduction in systemic vascular resistance and arterial blood pressure
4. Peripheral vasodilatation
5. Increased arteriovenous shunting[6]

The hyperdynamic circulation is a result of decreased systemic vascular resistance (SVR) and a compensatory increased cardiac output to maintain tissue perfusion. The clinical manifestations of hyperdynamic circulation include warm skin, spider angiomata, palmar erythema, and a bounding pulse.

The hyperdynamic circulation is thought to be caused by peripheral and splanchnic vasodilatation, which is secondary to increased production and activity of vasodilatory factors as well as decreased vascular reactivity to vasoconstrictors. This condition leads to reduction in the effective arterial blood volume,[5] which leads to a diminished renal blood flow in cirrhotic patients. This diminished flow in turn stimulates the

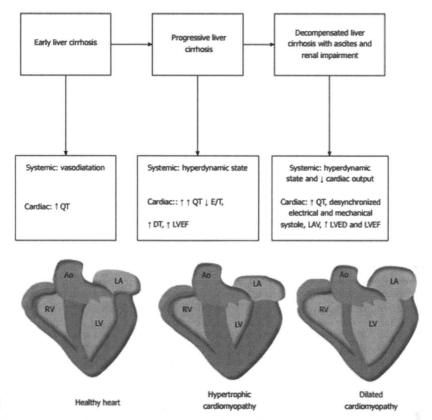

Fig. 1. Proposal of changes in cardiac output during the course of liver disease. Ao, aorta; DT, deceleration time; LA, left atrium; LAV, left atrial volume; LV, left ventricle; LVED, left ventricular end-diastolic volume; LVEF, left ventricular ejection fraction; RV, right ventricle. (*From* Fouad YM, Yehia R. Hepato-cardiac disorders. World J Hepatol 2014;6(1):44; with permission.)

renin-angiotensin-aldosterone system, the sympathetic nervous system, and release of antidiuretic hormone, resulting in renal artery vasoconstriction, sodium retention, and volume expansion.[7] Worsening liver disease results in progressive vasodilatation, making the hyperdynamic circulation and renal artery vasoconstriction more pronounced.[8,9]

Cirrhotic Cardiomyopathy

Chronic liver diseases may affect cardiac functions in the absence of other heart disease. Cirrhotic cardiomyopathy is a form of chronic cardiac dysfunction in patients with cirrhosis, characterized by blunted contractile responsiveness or systolic incompetence especially under conditions of stress, and/or diastolic dysfunction related to altered diastolic relaxation with electrophysiologic abnormalities in the absence of other known cardiac disease. The underlying mechanisms include downregulation of the beta-adrenergic receptors, increased circulating inflammatory mediators causing cardiac depression, increased myocardial fibrosis, and repolarization abnormalities.

Typical cirrhotic patients may undergo the following hemodynamic and pathologic changes: increased cardiac output, increased heart rate, reduced SVR, increased circulating volume, coronary artery disease, and cirrhotic cardiomyopathy. Although there is no single diagnostic test that can identify patients with cirrhotic cardiomyopathy, a combination of electrocardiogram (ECG), two-dimensional echocardiography, and various serum markers can be used to make the diagnosis.

Systolic dysfunction is the inability of the heart to meet its demand and generate sufficient arterial blood pressure and cardiac output. Systolic dysfunction can be unmasked in cirrhotic patients in conditions of stress, whether physical or pharmacologic, such as physical exercise and general anesthesia, or with vasoconstricting agents, because they increase SVR and increase afterload. As proposed by the 2005 World Congress of Gastroenterology, the diagnostic criteria for the systolic dysfunction component of cirrhotic cardiomyopathy includes a resting ejection fraction less than 55% and a blunted increase in cardiac output with exercise, volume challenge, or pharmacologic stimuli. The increased levels of nitric oxide and carbon monoxide produced in cirrhotic patients can exert a negative inotropic effect on the myocardium. Diastolic dysfunction has been found in 45% to 56% of cirrhotic patients.[5] Diastolic dysfunction in cirrhotic patients is attributable to increased stiffness of the myocardial wall caused by myocardial hypertrophy, fibrosis, and subendothelial edema. Hepatitis infection induces proliferative stimuli that may cause myocyte hypertrophy, because myocytes do not replicate but hypertrophy. Diastolic dysfunction is most likely to be problematic in situations in which the patient is volume overloaded and the stiff, hypertrophic left ventricle cannot accommodate the excess volume. The diagnostic criteria for the diastolic dysfunction component of cirrhotic cardiomyopathy includes echocardiographic findings of an E/A (ratio of the early [E] to late [A] ventricular filling velocities) ratio less than 1.0 (age corrected), prolonged deceleration time (>200 milliseconds), and a prolonged isovolumetric relaxation time (>80 milliseconds). In addition to the diagnostic criteria mentioned earlier, there are supportive criteria for cirrhotic cardiomyopathy. These criteria include electrophysiologic abnormalities, abnormal chronotropic response, electromechanical uncoupling/dyssynchrony, prolonged QTc interval, an enlarged left atrium, increased myocardial mass, increased brain natriuretic peptide (BNP) and pro-brain natriuretic peptide (pro-BNP) levels, and increased troponin level. Henricksen and colleagues found that both pro-BNP and BNP are positively correlated with not only the severity of cirrhosis but also the degree of cardiac dysfunction.[10] Furthermore, the more increased the BNP level, the more severe the interventricular septal wall thickness and left ventricular wall thickness.[5,11]

Electrophysiologic Abnormalities

The electrophysiologic abnormalities found in cirrhotic patients include QT interval prolongation, electrical and mechanical dyssynchrony, and chronotropic incompetence.[12–14] The prevalence of QT prolongation is as high as 60% in patients with advanced liver disease compared with the 5% prevalence in the general population, irrespective of the cause of the disease.[5] The presence of a prolonged QT interval predisposes patients to ventricular arrhythmias and cause sudden deaths in cirrhotic patients undergoing stressful procedures. Although the cause of the prolonged QT interval is unclear, various toxins that are at increased levels in cirrhosis can potentially exacerbate ion channel defects, thereby prolonging the QT interval. It has been found that the more prolonged the QT interval is, the more severe the disease is.[12] A study on cirrhotic patients revealed that those patients with a corrected QT (QTc) interval longer than 440 milliseconds had a significantly lower survival rate than those with normal QTc.[12]

Chronotropic incompetence is the failure of the heart rate to respond to physiologic and pharmacologic stimuli. Thus, factors that activate the sympathetic system, such as the Valsalva maneuver or physical exercise, do not produce an adequate increase in heart rate despite the presence of increased plasma norepinephrine levels. This defect is proportional to the severity of cirrhosis.[15] In addition, there can be a defect in electromechanical coupling in cirrhotic patients, such that there is asynchrony between electrical and mechanical systoles.

Coronary Artery Disease

Although it is established that the heart and liver interact and affect each other, the causality between liver cirrhosis and coronary artery disease (CAD) is uncertain. Recent literature estimates that the prevalence of CAD among cirrhotic patients ranges from 2.5% to 27.0%. There is controversy as to whether cirrhotic conditions accelerate or protect against CAD. The original belief was that liver disease carries a potential protective role against CAD. This belief has been supported by the potential protective role of coagulation abnormalities and thrombocytopenia, low serum cholesterol level, and low arterial blood pressure that are commonly seen in patients with liver cirrhosis.[16]

In contrast, other studies have suggested that liver cirrhosis does not serve a protective role against CAD and may even accelerate CAD. A 2014 study by An and colleagues[17] revealed that the prevalence of obstructive CAD was the same (approximately 8%) in both cirrhotic patients and their noncirrhotic counterparts, although cirrhotic patients were at higher risk of nonobstructive CAD, which has a more benign course. This study concluded that obstructive or nonobstructive CAD was not linked to liver function or coagulopathic status, but to theoretic cardiovascular risk factors such as older age, hypertension, diabetes, and alcohol-related cirrhosis. A 2010 study by Kalaitzakis and colleagues[16] concluded that patients with liver cirrhosis were not protected from CAD, and determined an association between alcoholic liver cirrhosis and older age and the occurrence of CAD. Patients with liver cirrhosis who had CAD were more likely to have cirrhosis secondary to alcohol than to cholestasis or hepatitis C. Alcohol cirrhosis was a significant CAD risk factor in cirrhotic patients, whereas hepatitis virus–related disease was not.[16]

The study by An and colleagues[17] revealed that all study subjects with liver cirrhosis had more extensive involvement of the coronary vessels compared with those without liver cirrhosis. Cirrhotic conditions may promote CAD because of the increased prevalence of moderate to severe coronary stenotic disorders found in up to 27% of patients with liver cirrhosis. This finding could be explained by (1) the growing incidence of liver cirrhosis secondary to nonalcoholic fatty liver disease in which patients frequently have metabolic syndrome and thereby increased risk of ischemic heart disease, and (2) patients with liver cirrhosis now living longer with the advancement of medicine.[17]

CAD has a significant unfavorable impact on mortality and morbidity in cirrhotic patients, especially following major surgery, such as liver transplant. Cardiovascular complications have been found to be the leading cause of non–graft-related posttransplant death. Furthermore, it is crucial to conduct a thorough assessment of cardiovascular risk and to prevent CAD and associated death in cirrhotic patients, especially preoperatively.[16,17] In summary, a thorough work-up of cirrhotic patients before surgery should be strongly considered.

Portopulmonary Hypertension

End-stage liver disease has a causal role in 2 main pulmonary syndromes: hepatopulmonary syndrome and portopulmonary hypertension (POPH). Hepatopulmonary syndrome is characterized by abnormal intrapulmonary vascular dilatation in patients with liver disease, leading to physiologic shunting, ventilation-perfusion mismatch, and hypoxemia.[18]

Chronic liver disease may be associated with remodeling of the pulmonary vasculature, which involves the following:

1. Vascular smooth muscle proliferation
2. Vasoconstriction
3. Intimal proliferation
4. Eventual fibrosis

This condition can result in pulmonary hypertension, which, when linked with portal hypertension, is termed POPH. Although the pathophysiology of POPH remains unclear, autoimmune disease and female gender have been deemed important risk factors.[19] POPH has been observed in patients with and without cirrhosis and is not related to the cause of the liver disease or the severity of the portal hypertension.[20]

Diagnostic criteria for POPH:

- Mean pulmonary artery pressure (mPAP) >25 mm Hg at rest
- Pulmonary vascular resistance (PVR) >240 dyn s.cm^{-5}

Clinical features of POPH:

- Right ventricular overload
- Right heart failure
- Hepatic congestion

POPH may be classified as mild (mPAP, 25–35 mm Hg), moderate (mPAP >35 and <45 mm Hg), and severe (mPAP >45 mm Hg). Although mild POPH is not associated with increased mortality at liver transplant, moderate and severe POPH are associated with significant mortality. Patients with moderate and severe pulmonary hypertension have a reduced 3-year survival after liver transplant compared with patients presenting with normal or mild pulmonary hypertension.[21] Therefore, it is important to address pulmonary hypertension before patients undergo liver transplant.

Right ventricular function is thought to be more important in perioperative mortality than the mPAP.[22] The clinical features of POPH affecting the heart include right ventricular overload and right heart failure. POPH burdens a right ventricle already exposed to physiologic stress during liver transplant. The success of a liver transplant depends on the right ventricle maintaining good function during and after the transplant despite the many dynamic changes involving cardiac output, volume, and PVR. Right ventricular dysfunction can threaten the viability of a graft. Thus, using transesophageal echocardiography (TEE) to assess the status of the right ventricle is advisable.[22]

ANESTHETIC IMPLICATIONS/MANAGEMENT
Preoperative Considerations and Testing

Preoperative evaluation of patients with liver disease should focus on the extent of liver dysfunction and effects on other organ systems. Being clinically latent, cirrhotic cardiomyopathy can be unmasked by physical or pharmacologic strain. Consequently, caution should be exercised in stressful procedures, such as large-volume paracentesis without adequate plasma volume expansion, transjugular intrahepatic portosystemic shunt insertion, peritoneovenous shunting, and surgery.[6] No specific treatment can be recommended for patients with cirrhotic cardiomyopathy. Heart failure should be treated as in noncirrhotic patients with sodium restriction, diuretics, and oxygen therapy when necessary.[23] Appropriate recommendations for preoperative angiotensin-converting enzyme (ACE) inhibitors and angiotensin antagonists in these patients is of increasing interest because of the risk of postinduction hypotension. A study by Comfere and colleagues[24] of 267 hypertensive patients undergoing surgery found that taking either an ACE inhibitor or angiotensin receptor blocker within 10 hours of surgery, compared with holding medication for at least 10 hours, increased the odds of moderate postinduction hypotension.

Cardiac studies done preoperatively should include ECG and also echocardiography if risk factors for left ventricular dysfunction, cardiomyopathy, valvular lesions, or pulmonary vascular disorder are present. If significant CAD is suspected, an exercise ECG, dynamic assessment of left ventricular function, or both may be helpful. Chest radiograph or ultrasonography may be useful for showing pleural effusions in need of drainage before operation. Lung function tests can be helpful to delineate any restrictive or obstructive pulmonary disease.[25]

Patient operative risk is dictated by severity of liver disease, coexisting medical diseases, and type of surgery (ie, upper abdominal, emergent, cardiac, and so forth). A preoperative transthoracic echocardiogram (TTE) should be performed routinely for the assessment of left ventricular, right ventricular, and valvular function. Volume status and symptoms of heart failure should be monitored and optimized before any surgery.[26] The literature suggests that carvedilol is the optimal choice for beta-blockade in patients with end-stage liver disease (ESLD), because it has been shown to cause a reduction in portal pressure through decreased splanchnic blood flow and decreased portocollateral resistance.[27,28] Given that left ventricular hypertrophy and hyperdynamic systolic function in ESLD may result in hemodynamically significant left ventricular outflow tract obstruction (LVOTO), TTE can also be used to assess and evaluate LVOTO.[23,29] In addition, an assessment for pericardial fluid and tamponade physiology is an important part of the preoperative TTE in patients with ESLD because these patients can develop pericardial effusions resulting in cardiac tamponade, especially in cases of hepatitis C infection and cryoglobinuria. A complete bedside assessment and physical examination is also indicated to accurately diagnose tamponade in these patients.

Preoperative echocardiography is useful to calculate pulmonary artery systolic pressure (PASP). If the PASP is increased or if there is right ventricular dysfunction, right-side heart catheterization should be performed. PASP values of 45 to 50 mm Hg and/or right ventricular dysfunction are usually used for screening POPH.[30] Right-heart catheterization should be performed to gauge the mean pulmonary artery pressure, pulmonary capillary wedge pressure, and transpulmonary gradient because 5% to 10% of ESLD candidates have POPH. A preoperative mPAP of 35 to 50 mm Hg has been associated with a 50% risk of mortality after liver transplant in patients with POPH,[31] and mortality approached 100% among patients with POPH and mPAP greater than or equal to 50 mm Hg.[32] Thus, POPH warrants perioperative management by a specialist versed in pulmonary hypertension and often involves treatment with pulmonary vasodilators such as epoprostenol, sildenafil, or nitric oxide.

Given that patients with ESLD are at risk for the development of CAD, stress testing of patients with ESLD can be informative. Coronary angiography is the gold standard for detecting CAD.[23] Transesophageal echocardiography and/or pulmonary artery catheterization may be used intraoperatively to allow for real-time hemodynamic monitoring and assessment of volume status. Dobutamine stress echocardiography has been found to have a negative predictive value of 85% in patients with ESLD.[33,34] The predictive value of nuclear single-photon emission computed tomography (SPECT) stress imaging is limited by the chronic vasodilatory state shown by patients with ESLD.[35] The specificity of abnormal SPECT findings for obstructive CAD by coronary angiography is only 61%.[36] Cardiac MRI can also be used for detection of ischemia; both perfusion and wall motion can be detected during stress and at rest.[37] QTc prolongation is common in patients with ESLD, and thus a preoperative ECG is strongly indicated. Although a prolonged QTc is not a contraindication to surgery, it should trigger a search for reversible causes, such as electrolyte disturbance (eg, hypokalemia or hypomagnesemia) or the use of QT interval–prolonging drugs.[24] Torsades de pointes is a rare, life-threatening arrhythmia usually associated with a long QT interval, and can be caused by hypomagnesemia and hypokalemia, conditions often seen in alcoholic patients. Thus, especially when treating patients with alcoholic cirrhosis, it is important to maintain normal electrolyte levels.[38]

It is important to assess the risks of anesthesia and surgery in patients with liver disease. The risk of surgery in patients with cirrhosis depends on the severity of the disease, the clinical setting, and the type of surgical procedure. In addition, perioperative events, such as hypotension, sepsis, or the administration of hepatotoxic drugs, can further exacerbate injury to the liver. The Child-Turcotte-Pugh (CTP) score or Child-Pugh class has been the principal predictor of operative risk in patients with cirrhosis, but more recently studies have suggested that the Model for End-Stage Liver Disease (MELD) score may be superior.[39] The Child-Pugh class is assigned based on bilirubin level, albumin level, prothrombin time (PT), ascites, and encephalopathy. The MELD score predicts severity based on serum creatinine level, total bilirubin level, and PT/International Normalized Ratio (INR). A study by Teh and colleagues[40] showed that surgical patients with a MELD score of 7 or less had a mortality of 5.7%, patients with a MELD score of 8 to 11 had a mortality of 10.3%, and patients with a MELD score of 12 to 15 had a mortality of 25.4%. In cirrhotic patients who undergo abdominal surgery, CTP classes A, B, and C are associated with mortality of 10%, 30% to 31%, and 76% to 82%, respectively.[41] In patients with cirrhosis, cardiac surgery that requires cardiopulmonary bypass has an increased perioperative risk. A 2004 study of cirrhotic patients who underwent elective cardiac surgery (coronary artery bypass grafting, valve surgery, or pericardiectomy) showed a strong association between CTP score and postoperative mortality, such that patients with a CTP score of 8 or higher had significantly higher postoperative mortality than those with a CTP score less than 8.[42]

Intraoperative Management

Elective surgery should only be considered in patients who have well-compensated chronic liver disease.[43] Emergency surgery warrants urgent optimization of the patient, with close consideration of the patient's intravascular volume status, coagulation function, neurologic status, and the presence/absence of infection.[24] Both neuraxial and regional anesthesia could be considered in patients with hepatic failure.

Coagulopathy should be considered as a contraindication to some types of regional anesthesia.

Sedative premedication should be used judiciously in patients with liver disease because it may precipitate encephalopathy. The half-life of midazolam is prolonged because of reduced clearance and reduced protein binding, resulting in prolonged duration of action and enhanced sedative effect, especially after multiple doses or a continuous infusion.

All patients should receive standard monitoring (as recommended by the American Society of Anesthesiologists), but, for major surgery, both arterial and central venous pressure monitoring should be strongly considered. TEE may be helpful in certain patients, but probe placement is relatively contraindicated in patients with significant esophageal varices or recent banding, as are the insertion of nasogastric tubes and esophageal temperature probes. A pulmonary artery catheter may be required in patients with varices. An intra-arterial catheter allows regular monitoring of arterial blood gases; lactate, glucose, and electrolyte levels; and coagulation status. Monitoring of core body temperature, neuromuscular block, and urine output is also recommended.[24]

The goals of intraoperative management include maintenance of adequate hepatic blood flow and oxygen delivery. General anesthesia reduces total hepatic blood flow, especially the contribution of the hepatic artery. Studies showed that, in healthy volunteers, hepatic blood flow decreases by 35% to 42% in the first 30 minutes following anesthesia induction. In patients with hepatic dysfunction, especially cirrhosis, compensation for reduced portal blood flow does not occur under anesthesia, which may cause further hepatic dysfunction, and difficulty in perioperative management.[6]

When inducing patients with liver disease, the oxygen supply-demand relationship should be considered. The goal is to maintain adequate pulmonary ventilation and cardiovascular function. For this reason, cardiac output, blood volume, and perfusion pressures should be kept near the patient's baseline range. Arterial hypotension may be drug induced or caused by inadequate blood volume replacement or excess delivery of inhalational anesthetics. Investigations have shown that the outcomes of these effects are vasodilation and a reduction in perfusion pressure, plus a decline in blood velocity.[6] Intravenous anesthetics have a modest impact on hepatic blood flow but no clinically significant adverse impact on postoperative liver function if the mean arterial pressure is adequately maintained intraoperatively. Intravenous anesthetics have different effects on hepatic blood flow. Propofol has a significant vasodilatory effect because it increases total hepatic blood flow in both hepatic arterial and portal venous circulation.[44,45] In contrast, etomidate and thiopental decrease hepatic blood flow, either from increasing hepatic arterial vascular resistance or from reduced cardiac output and/or blood pressure.[46] Ketamine has little impact on hepatic blood flow.[47] Dexmedetomidine, an alpha2-adrenergic agonist with sedative and analgesic properties, is metabolized primarily by the liver and thus dose adjustments must be made in patients with significant hepatic dysfunction.[48] Among intravenous anesthetic agents, propofol is often a good choice in patients with liver disease. It has a short half-life even in patients with decompensated cirrhosis.[6] Patients with hepatic dysfunction are more sensitive to the sedative and cardiorespiratory depressant effects of propofol, thus the dose should be reduced.

There is an apparent resistance to nondepolarizing neuromuscular blockers (NMBs) in patients with liver disease, which may be caused by an increased volume of distribution, altered protein binding, or impaired biliary excretion. Atracurium and cisatracurium are suitable NMBs that have been recommended as the agents of choice because they rely on neither the liver nor kidney for excretion. Atracurium and its isomer cisatracurium undergo Hoffman degradation followed by ester hydrolysis. Clinical duration of actions of atracurium and cisatracurium have been shown to be similar to those in normal patients.[49,50] However, it has been found that, because of a larger volume of distribution, distribution half-lives are shorter in patients with severe hepatorenal dysfunction compared with normal individuals. In patients with liver disease and edema, neuromuscular blocking agent doses must be augmented because fluid retention increases the volume of distribution. Neuromuscular blocking agents that are metabolized by the liver, such as vecuronium and rocuronium, which are steroid-based NMBs, have a slower onset and longer duration of action in severe liver disease. Liver disease reduces plasma cholinesterase activity, and prolonged neuromuscular blockade has been reported after succinylcholine administration. As in all cases, it is advisable to monitor neuromuscular function.

The literature shows that, among the inhalation anesthetics, halothane (although now rarely used) should be avoided because maintaining hepatic blood flow is critical in hepatic patients, and halothane has the most dramatic effect in reducing hepatic arterial blood flow, oxygen supply, and postoperative hepatic dysfunction of all the inhalation anesthetics. In addition, halothane administration carries the risk of immunologically mediated severe postoperative halothane hepatitis.[6,30] Isoflurane, desflurane, and sevoflurane have consistently been shown to better preserve hepatic blood flow and function. Newer volatile anesthetics, such as sevoflurane and desflurane, have not been studied to the same extent as older agents but a few indirect comparisons of sevoflurane and desflurane with enflurane and halothane suggest that sevoflurane and desflurane undergo less hepatic metabolism, and that sevoflurane could have some advantages compared with the other volatile anesthetics.

In patients with pulmonary hypertension, regional anesthesia, including peripheral nerve blocks and epidurals, can be considered. For moderate to severe pulmonary hypertension, spinal anesthesia is contraindicated because of the chance for abrupt alterations in SVR and preload. Advantages include avoiding increases in PVR by preventing hypoxemia, acidosis, hypercarbia, and pain. In patients with POPH, SVR should be maintained because a reduction in SVR leads to a reduction in cardiac output as PVR is fixed. Myocardial depressants should be avoided and myocardial contractility should be maintained.

Opioids have been successfully used in patients with hepatic and cardiac disease. However, certain pharmacologic consequences, such as delayed drug clearance and prolonged half-life, should be considered. Drugs such as morphine, meperidine, benzodiazepines, and barbiturates should be used with caution because of their dependence on the liver for metabolism. In general, the doses of these agents should be decreased by 50%. Morphine has significantly reduced metabolism in patients with advanced cirrhosis, and thus has potentially prolonged and exaggerated sedative and respiratory depressant effects. In patients with associated renal failure, accumulation of the active metabolite morphine-6-glucuronide occurs. In general, it is strongly advised to avoid morphine in patients with decompensated liver failure because it may precipitate hepatic encephalopathy. Although fentanyl is also metabolized by the liver, fentanyl elimination is not appreciably altered in patients with cirrhosis; fentanyl does not have an active metabolite and is renally excreted.[51] For these reasons, fentanyl is considered the opioid of choice in these patients because, when used in moderate doses, it does not decrease hepatic oxygen and blood supply, nor does it prevent increases in hepatic oxygen requirements.[52,53] Unlike fentanyl, alfentanil's half-life is almost double in patients with cirrhosis.[54] The elimination of remifentanil in unchanged in patients with liver disease because it undergoes hydrolysis by blood and tissue esterases.[55] As a general rule, all long-acting narcotics and sedatives should be avoided in patients with cirrhosis and/or cardiac disease.

Patients with liver disease tend to have several baseline cardiovascular abnormalities, including decreased SVR and increased cardiac index, which may further affect hepatic blood flow. Catecholamine and other neurohormonal responses are impaired in patients with liver disease; therefore, intraoperative hypovolemia or hemorrhage may not trigger adequate compensatory mechanisms. Anesthetics causing sympathetic blockade further blunt this response, which may be further impaired when patients with varices are being maintained on beta-adrenergic blockers. The result of this reduction in hepatic perfusion is a drastic loss of their remaining marginal hepatic function.[56]

As discussed earlier, ESLD can be associated with left ventricular hypertrophy and hyperdynamic systolic function, which could result in a hemodynamically significant LVOTO. Patients with LVOTO can have poor tolerance of the hemodynamic stresses associated with anesthesia and surgery, thus it is crucial to monitor these patients carefully intraoperatively and have the following goals: avoidance of tachycardia, limited use of inotropic agents, and TEE-guided volume administration.[23]

It is crucial to recognize the extrahepatic manifestations of liver disease, namely the hematologic changes. With severe hepatic dysfunction comes a marked reduced capability to synthesize clotting factors, particularly the vitamin K–dependent factors II, VII, IX, and X. This coagulopathy results in increased PT and activated partial thromboplastin time. It is also common to have thrombocytopenia and platelet dysfunction. Anemia in these patients can be caused by multiple processes, including chronic blood loss from the gastrointestinal tract, hypersplenism-induced hemolysis, chronic disease, and malnutrition. Bleeding during surgery in patients with hepatic and cardiac dysfunction can result from acquired coagulation disturbances, or from surgical causes. Note that the preoperative INR may not predict intraoperative blood loss, and the utility of fresh frozen plasma (FFP) administration to correct abnormal INR values is controversial because the volume load associated with FFP transfusions may increase bleeding.[57] A useful test that can be done intraoperatively to assess coagulation status is the thromboelastograph (TEG), which provides information on the rate and strength of clot formation. By detecting intraoperative hypercoagulability, the TEG may act to facilitate specific goal-directed therapy.

Postoperative Management

Vigilance and careful monitoring are essential in the postoperative course because surgery and anesthesia can worsen hepatic and cardiac function. Postoperatively, there is potential for renal dysfunction, worsening hepatic dysfunction, and new or worsening coagulopathy. Invasive cardiovascular monitoring and careful fluid management are continued to avoid the development of postoperative renal failure. Monitoring of coagulation and also maintaining vigilance for signs of postoperative bleeding should be continued.

Regarding postoperative pain management, regional anesthesia should be considered whenever appropriate because it reduces the need for systemic analgesia, but once again the patient's coagulation status must be considered. The literature suggests that epidural analgesia should be considered with extreme caution and only if the INR is less than 1.5 and the platelet count is sufficiently preserved. Thoracic epidurals may be beneficial for liver resections, in which the catheter is typically placed at the T6 to T9 space. The transverse abdominis plane block or local nerve infiltration is beneficial in these patients when appropriate. Patient-controlled analgesia using fentanyl has been shown to be well tolerated in patients with liver disease. Nonsteroidal antiinflammatory drugs (NSAIDs) should be avoided because they increase the risk of gastrointestinal bleeding, platelet dysfunction, and renal toxicity. In contrast with NSAIDs, acetaminophen is not associated with platelet impairment, gastrointestinal toxicity, or nephrotoxicity, but it has the potential for further hepatic toxicity.[58]

Patients with cardiac and hepatic dysfunction often require multiple blood transfusions intraoperatively, and this can increase the levels of unconjugated bilirubin because approximately 10% of stored whole blood undergoes hemolysis within 24 hours of transfusion. Each half to full unit of blood stored in citrate phosphate dextrose adenine yields 7.5 mg of hemoglobin, which is then converted to approximately 250 mg of bilirubin. This process can potentially overwhelm the liver's ability to conjugate and excrete bilirubin.

SUMMARY

Anesthesia and surgery in patients with hepatic and cardiac dysfunction poses a formidable challenge for all physicians involved. It is imperative to optimize these patients using targeted interventions perioperatively to prevent complications and improve outcomes. Perioperative management of these patients requires that careful attention be paid to the potential complications of cardiac disease, liver disease, and the disease processes that overlap between the two.

REFERENCES

1. Garrison RN, Cryer HM, Howard DA, et al. Clarification of risk factors for abdominal operations in patients with hepatic cirrhosis. Ann Surg 1984;199(6):648–55.
2. del Olmo JA, Flor-Lorente B, Flor-Civera B, et al. Risk factors for nonhepatic surgery in patients with cirrhosis. World J Surg 2003;27(6):647–52.
3. Decker RC, Foley JR, Moore TJ. Perioperative management of the patient with cardiac disease. J Am Acad Orthop Surg 2010;18(5):267–77.
4. Al-Hamoudi WK. Cardiovascular changes in cirrhosis: pathogenesis and clinical implications. Saudi J Gastroenterol 2010;16:145–53.
5. Fouad YM, Yehia R. Hepato-cardiac disorders. World J Hepatol 2014;6(1):41–54.
6. Rahimzadeh P, Safari S, Faiz SH, et al. Anesthesia for patients with liver disease. Hepat Mon 2014;14(7):e19881.
7. Wong F, Sniderman K, Blendis L. The renal sympathetic and renin-angiotensin response to lower body negative pressure in well-compensated cirrhosis. Gastroenterology 1998;115:397–405.
8. Mψller S, Henriksen JH, Bendtsen F. Pathogenetic background for treatment of ascites and hepatorenal syndrome. Hepatol Int 2008;2:416–28.
9. Mackelaite L, Alsauskas ZC, Ranganna K. Renal failure in patients with cirrhosis. Med Clin North Am 2009;93:855–69.
10. Jimenez W, Arroyo V. Origins of cardiac dysfunction in cirrhosis. Gut 2003;52:1511–7.
11. Yildiz R, Yildirim B, Karincaoglu M, et al. Brain natriuretic peptide and severity of disease in non-alcoholic cirrhotic patients. J Gastroenterol Hepatol 2005;20:1115–20.
12. Bernardi M, Calandra S, Colantoni A, et al. Q-T interval prolongation in cirrhosis: prevalence, relationship with severity, and etiology of the disease and possible pathogenetic factors. Hepatology 1998;27(1):28–34.
13. Henriksen JH, Fuglsang S, Bendtsen F, et al. Dyssynchronous electrical and mechanical systole in patients with cirrhosis. J Hepatol 2002;36:513–20.

14. Kelbaek H, Rabol A, Brynjolf I, et al. Haemodynamic response to exercise in patients with alcoholic liver cirrhosis. Clin Physiol 1987;7:35–41.
15. Wong F. Cirrhotic cardiomyopathy. Hepatol Int 2009;3(1):294–304.
16. Kalaitzakis E, Rosengren A, Skommevik T, et al. Coronary artery disease in patients with liver cirrhosis. Dig Dis Sci 2010;55(2):467–75.
17. An J, Shim JH, Kim SO, et al. Prevalence and prediction of coronary artery disease in patients with liver cirrhosis. a registry-based matched case–control study. Circulation 2014;130:1353–62.
18. Hoeper MM, Krowka MJ, Strassburg CP. Portopulmonary hypertension and hepatopulmonary syndrome. Lancet 2004;363:1461–8.
19. Kawut SM, Krowka MJ, Trotter JF, et al. Clinical risk factors for portopulmonary hypertension. Hepatology 2008;48:196–203.
20. Aldenkortt F, Aldenkortt M, Caviezel L, et al. Portopulmonary hypertension and hepatopulmonary syndrome. World J Gastroenterol 2014;20(25):8072–81.
21. Ramsay MAE, Simpson BR, Nguyen AT, et al. Severe pulmonary hypertension in liver transplant candidates. Liver Transpl Surg 1997;3:494–500.
22. Ramsay M. Portopulmonary hypertension and right heart failure in patients with cirrhosis. Curr Opin Anaesthesiol 2010;23(2):145–50.
23. Moller S, Henrickesen JH. Cardiovascular complications of cirrhosis. Gut 2008; 57(2):268–78.
24. Comfere T, Sprung J, Kumar MM, et al. Angiotensin system inhibitors in a general surgical population. Anesth Analg 2005;100:636.
25. Vaja R, McNicol L, Sisley I. Anaesthesia for patients with liver disease. Cont Educ Anaesth Crit Care Pain 2010;10(1):15–9.
26. Raval Z, Harinstein ME, Skaro AI, et al. Cardiovascular risk assessment of the liver transplant candidate. J Am Coll Cardiol 2011;58(3):223–31.
27. Tripathi D, Hayes PC. The role of carvedilol in the management of portal hypertension. Eur J Gastroenterol Hepatol 2010;22:905–11.
28. Lin HC, Huang YT, Wei HC, et al. Hemodynamic effects of one week carvedilol administration on cirrhotic rats. J Gastroenterol 2006;41:361–8.
29. Maraj S, Jacobs LE, Maraj R, et al. Inducible left ventricular outflow tract gradient during dobutamine stress echocardiography: an association with intraoperative hypotension but not a contraindication to liver transplantation. Echocardiography 2004;21:681–5.
30. Dalal A, Lang JD Jr. Anesthetic considerations for patients with liver disease. In: Abdeldayem H, editor. Hepatic Surgery. Intech; 2013. Available at: http://www. intechopen.com/books/hepatic-surgery/anesthetic-considerations-for-patients-with-liver-disease.
31. Swanson KL, Wiesner RH, Nyberg SL, et al. Survival in portopulmonary hypertension: Mayo Clinic experience categorized by treatment subgroups. Am J Transplant 2008;8:2445–53.
32. Martinez-Palli G, Taura P, Balust J, et al. Liver transplantation in high-risk patients: hepatopulmonary syndrome and portopulmonary hypertension. Transplant Proc 2005;37:3861–4.
33. Williams K, Lewis JF, Davis G, et al. Dobutamine stress echocardiography in patients undergoing liver transplantation evaluation. Transplantation 2000;69: 2354–6.
34. Donovan CL, Marcovitz PA, Punch JD, et al. Two-dimensional and dobutamine stress echocardiography in the preoperative assessment of patients with end-stage liver disease prior to orthotopic liver transplantation. Transplantation 1996;61:1180–8.

35. Davidson CJ, Gheorghiade M, Flaherty JD, et al. Predictive value of stress myocardial perfusion imaging in liver transplant candidates. Am J Cardiol 2002;89:359–60.

36. Aydinalp A, Bal U, Atar I, et al. Value of stress myocardial perfusion scanning in diagnosis of severe coronary artery disease in liver transplantation candidates. Transplant Proc 2009;41:3757–60.

37. Nandalur KR, Dwamena BA, Choudhri AF, et al. Diagnostic performance of stress cardiac magnetic resonance imaging in the detection of coronary artery disease: a meta-analysis. J Am Coll Cardiol 2007;50:1343–53.

38. Nakasone H, Sugama R, Sakugawa H, et al. Alcoholic liver cirrhosis complicated with torsade de pointes during plasma exchange and hemodiafiltration. J Gastroenterol 2001;36(8):564–8.

39. O'Leary JG, Friedman LS. Predicting surgical risk in patients with cirrhosis: from art to science. Gastroenterology 2007;132:1609.

40. Teh SH, Nagorney DM, Stevens SR, et al. Risk factors for mortality after surgery in patients with cirrhosis. Gastroenterology 2007;132:1261–9.

41. Mansour A, Watson W, Shayani V, et al. Abdominal operations in patients with cirrhosis: still a major surgical challenge. Surgery 1977;122:730–5.

42. Suman A, Barnes DS, Zein NN, et al. Predicting outcome after cardiac surgery in patients with cirrhosis: a comparison of Child-Pugh and MELD scores. Clin Gastroenterol Hepatol 2004;2:719–23.

43. Maze M, Bass NM. Anaesthesia and the hepatobiliary system. Anesthesia. 5th edition. Philadelphia: Churchill Livingstone; 2000. p. 1960–72.

44. Carmichael FJ, Crawford MW, Khayyam N, et al. Effect of propofol infusion on splanchnic hemodynamics and liver oxygen consumption in the rat. Anesthesiology 1993;79:1051–60.

45. Wouters PF, Van de Velde MA, Marcus MA, et al. Hemodynamic changes during induction of anesthesia with eltanolone and propofol in dogs. Anesth Analg 1995; 81:125–31.

46. Thompson IA, Fitch W, Hughes RL, et al. Effects of certain IV anesthetics on liver blood flow and hepatic oxygen consumption in the greyhound. Br J Anaesth 1986;58:69–80.

47. Thompson IA, Fitch W, Campbell D, et al. Effects of ketamine on liver blood flow and hepatic oxygen consumption: studies in the anesthetized greyhound. Acta Anaesthesiol Scand 1988;32:10–4.

48. Baughman VL, Cunningham FE, Layden T. Pharmacokinetic/pharmacodynamic effects of dexmedetomidine in patients with hepatic failure. Anesth Analg 2000; 90(Suppl):S391. p. 4–5.

49. De Wolf AM, Freeman JA, Scott VL, et al. Pharmacokinetics and pharmacodynamics of cisatracurium in patients with end-stage liver disease undergoing liver transplantation. Br J Anaesth 1996;76:624–8.

50. Ward S, Neill EA. Pharmacokinetics of atracurium in acute hepatic failure (with acute renal failure). Br J Anaesth 1983;55:1169–72.

51. Haberer JP, Schoeffler P, Couderc E, et al. Fentanyl pharmacokinetics in patients with cirrhosis. Br J Anaesth 1982;54(12):1267–70.

52. Hoetzel A, Ryan H, Schmidt R. Anesthetic considerations for the patient with liver disease. Curr Opin Anaesthesiol 2012;25(3):340–7.

53. Kiamanesh D, Rumley J, Moitra VK. Monitoring and managing hepatic disease in anaesthesia. Br J Anaesth 2013;111(Suppl 1):i50–61.

54. Ferrier C, Marty J, Bouffard Y, et al. Alfentanil pharmacokinetics in patients with cirrhosis. Anesthesiology 1985;62:480–4.

55. Dershwitz M, Hoke JF, Rosow CE, et al. Pharmacokinetics and pharmacody-namics of remifentanil in volunteer subjects with severe liver disease. Anesthesiology 1996;84:812–20.
56. O'Glasser AY, Haranath S, Conjeevaram H, et al. Perioperative management of the patient with liver disease. Medscape 2015.
57. Massicote L, Capitanio U, Beaulieu D, et al. Independent validation of a model predicting the need for RBC transfusion in liver transplantation. Transplantation 2009;88:386–91.
58. Benson GD, Koff RS, Tolman KG. The therapeutic use of acetaminophen in patients with liver disease. Am J Ther 2005;12(2):133–41.

Anesthesia for Patients with Traumatic Brain Injuries

Bishwajit Bhattacharya, MD, FACS, Adrian A. Maung, MD, FACS, FCCM*

KEYWORDS

- Traumatic brain injury • Management • Anesthesia • Perioperative

KEY POINTS

- Traumatic brain injury is one of the leading causes of morbidity and mortality worldwide, especially in younger age groups.
- Long-term outcomes after traumatic brain injury are influenced by the initial medical management, including in the perioperative arena.
- Traumatic brain injury is commonly divided into primary and secondary brain injury. Although primary brain injury occurs before medical attention at the time of the initial trauma, secondary brain injury can be decreased through optimal evidence-based medical management.
- Even brief episodes of hypotension and hypoxemia should be avoided because they have been associated with worse outcomes. Appropriate airway management is therefore crucial.
- An algorithmic approach should be used to maintain intracranial pressure less than 20 mm Hg and cerebral perfusion pressure between 50 and 70 mm Hg.

INTRODUCTION

Traumatic brain injury (TBI) is one of the leading causes of morbidity and mortality in the United States. It is estimated that there are 2.5 million new TBI cases every year in the United States alone, with an estimated economic burden of $60 billion a year.[1,2] It is also estimated that by the year 2020 TBI may surpass many diseases as the leading cause of death worldwide because of the increasing use of motor vehicles in developing countries.[3]

Conflicts of Interest: None.
Disclosures: None.
Section of General Surgery, Trauma & Surgical Critical Care, Department of Surgery, 330 Cedar Street, BB 310, New Haven, CT 06510, USA
* Corresponding author.
E-mail address: adrian.maung@yale.edu

Anesthesiology Clin 34 (2016) 747–759
http://dx.doi.org/10.1016/j.anclin.2016.06.009   anesthesiology.theclinics.com
1932-2275/16/© 2016 Elsevier Inc. All rights reserved.

TBI can vary in a spectrum of significance ranging from mild concussions with no long-term sequelae to severe nonsurvivable injuries. Although the outcome after TBI depends on the severity of the original injury, the initial and subsequent medical care can significantly affect the ultimate recovery. Health care practitioners providing anesthesia to patients with TBI in the operating room can influence the eventual outcome, which may not be apparent for months or even years after the encounter, by providing optimal evidence-based medical management that prevents additional brain injury.

CLASSIFICATION

The severity of TBI can classified by a quick and reproducible neurologic examination: the Glasgow Coma Scale (GCS). The GCS score is based on 3 components (1) eye opening, (2) verbal communication, and (3) motor function (**Table 1**). Patients can score a minimum of 1 point on each section with a minimal total score of 3 and a maximal score of 15. Intubated patients are distinguished by adding the suffix T and can only have a maximum score of 11T because of the inability to verbally communicate. The GCS stratification can be used to triage patients to the appropriate level of trauma system activation and can also help guide work-up based on the likelihood of TBI. TBI with a GCS score of 3 to 8 is classified as severe, 9 to 12 as moderate, and 13 to 15 as mild. According to advanced trauma life support guidelines, patients with a GCS of 8 or less should be intubated for airway protection.[4]

However, the GCS score has been criticized for interuser variability, which may be experience dependent.[5–7] Confounding factors, such as facial trauma, intoxication, and intubation, may also diminish the reliability of its tabulation.[8] Despite these limitations, GCS score has been shown in multiple studies to be a valid prognosticator of survival and outcome.[9–14]

Table 1 GCS score	
Eye Opening	
Spontaneous	4
In response to speech	3
In response to pain	2
None	1
Verbal Response	
Oriented	5
Confused	4
Inappropriate words	3
Incomprehensible sounds	2
None	1
Motor Response	
Obeying	6
Localization to pain	5
Withdrawing in response to pain	4
Flexor response (decorticate)	3
Extensor response (decerebrate)	2
None	1

TBI is a broad term that represents a variety of 1 or more pathologic injuries identified on head computed tomography (CT) (**Table 2**). Some anatomic injuries are not readily seen on CT scans and require MRI imaging; in particular, diffuse axonal injury, which has been associated with worse functional prognosis.[15,16]

PATHOPHYSIOLOGY

The disorder in TBI is commonly considered to be caused by 2 separate but related events: primary and secondary injury. Although primary brain injury occurs at the time of the initial trauma as a result of the external forces being transmitted to the intracranial structures, secondary brain injury occurs hours to days after the injury, partly because of histopathologic and molecular changes initiated by the initial trauma.

Table 2
Various pathologic injuries in TBI

Diagnosis	Disorder	CT Findings	Notes
Epidural hematoma	Arterial bleeding into the space between the inner table of the skull and the dura	Hyperdense mass with biconvex layers. Does not cross cranial suture lines	Patients classically present with a lucid interval and proceed to deteriorate in mental status
Subdural hematoma	Tearing of the bridging veins or small arteries causing bleeding into the layer between the inner dura and the surface of the brain	High-density crescentic collection across the hemispheric convexity	—
Subarachnoid hemorrhage	Disruption of vessels leading to bleeding in the subarachnoid space	Hyperdense lesions that conform to the sulci and cisterns	Can also occur because of aneurysmal rupture
Cerebral contusion	Punctate areas of hemorrhage and necrosis	May or may not appear on initial CT scans	Often associated with other injuries
Intraparenchymal hemorrhage	Areas of hemorrhage in brain parenchyma	Hyperdense lesions in the parenchyma	Often associated with other injuries
Intraventricular hemorrhage	Hemorrhage within the ventricular system	Hyperdense lesion within the ventricles	Most commonly as a result of other intracerebral or subarachnoid hemorrhage
Diffuse axonal injury	Shear injury between gray and white matter, commonly as a result of sudden deceleration	Not readily seen on initial CT scan unless severe	Better seen on MRI May be responsible for many cognitive deficits

Episodes of hypotension and hypoxemia have also been linked with secondary brain injury. Although the exact pathways are not fully known, inflammatory changes, cell apoptosis, electrolyte disturbances, and tissue ischemia have been implicated along with increased cerebral edema and intracranial pressure (ICP).

According to the Monroe-Kelli hypothesis, even though the total volume inside the rigid skull is fixed, the volume of the individual components (blood, cerebrospinal fluid [CSF], and brain parenchyma) can vary.[17] An increase in the volume of one component thus results in the decrease of one or both of the others. After TBI, the increased volume caused by extra-axial bleeding and/or parenchymal tissue edema is initially compensated by a decrease in CSF volume. However, this compensation is limited, and further increases in the space-occupying lesion result in increased ICP. As ICP increases, the blood inflow into the skull is restricted, leading to tissue ischemia.

Cerebral perfusion pressure (CPP) = Mean arterial pressure (MAP) − ICP

The increased ICP is also transmitted to the brain parenchyma and can cause herniation across natural orifices, such as the foramen magnum (uncal herniation), or rigid membranes (eg, falx). This movement can compress vital structures and lead to further tissue injury and death. For example, uncal herniation leads to brainstem compression, loss of the brainstem reflexes, and death.

PREVENTION OF SECONDARY INJURY

Primary brain injury can only be mitigated through injury prevention and engineering of safety equipment. Medical management of TBI therefore focuses on preventing secondary injury to viable brain tissue by controlling ICP and ensuring adequate perfusion and oxygen delivery as well as preventing other commonly associated complications. Both hypotension and hypoxemia have been associated with increased morbidity and mortality in TBI.[18–22]

INTRACRANIAL PRESSURE/CEREBRAL PERFUSION PRESSURE MANAGEMENT

The Brain Trauma Foundation published evidence-based *Guidelines for the Management of Severe Traumatic Brain Injury* in 2007.[23] The management, whether in the intensive care unit or in the operating room, includes maintaining appropriate cerebral blood flow and oxygenation to avoid secondary brain injury. In the past, this therapy was directed toward the management of ICP but more recently there has been a shift toward a strategy of also maintaining adequate CPP (**Box 1**). ICP monitoring is used to guide both strategies; however, a recent randomized multicenter trial (BEST:TRIP [Benchmark Evidence From South American Trials: Treatment of Intracranial Pressure]) and a published meta-analysis have raised concerns that intensive ICP monitoring does not provide additional benefits.[24,25]

Common targets of TBI management are maintaining ICP less than 20 mm Hg and cerebral perfusion pressure between 50 and 70 mm Hg.[23] Aggressive therapy to increase CPP to more than 70 mm Hg has been linked to increased incidence of acute respiratory distress syndrome and other adverse events. Brain tissue oxygen tension monitoring can also be used as a marker for resuscitation with a treatment threshold of an oxygen tension level less than 15 mm Hg.[23,26]

Initial management to decrease ICP includes simple techniques to promote cerebral venous drainage by head-of-bed elevation to 30° as well as keeping the neck in a neutral position and ensuring that the cervical collar is not too tight. Reverse Trendelenburg position can be used intraoperatively if head-of-bed elevation is not feasible.[27]

Box 1
Management strategies for increased ICP

- Elevate head of bed more than 30° (be aware of any spinal precautions)

- Position head midline

- Ensure that the cervical collar is not too tight and no occlusive dressings are present that may impair venous drainage

- Implement appropriate sedation and analgesia
  - Propofol drip
  - Fentanyl drip
  - Titrate to Richmond Agitation-Sedation Scale −4 to −5

- Hyperosmolar therapy
  - Monitor serum Na and osmolality
  - Mannitol: bolus of 0.25 to 1 g/kg (avoid in hypotensive patients)
  - 3% sodium chloride: bolus of 250 mL over 30 minutes via central access
  - 23.4% sodium chloride: 30 mL over 15 minutes via central access

- CSF drainage via an external ventricular drain

- Increase MAP with pressors to maintain CPP (50–70 mg Hg)

- Surgical management
  - Evacuation of extra-axial blood collections
  - Decompressive craniectomy

Sedation is often used to reduce ICP and cerebral metabolic demand as well as to blunt the effects of tachycardia and hypertension. Propofol is commonly used in the intensive care setting because of its quick onset and short duration of action, which facilitates frequent neurologic assessment. However, there is no conclusive evidence that one agent is more efficacious than another in improving Glasgow Outcome Scale scores, mortality, ICP, or CPP.[28,29] Propofol has also been associated in rare instances with propofol infusion syndrome; risk factors for this syndrome include young age, TBI, high doses, and prolonged (>48 hours) use.[30] Sedatives may also induce hypotension and cerebral vasodilation and thus exacerbate cerebral hypoperfusion. Barbiturates have been traditionally used as third-line agents for refractory intracranial hypertension to induce barbiturate coma but there is no clear clinical evidence to support this practice.[31] High-dose barbiturates also cause hypotension in more than 25% of patients.

Hyperosmolar medications can decrease ICP by creating an osmolar gradient that draws water across the blood-brain barrier into the intravascular space and thus decreases the interstitial volume. Commonly used agents include mannitol and hypertonic saline. Although definitive data are lacking, hypertonic saline has been observed in small trials to have some advantage compared with mannitol in reducing ICP and improving outcomes.[32] In addition to the osmolar effect, mannitol may also promote cerebral blood flow by temporarily reducing blood viscosity. It is generally dosed 0.25 to 1 g/kg every 4 to 6 hours but becomes less effective with repeat dosing. Serum osmolality should be measured serially during mannitol therapy to maintain it at less than 320 mOsm/L and caution should be used in hypovolemic patients because of its diuretic effects. Hypertonic saline is available in a variety of concentrations (1.5%–23.4%) with concentrations 3% or higher requiring administration via central venous access. Bolus administration seems to be superior to continuous infusion.[32] Although the ideal serum sodium concentration is not well established, clinicians commonly target levels of 150 to 160 mEq/L. The effects of intravascular administration of hyperosmolar agents changes in the presence of a rupture in the blood-brain barrier, which is frequently present in patients with TBI.

Mechanical ventilation should be adjusted to prevent hypoxemia and maintain normocarbia (goal $Paco_2$ 35–40 mm Hg). Both hypocarbia and hypercarbia can have deleterious effects. Hyperventilation induces cerebral vasoconstriction, resulting in not only decreased ICP but also decreased cerebral blood flow leading to secondary ischemia and worse outcomes.[33] It can be used briefly as a temporizing measure in patients with evidence of herniation while other therapies are being implemented.

Although decreasing ICP is first-line therapy, hemodynamic support with pressors is sometimes used to maintain CPP by increasing the MAP. Norepinephrine is the preferred agent because of its hemodynamic profile, although it may cause reflex bradycardia.[34] However, artificial increase of CPP to more than 70 mm Hg has been linked with increased complications and is not recommended.

Hypovolemia should be corrected before the initiation of pressors. Isotonic normal saline should be used because hypotonic saline can exacerbate cerebral edema and the use of albumin in patients with TBI may be harmful as well.[35] In patients with polytrauma, hypovolemia may be caused by acute blood loss. Patients with acute blood loss anemia should be transfused with blood products to correct hemorrhagic hypovolemia and may require procedures to stop the source of ongoing hemorrhage. Transfusion triggers for critically ill patients are typically hemoglobin level less than 7 g/dL and patients with TBI do not seem to have improved neurologic outcome if transfused to a higher hemoglobin target.[36,37]

In addition to the medical therapy described earlier, several surgical options may be appropriate in the management of TBI. CSF drainage via an external ventricular drain, which can be placed at the bedside in the intensive care unit, can be used to reduce ICP; continuous rather than intermittent drainage of CSF may be more effective.[38] Surgical drainage of space-occupying extra-axial lesions such as subdural or epidural hematomas also decreases ICP. Decompressive craniectomy, an operation in which a portion of the skull is removed to allow the brain to herniate outward, has been used for some patients with uncontrolled intracranial hypertension. A randomized trial (DECRA [Decompressive Craniectomy] trial) published in 2011, which showed decreased ICP but more unfavorable outcomes in the decompressive craniectomy group, has stimulated extensive discussion regarding the proper role of this procedure.[39] However, the DECRA trial had significant limitations and has left many questions unanswered; questions that may be answered by another trial of 400 patients that has recently completed enrollment.[40]

MONITORING DEVICES

Various technologies are available to assist in ICP/CPP management. ICP can be monitored through 2 categories of devices. One type, which is commonly referred to as bolt, is only able to measure the pressure, whereas a second type (ventriculostomy, or external ventricular drain) is able to both measure ICP and also drain CSF as a therapeutic maneuver to decrease the ICP. The Brain Trauma Foundation recommends that all patients with salvageable severe brain injury (GCS 3–8) with a CT scan abnormality should have an ICP monitor.[23] However, this recommendation is controversial because studies have questioned whether ICP monitoring improves outcomes.[41–44]

Continuous or intermittent jugular venous oximetry can be used as a surrogate for cerebral oxygen use. A catheter is placed retrograde into the jugular vein with the tip at the jugular bulb (level of the mastoid on a plain film). The blood obtained at this level is a sample of mixed cerebral blood. Jugular venous oxygen saturation is an indirect measure of the balance between cerebral blood supply and metabolic demand. Normal jugular venous oxygen saturation is 60% to 70%. A decrease in the saturation suggests an imbalance between oxygen delivery and oxygen demand (the brain has to extract more oxygen to compensate for the deficiency in the delivery). This condition may arise from a variety of causes, including hypotension, vasospasm, increased ICP, decreased CPP, and/or cardiopulmonary insufficiency.[45] There are several limitations with the use of jugular venous oximetry, including sampling errors from either catheter malposition or possible nondrainage from infarcted territories. A high incidence of false-positive desaturation episodes has also been observed in studies.[46]

Near-infrared spectroscopy (NIRS) is a noninvasive cerebral oxygen monitoring technique. Near-infrared wavelengths of light are able to penetrate the skull and are absorbed differently by oxygenated and deoxygenated hemoglobin as well as cytochrome aa_3 within brain parenchyma. Their relative concentrations can therefore be measured by using spectroscopy applied to the forehead. NIRS has been reported to be more sensitive in detecting episodes of jugular venous desaturation compared with jugular oximetry.[47] However, the accuracy of NIRS can be limited by brain tissue edema and inaccuracies in distinguishing oxygenation changes in intracranial versus extracranial tissues. Studies of outcomes of the use of tissue oxygenation versus ICP monitors have provided mixed results.[48–50]

Brain tissue oxygenation monitoring is an invasive approach to monitoring the brain tissue oxygen partial pressure by introducing a catheter into brain parenchyma via a surgical site or a bolt. Research to validate this technique is ongoing. A more elaborate way to monitor the metabolic state of the brain is to measure metabolites of the brain via microdialysis. A catheter is introduced into the parenchyma and perfused with a physiologic solution. Numerous metabolites such as glucose, lactate, pyruvate, inflammatory markers, and neurotransmitters can be measured using this technique. The ratio of metabolites, in particular the lactate/pyruvate ratio, has been shown to correlate with severity of injury.[45]

INTRAOPERATIVE MANAGEMENT

Patients with TBI commonly require operative management of other concomitant injuries and occasionally of the brain injury. A well-planned and well-executed intraoperative anesthetic management is crucial to avoid secondary brain injury. An early secure airway is essential to maintain adequate oxygenation. Patients with trauma who require emergent intubation for depressed GCS or emergent operative intervention should undergo rapid sequence intubation. All patients with trauma should be assumed to have unstable cervical injuries and a full stomach until proved otherwise. Patients should be intubated by maintaining a manual inline stabilization of the cervical spine. The need for a difficult airway algorithm should be anticipated, especially in patients with facial or neck trauma. Nasal tubes (endotracheal or gastric) should be avoided in patients with skull base fractures or coagulopathy.

Induction is usually performed with etomidate to avoid hypotension, although there are concerns for possibly inducing adrenal insufficiency.[51] Other agents, such as propofol and thiopental, should be used with caution, especially in hypovolemic or hypotensive patients, because of their suppressive effect on the cardiovascular system. Ketamine has traditionally been avoided in patients with TBI because of its ability to increase cerebral blood flow and thus increase ICP. However, more recent studies have challenged this dictum.[52] Short-acting paralytic agents are usually chosen for intubation. Hypotonic fluids should be avoided, as discussed earlier, because they can worsen cerebral edema.

All volatile agents decrease cerebral oxygen metabolic rate but may cause cerebral vasodilation and increased ICP, although the effect is likely to be low at concentrations less than 1 minimum alveolar concentration.[53] Nitrous oxide should be avoided because it is a cerebral vasodilator and may increase ICP. Certain anesthetic agents may be beneficial in TBI. Isoflurane has been shown in animal studies to have a neuro-protective effect by inhibiting the apoptosis cytokine cascade.[54,55] Similarly, other animal studies have shown a theoretic benefit of xenon as a general anesthetic by acting as an N-methyl-D-aspartate (NMDA) antagonist that prevents ischemic and excitotoxic injury.[56] Other more conventional agents also have purported benefits in the setting of TBI. Propofol may act as a cerebral protector because of its ability to suppress brain electrical activity and preserve cerebral pressure autoregulation. In addition, it may also act as an antioxidant agent that protects against additional neuroinjury.

PERIOPERATIVE CARE

Anesthesia teams caring for patients with TBI should also be aware of the other therapies that may be used in this population.

Seizures

Up to 30% of patients with severe TBI develop early (within 7 days) posttraumatic seizures. Prophylactic antiepileptic drugs have been shown to reduce the incidence of the early, but not late, seizures. Common regimens include a 7-day to 14-day course of phenytoin or levetiracetam. Development of seizures can cause an increase in cerebral metabolism, which, coupled with the increase in ICP and decreased cerebral blood flow, can exacerbate secondary brain injury.[23] Treatment of seizures is similar to the management in patients without TBI.

Endocrine

Both hyperglycemia and hypoglycemia have been associated with worse outcomes after TBI.[57] Hyperglycemia has been shown to contribute to metabolic acidosis and increased oxidative radicals that ultimately lead to neuron death. However, intense glucose therapy (goal, 80–120 mg/dL) has become contentious because it has been linked to increased incidence of hypoglycemic episodes.[58] Current recommendation for critically ill patients in general is to target a glucose level less than 180 mg/dL, but this may vary depending on the patient population as well as the presence of pre-existing diabetes.[59,60] Both intermittent and continuous insulin infusion can be used, depending on the glucose levels.

Although glucocorticoids have been used in the past for the treatment of TBI, more recent studies have shown that steroids in this population are associated with more harm than benefit. The CRASH (Corticosteroid Randomization After Significant Head Injury) trial, which randomized 10,008 patients with TBI to 48 hours of steroids or placebo, revealed an increased risk of death in the steroid group at 2 weeks (Relative Risk [RR], 1.18) and 6 months (RR, 1.15) independent of injury severity.[61,62]

Hematological

Patients with trauma are at an increased risk for developing venous thromboembolisms; however, the presence of TBI may represent a relative contraindication to pharmacologic prophylaxis because of concerns for potentially exacerbating the bleeding. There is currently wide variability in clinical practice in the timing and use of pharmacologic venous thromboembolism prophylaxis. Patients with TBI may also be on antiplatelet and/or anticoagulation agents before injury, and TBI may induce coagulopathy that will need to be corrected in the perioperative state. Although anemia is common in severely injured patients with trauma, including those with TBI, transfusion of red blood cells above a hemoglobin of 7 g/dL has been associated with an increased incidence of adverse events without any improvement in neurologic outcomes.[37]

In the setting of TBI, patients who are on antiplatelet or anticoagulation therapy for cardiovascular comorbidities may require quick and effective reversal of the agents. In addition to warfarin, clinicians are now encountering more patients who are anticoagulated with newer-generation factor Xa inhibitors and direct thrombin inhibitors. Although these drugs are more convenient for patients because they do not require blood level monitoring, the activity of these drugs cannot be quantified by routine hematologic laboratory tests and readily available antidotes are just coming on the market. Fresh frozen plasma, which is the mainstay for the reversal of warfarin, is not beneficial in the reversal of the factor Xa inhibitors. Administration of prothrombin complex concentrate may have some utility in the reversal of these agents. The direct thrombin inhibitor is renally excreted and emergent dialysis has been used in instances of life-threatening hemorrhage. A direct inhibitor for dabigatran was approved by the US Food and Drug Administration in October 2015.

Pharmacy

Agitation and delirium are common after TBI and often require multimodal therapy, including narcotics, benzodiazepines, antipsychotic agents, clonidine, methadone, and/or dexmedetomidine. β-Blockers, most commonly propranolol, are used not only for their sedative effects but also to block excess catecholamines. Their administration has been linked to improved survival and outcomes.[63,64] A course of amantadine, a weak antagonist of the NMDA-type glutamate receptor used in Parkinson disease and for the treatment of influenza (before the development of widespread resistance), has also been shown to accelerate functional neurologic recovery.[65]

Temperature Management

Temperature should be carefully controlled because hyperthermia increases cerebral metabolism and possibly aggravates secondary brain injury. Management strategies include antipyretic medications, external surface cooling devices, as well as endovascular temperature management catheters.

Therapeutic hypothermia has shown promise in improving neurologic outcomes in patients following cardiac arrest. It was therefore hypothesized that therapeutic hypothermia may also benefit the traumatically injured brain by slowing the inflammatory cascade following injury, thus preventing reperfusion injury and directly decreasing ICP. Although studies have shown the ability of induced hypothermia (32°C–35°C) to reduce ICP, it does not seem to have any significant outcome benefit to patients with TBI and has increased risk of infectious complications.[66] The currently available studies that have shown improved outcomes are of low quality[67] and thus induced hypothermia in patients with TBI currently should be reserved for research studies.[66,68]

MULTIPLE INJURED PATIENTS WITH TRAUMA AND PRIORITIES OF SURGERIES

Patients with severe TBI often have other injuries that may require operative intervention. Life-threatening intra-abdominal or intrathoracic bleeding typically take precedence over neurosurgical interventions, although ideally the 2 teams (eg, trauma and neurosurgery) would perform simultaneous operations. If the patient has intracranial hypertension, limb-threatening injuries should be addressed with abbreviated damage-control operations rather than definitive repair. Less urgent procedures, especially if they may potentially result in significant blood loss or hypotension, should be postponed. The overall goal is to balance the need for the surgical procedure with the risk of inducing secondary brain injury.

SUMMARY

TBI represents a wide spectrum of disease and disease severity. Because the primary brain injury occurs before the patient enters the health care system, medical interventions seek principally to prevent secondary injury. Anesthesia teams that provide care for patients with TBI both in and out of the operating room should be aware of the specific therapies and needs of this unique and complex patient population.

REFERENCES

1. Frieden T, Houry D, Baldwin G. Report to Congress on traumatic brain injury in the United States: epidemiology and rehabilitation. Atlanta (GA): National Center for Injury Prevention and Control; Division of Unintentional Injury Prevention; 2014.
2. Finkelstein E, Corso P, Miller T. The incidence and economic burden of injuries in the United States. New York: Oxford University Press; 2006.
3. Hyder AA, Wunderlich CA, Puvanachandra P, et al. The impact of traumatic brain injuries: a global perspective. NeuroRehabilitation 2007;22(5):341–53.
4. ATLS Subcommittee, American College of Surgeons' Committee on Trauma, International ATLS working group. Advanced trauma life support ATLS student course manual 9th ed. Chicago (IL): American College of Surgeons; 2012.
5. Lindsay KW, Teasdale GM, Knill-Jones RP. Observer variability in assessing the clinical features of subarachnoid hemorrhage. J Neurosurg 1983;58(1):57–62.
6. Rowley G, Fielding K. Reliability and accuracy of the Glasgow Coma Scale with experienced and inexperienced users. Lancet 1991;337(8740):535–8.
7. Teasdale G, Knill-Jones R, van der Sande J. Observer variability in assessing impaired consciousness and coma. J Neurol Neurosurg Psychiatry 1978;41(7): 603–10.
8. Fischer J, Mathieson C. The history of the Glasgow Coma Scale: implications for practice. Crit Care Nurs Q 2001;23(4):52–8.
9. Ritchie PD, Cameron PA, Ugoni AM, et al. A study of the functional outcome and mortality in elderly patients with head injuries. J Clin Neurosci 2000;7(4):301–4.
10. Tornetta P 3rd, Mostafavi H, Riina J, et al. Morbidity and mortality in elderly trauma patients. J Trauma 1999;46(4):702–6.
11. Meredith W, Rutledge R, Fakhry SM, et al. The conundrum of the Glasgow Coma Scale in intubated patients: a linear regression prediction of the Glasgow verbal score from the Glasgow eye and motor scores. J Trauma 1998;44(5):839–44 [discussion: 844–5].
12. Meredith W, Rutledge R, Hansen AR, et al. Field triage of trauma patients based upon the ability to follow commands: a study in 29,573 injured patients. J Trauma 1995;38(1):129–35.
13. Kuhls DA, Malone DL, McCarter RJ, et al. Predictors of mortality in adult trauma patients: the physiologic trauma score is equivalent to the trauma and injury severity score. J Am Coll Surg 2002;194(6):695–704.
14. Kilaru S, Garb J, Emhoff T, et al. Long-term functional status and mortality of elderly patients with severe closed head injuries. J Trauma 1996;41(6):957–63.

15. Paterakis K, Karantanas AH, Komnos A, et al. Outcome of patients with diffuse axonal injury: the significance and prognostic value of MRI in the acute phase. J Trauma 2000;49(6):1071–5.

16. Chelly H, Chaari A, Daoud E, et al. Diffuse axonal injury in patients with head injuries: an epidemiologic and prognosis study of 124 cases. J Trauma 2011;71(4): 838–46.

17. Mokri B. The Monro-Kellie hypothesis: applications in CSF volume depletion. Neurology 2001;56(12):1746–8.

18. Chesnut RM, Marshall LF, Klauber MR, et al. The role of secondary brain injury in determining outcome from severe head injury. J Trauma 1993;34(2):216–22.

19. McHugh GS, Engel DC, Butcher I, et al. Prognostic value of secondary insults in traumatic brain injury: results from the IMPACT study. J Neurotrauma 2007;24(2): 287–93.

20. Franschman G, Peerdeman SM, Andriessen TM, et al. Effect of secondary prehospital risk factors on outcome in severe traumatic brain injury in the context of fast access to trauma care. J Trauma 2011;71(4):826–32.

21. Brenner M, Stein D, Hu P, et al. Association between early hyperoxia and worse outcomes after traumatic brain injury. Arch Surg 2012;147(11):1042–6.

22. Brain Trauma Foundation, American Association of Neurological Surgeons, Congress of Neurological Surgeons, et al. Guidelines for the management of severe traumatic brain injury. I. Blood pressure and oxygenation. J Neurotrauma 2007;24(Suppl 1):S7–13.

23. Brain Trauma Foundation, American Association of Neurological Surgeons, Congress of Neurological Surgeons. Guidelines for the management of severe traumatic brain injury. J Neurotrauma 2007;24(Suppl 1):S1–106.

24. Chesnut RM, Temkin N, Carney N, et al. A trial of intracranial-pressure monitoring in traumatic brain injury. N Engl J Med 2012;367(26):2471–81.

25. Yuan Q, Wu X, Sun Y, et al. Impact of intracranial pressure monitoring on mortality in patients with traumatic brain injury: a systematic review and meta-analysis. J Neurosurg 2015;122(3):574–87.

26. Prabhakar H, Sandhu K, Bhagat H, et al. Current concepts of optimal cerebral perfusion pressure in traumatic brain injury. J Anaesthesiol Clin Pharmacol 2014;30(3):318–27.

27. Tankisi A, Rolighed Larsen J, Rasmussen M, et al. The effects of 10 degrees reverse Trendelenburg position on ICP and CPP in prone positioned patients subjected to craniotomy for occipital or cerebellar tumours. Acta Neurochir (Wien) 2002;144(7):665–70.

28. Gu JW, Yang T, Kuang YQ, et al. Comparison of the safety and efficacy of propofol with midazolam for sedation of patients with severe traumatic brain injury: a meta-analysis. J Crit Care 2014;29(2):287–90.

29. Roberts DJ, Hall RI, Kramer AH, et al. Sedation for critically ill adults with severe traumatic brain injury: a systematic review of randomized controlled trials. Crit Care Med 2011;39(12):2743–51.

30. Kam PC, Cardone D. Propofol infusion syndrome. Anaesthesia 2007;62(7): 690–701.

31. Roberts I, Sydenham E. Barbiturates for acute traumatic brain injury. Cochrane Database Syst Rev 2012;(12):CD000033.

32. Hinson HE, Stein D, Sheth KN. Hypertonic saline and mannitol therapy in critical care neurology. J Intensive Care Med 2013;28(1):3–11.

33. Muizelaar JP, Marmarou A, Ward JD, et al. Adverse effects of prolonged hyperventilation in patients with severe head injury: a randomized clinical trial. J Neurosurg 1991;75(5):731–9.

34. Perez-Barcena J, Llompart-Pou JA, O'Phelan KH. Intracranial pressure monitoring and management of intracranial hypertension. Crit Care Clin 2014;30(4): 735–50.

35. SAFE Study Investigators, Australian and New Zealand Intensive Care Society Clinical Trials Group, Australian Red Cross Blood Service, et al. Saline or albumin for fluid resuscitation in patients with traumatic brain injury. N Engl J Med 2007; 357(9):874–84.

36. Retter A, Wyncoll D, Pearse R, et al. Guidelines on the management of anaemia and red cell transfusion in adult critically ill patients. Br J Haematol 2013;160(4): 445–64.

37. Robertson CS, Hannay HJ, Yamal JM, et al. Effect of erythropoietin and transfusion threshold on neurological recovery after traumatic brain injury: a randomized clinical trial. JAMA 2014;312(1):36–47.

38. Nwachuku EL, Puccio AM, Fetzick A, et al. Intermittent versus continuous cerebrospinal fluid drainage management in adult severe traumatic brain injury: assessment of intracranial pressure burden. Neurocrit Care 2014;20(1):49–53.

39. Cooper DJ, Rosenfeld JV, Murray L, et al. Decompressive craniectomy in diffuse traumatic brain injury. N Engl J Med 2011;364(16):1493–502.

40. Hutchinson PJ, Corteen E, Czosnyka M, et al. Decompressive craniectomy in traumatic brain injury: the randomized multicenter RESCUEicp study (www.RESCUEicp.com). Acta Neurochir Suppl 2006;96:17–20.

41. Talving P, Karamanos E, Teixeira PG, et al. Intracranial pressure monitoring in severe head injury: compliance with Brain Trauma Foundation guidelines and effect on outcomes: a prospective study. J Neurosurg 2013;119(5):1248–54.

42. Cremer OL, van Dijk GW, van Wensen E, et al. Effect of intracranial pressure monitoring and targeted intensive care on functional outcome after severe head injury. Crit Care Med 2005;33(10):2207–13.

43. Tang A, Pandit V, Fennell V, et al. Intracranial pressure monitor in patients with traumatic brain injury. J Surg Res 2015;194(2):565–70.

44. MacLaughlin BW, Plurad DS, Sheppard W, et al. The impact of intracranial pressure monitoring on mortality after severe traumatic brain injury. Am J Surg 2015; 210(6):1082–7.

45. Bhatia A, Gupta AK. Neuromonitoring in the intensive care unit. II. Cerebral oxygenation monitoring and microdialysis. Intensive Care Med 2007;33(8): 1322–8.

46. Sheinberg M, Kanter MJ, Robertson CS, et al. Continuous monitoring of jugular venous oxygen saturation in head-injured patients. J Neurosurg 1992;76(2): 212–7.

47. Kirkpatrick PJ, Smielewski P, Czosnyka M, et al. Near-infrared spectroscopy use in patients with head injury. J Neurosurg 1995;83(6):963–70.

48. Narotam PK, Morrison JF, Nathoo N. Brain tissue oxygen monitoring in traumatic brain injury and major trauma: outcome analysis of a brain tissue oxygen-directed therapy. J Neurosurg 2009;111(4):672–82.

49. Green JA, Pellegrini DC, Vanderkolk WE, et al. Goal directed brain tissue oxygen monitoring versus conventional management in traumatic brain injury: an analysis of in hospital recovery. Neurocrit Care 2013;18(1):20–5.

50. Martini RP, Deem S, Yanez ND, et al. Management guided by brain tissue oxygen monitoring and outcome following severe traumatic brain injury. J Neurosurg 2009;111(4):644–9.
51. Cohan P, Wang C, McArthur DL, et al. Acute secondary adrenal insufficiency after traumatic brain injury: a prospective study. Crit Care Med 2005;33(10):2358–66.
52. Chang LC, Raty SR, Ortiz J, et al. The emerging use of ketamine for anesthesia and sedation in traumatic brain injuries. CNS Neurosci Ther 2013;19(6):390–5.
53. Engelhard K, Werner C. Inhalational or intravenous anesthetics for craniotomies? Pro inhalational. Curr Opin Anaesthesiol 2006;19(5):504–8.
54. McAuliffe JJ, Joseph B, Vorhees CV. Isoflurane-delayed preconditioning reduces immediate mortality and improves striatal function in adult mice after neonatal hypoxia-ischemia. Anesth Analg 2007;104(5):1066–77, tables of contents.
55. Segal N, Matsuura T, Caldwell E, et al. Ischemic postconditioning at the initiation of cardiopulmonary resuscitation facilitates functional cardiac and cerebral recovery after prolonged untreated ventricular fibrillation. Resuscitation 2012; 83(11):1397–403.
56. Coburn M, Maze M, Franks NP. The neuroprotective effects of xenon and helium in an in vitro model of traumatic brain injury. Crit Care Med 2008;36(2):588–95.
57. Liu-DeRyke X, Collingridge DS, Orme J, et al. Clinical impact of early hyperglycemia during acute phase of traumatic brain injury. Neurocrit Care 2009;11(2): 151–7.
58. Bilotta F, Caramia R, Cernak I, et al. Intensive insulin therapy after severe traumatic brain injury: a randomized clinical trial. Neurocrit Care 2008;9(2):159–66.
59. Clain J, Ramar K, Surani SR. Glucose control in critical care. World J Diabetes 2015;6(9):1082–91.
60. Abdelmalak BB, Lansang MC. Revisiting tight glycemic control in perioperative and critically ill patients: when one size may not fit all. J Clin Anesth 2013; 25(6):499–507.
61. Roberts I, Yates D, Sandercock P, et al. Effect of intravenous corticosteroids on death within 14 days in 10008 adults with clinically significant head injury (MRC CRASH trial): randomised placebo-controlled trial. Lancet 2004; 364(9442):1321–8.
62. Edwards P, Arango M, Balica L, et al. Final results of MRC CRASH, a randomised placebo-controlled trial of intravenous corticosteroid in adults with head injury-outcomes at 6 months. Lancet 2005;365(9475):1957–9.
63. Schroeppel TJ, Sharpe JP, Magnotti LJ, et al. Traumatic brain injury and beta-blockers: not all drugs are created equal. J Trauma Acute Care Surg 2014; 76(2):504–9 [discussion: 509].
64. Zangbar B, Khalil M, Rhee P, et al. Metoprolol improves survival in severe traumatic brain injury independent of heart rate control. J Surg Res 2016;200(2): 586–92.
65. Giacino JT, Whyte J, Bagiella E, et al. Placebo-controlled trial of amantadine for severe traumatic brain injury. N Engl J Med 2012;366(9):819–26.
66. Andrews PJ, Sinclair HL, Rodriguez A, et al. Hypothermia for intracranial hypertension after traumatic brain injury. N Engl J Med 2015;373(25):2403–12.
67. Crossley S, Reid J, McLatchie R, et al. A systematic review of therapeutic hypothermia for adult patients following traumatic brain injury. Crit Care 2014; 18(2):R75.
68. Georgiou AP, Manara AR. Role of therapeutic hypothermia in improving outcome after traumatic brain injury: a systematic review. Br J Anaesth 2013;110(3): 357–67.

Anesthesia for Patients with Concomitant Sepsis and Cardiac Dysfunction

Abed Abubaih, MD, Charles Weissman, MD*

KEYWORDS

- Sepsis • Septic shock • Cardiac dysfunction • Physiologic monitoring
- Sepsis-induced cardiac dysfunction • Coronary artery disease • Vasopressors
- Inotropic agents

KEY POINTS

- Cardiac dysfunction in patients with sepsis may be caused by the sepsis itself or preexisting cardiac disease.
- Anesthetic management in patients with severe sepsis or septic shock with concomitant cardiac disease involves optimizing hemodynamic and metabolic functions.
- Among the aims of managing these patients is preventing further organ damage, such as using protective ventilation to prevent or reduce lung injury.
- Increased mortality is caused by the inability of patients with septic shock with concomitant cardiac disease to adequately compensate for the sepsis-induced cardiovascular changes.

INTRODUCTION

Patients suffering from sepsis and septic shock often undergo surgery to treat the source of their sepsis or a complication thereof. Anesthetizing such patients is challenging especially if there is concurrent cardiac dysfunction. Sepsis is associated with cardiac dysfunction under a variety of circumstances (**Box 1**). Therefore, anesthesiologists faced with a patient with sepsis with concurrent cardiac dysfunction must be cognizant of the patient's cardiac status and the cause of the cardiac problem so that they can appropriately tailor their anesthetic management and physiologic monitoring.

Cardiac Dysfunction Attributable to Sepsis

Although sepsis is usually associated with a hyperdynamic state (elevated cardiac output in face of reduced systemic vascular resistance), there is often underlying

Department of Anesthesiology and Critical Care Medicine, Hadassah – Hebrew University Medical Center, Hebrew University – Hadassah School of Medicine, Jerusalem, Israel
* Corresponding author. Hadassah-Hebrew University Medical Center, Kiryat Hadassah, POB 12000, Jerusalem 91120, Israel.
E-mail address: charles@hadassah.org.il

Anesthesiology Clin 34 (2016) 761–774
http://dx.doi.org/10.1016/j.anclin.2016.06.010
1932-2275/16/© 2016 Elsevier Inc. All rights reserved.
anesthesiology.theclinics.com

Box 1

Sepsis and concomitant cardiac dysfunction

1. Cardiac dysfunction secondary to the sepsis itself (sepsis-induced cardiac dysfunction).

2. Preexisting cardiac dysfunction (eg, chronic heart failure, ischemic heart disease) in the patient with sepsis.

3. Combined acute cardiac disease and sepsis-induced cardiac dysfunction (eg, bacterial endocarditis and septic shock).

4. The stress of sepsis and septic shock (eg, hypotension, tachycardia) causing cardiac dysfunction (eg, myocardial ischemia and infarction).

---

disordered myocardial function (**Box 2**). Compensatory mechanisms, such as tachycardia and left ventricular dilation, attempt to compensate for this myocardial dysfunction. When these compensatory mechanisms fail and/or cardiac filling decreases substantially, septic shock ensues. In some patients, a hypodynamic (low cardiac output) state is found, with 25% of adult patients having relatively low cardiac outputs even after fluid resuscitation.[1] Merx and Weber[2] found that the survival rate decreased in patients with sepsis with cardiac dysfunction (septic cardiomyopathy).

Preexisting Cardiac Dysfunction in the Patient with Sepsis

Not only can sepsis itself cause cardiovascular dysfunction, but preexisting cardiac conditions can be exacerbated by sepsis and its treatment. A significant cardiac history, defined as prior myocardial infarction, abnormal treadmill report, nuclear medicine study, or coronary angiogram, or history of congestive heart failure or arrhythmia requiring treatment, was associated with increased mortality in severe sepsis and septic shock.[3]

Box 2

Cardiac dysfunction associated with sepsis

1. Reduced global left ventricular systolic function.

2. Decreased global longitudinal peak strain.

3. Depressed left ventricular ejection fraction (LVEF) (20%–60% of patients with septic shock).

4. Left ventricular dilatation.

5. Left ventricular diastolic dysfunction.[40]

6. Right ventricular systolic dysfunction.[41]

- Patients with sepsis with either systolic or diastolic dysfunction or a combination of both have higher mortality than those diagnosed with sepsis but without diastolic or systolic dysfunction. However, left ventricular systolic dysfunction associated with sepsis when defined as low LVEF is neither a sensitive nor a specific predictor of mortality.[42]

- Sepsis-associated cardiac dysfunction is reversible in survivors.

- Attenuation of the adrenergic response at the cardiomyocyte level likely explains the reduced response to exogenously administered catecholamines.

- Catecholamine-mediate myocardial injury may possibly occur in addition to septic (inflammatory)-mediated myocardial depression.

Preexisting coronary artery disease is especially problematic. For example, among patients with sepsis admitted to an emergency department, factors associated with progression to septic shock within 4 and 48 hours of arrival included female gender, nonpersistent hypotension, bands greater than or equal to 10%, serum lactate concentrations greater than or equal to 4.0 mmol/L, and a history of coronary artery disease.[4] Moreover, among patients with coronary artery disease the tachycardia and hypotension that occurs during septic shock can cause or exacerbate myocardial ischemia, whereas some vasopressors, such as epinephrine, used to treat hypotension can further exacerbate ischemia.[5] Dopamine, with its tendency to cause tachycardia, is especially problematic. Unlike dopamine and epinephrine, norepinephrine and vasopressin should produce less tachycardia and thus less myocardial ischemia. In a prospective randomized study of patients with septic shock there were no significant differences in troponin and creatinine kinase concentrations and electrocardiograms between those treated with vasopressin or norepinephrine.[6]

Preexisting heart failure is a mortality risk factor during the first 24 hours after admission for severe sepsis and septic shock.[7] It is also a risk factor for developing septic shock.[8] Similarly, congestive heart failure was a risk factor for mortality from nosocomial infections and among intensive care unit (ICU) patients.[9,10] Furthermore, chronic heart failure was also a risk factor for early (<3 days) mortality from sepsis.[11]

Underlying valvular disease can complicate sepsis and septic shock by impairing compensation for the hemodynamics demands of distributive shock. Therefore, treatment must include reducing the effects of the valvular lesion, such as percutaneous balloon mitral valvotomy in critical mitral stenosis.[12]

Noncardiac pulmonary hypertension, such as caused by chronic obstructive pulmonary disease, interstitial lung disease, or portopulmonary hypertension, is also a mortality risk factor in severe sepsis and septic shock. The severity of the pulmonary hypertension, new-onset atrial fibrillation/flutter (AF), and longer duration vasopressor support were associated with poor outcomes.[13] Moreover, sepsis itself might contribute to the pulmonary hypertension thus exacerbating the situation in patients with preexisting elevated pulmonary artery pressures.[14]

Combined Acute Cardiac Disease and Sepsis-Induced Cardiac Dysfunction

Bacterial endocarditis often combines acute cardiac dysfunction with sepsis/sepsis shock. Although systemic embolic events occur frequently in infective endocarditis, coronary embolization remains an uncommon cause of ST elevation myocardial infarction.[15] In acute native mitral valve endocarditis, patients with septic shock had more than 3.8 times greater risk of death than those with cardiogenic shock. This greater risk rose to more than four times versus patients without shock. Additionally, patients with septic shock had 4.2 times and 4.3 times higher risk of complications compared with patients with cardiogenic shock and without shock.[16] The conclusions were that valve-replacement surgery should be performed before septic shock intervenes.[16]

Sepsis and Septic Shock Causing Cardiac Dysfunction

In patients with sepsis with coexisting and possibly undiagnosed coronary artery disease, myocardial ischemia or infarction secondary to the coronary artery disease can occur as the results of the stresses of the sepsis, subsequent surgery, acidosis, and hypoxemia.[2] Precipitating events include hemodynamic changes and sepsis-induced microvascular dysfunction.[2]

Disseminated intravascular coagulopathy and stress-induced hypercoagulable state likely contribute to the development of myocardial ischemia or infarction associated with sepsis. Ischemic cardiac disease (myocardial infarction, unstable angina, cardiac arrest, or congestive heart failure) in critically ill medical patients is linked to increased mortality. When compared with critically ill medical patients without elevated serum concentrations of cardiac troponin I, those with elevated blood levels had greater hospital mortality.[17] This increased ICU and hospital mortality was also seen in critically ill patients with severe sepsis and elevated serum troponin concentrations. Yet, cardiac troponin did not independently predict hospital mortality.[18] Similarly, another study of patients with severe sepsis and septic shock showed that preexisting cardiac disease, and not troponin I elevation, was associated with increased mortality.[3] Furthermore, most patients with sepsis-associated troponin do not have a prior history of coronary artery disease.[19]

Among the cardiac problems that occur with sepsis is takotsubo syndrome or cardiomyopathy, an acquired and reversible syndrome. It is characterized by apical ballooning and base hypercontractility likely triggered by emotional and physical stresses causing a hyperadrenergic state. However, managing takotsubo syndrome in septic critically ill patients may be challenging because exogenous catecholamines used for circulatory support might further worsen the cardiomyopathy. This might require reducing or stopping the catecholamines. The calcium channel sensitizer, levosimendan, might be an alternative treatment.[20]

Why Does Concomitant Cardiac Dysfunction Increase Mortality in Sepsis?

The problem often encountered in patients with sepsis with underlying cardiac disease is the inability to compensate for the vasodilatory pathology. Such patients might not tolerate tachycardia either because it causes myocardial ischemia or prevents adequate cardiac filling. Some patients might not even be able to substantially increase heart rate. Furthermore, the ability of the left ventricle to undergo dilation might be compromised because of left ventricular hypertrophy, right ventricular dilation, and/or diastolic dysfunction. The inability to dilate the left ventricle is associated with reduced survival. Furthermore, sepsis-induced depression of the function of an already dysfunctional left or right ventricle can result in a hypodynamic state unable, even with inotropic and vasopressor support, to overcome the peripheral vasodilated condition, thus resulting in shock refractory to contemporary treatments.

MANAGEMENT GOALS

The initial hours (golden hours) of clinical management of severe sepsis represent an opportunity to decrease morbidity and mortality. Rapid clinical evaluation, timely resuscitation, early effective antimicrobial therapy and, if indicated, surgery, are key management to improved patient outcome. Anesthesiologists play a central role in the multidisciplinary management of patients with severe sepsis including ICU care and intraoperative management for emergency surgery. The timely administration of appropriate intravenous antimicrobial therapy is crucial when caring for patients with severe sepsis who may require source control surgery. Preoperative resuscitation, aimed at optimizing major organ perfusion/function, includes judicious use of fluids, vasopressors, and inotropes. Intraoperative anesthesia management requires attention to multiple issues (**Box 3**). Postoperative care overlaps with the ongoing management of the severe sepsis. These patients are by definition high risk and require much support along with experienced and skillful decision-making to optimize their chances of a favorable outcome.

Box 3
Considerations when anesthetizing a patient with severe sepsis or septic shock with cardiac dysfunction

1. Assess the current cardiovascular state to determine myocardial performance. This is achieved using focused transthoracic echocardiography; assessing hemodynamic state with invasive monitoring; and examining the electrocardiogram to determine whether there is systemic vasodilation, ischemia systolic failure, diastolic dysfunction, relative hypovolemia, hypervolemia, and/or right ventricle failure.

2. Intraoperative monitoring should be tailored to the patient's hemodynamic state and can include continuous intra-arterial monitoring, central venous pressure monitoring, transesophageal echocardiographic monitoring, pulmonary arterial catheter monitoring of pulmonary artery and pulmonary capillary wedge pressures, and continuous cardiac output trending. A urinary catheter should be in place to facilitate urine output monitoring.

3. Attempt to restore cardiovascular stability using vasopressor or inotropic drugs before anesthesia induction and adjust intraoperatively as necessary. The aim should be a mean arterial pressure of 70 to 75 mm Hg. Higher mean arterial pressures should be considered in patients with hypertension, especially if poorly controlled or uncontrolled.

4. Choose the safest induction agent and use as little as possible to provide conditions for intubation.

5. Select an anesthetic maintenance regimen that provides hemodynamic stability. If necessary, increase or add vasoactive agents to maintain blood pressure and peripheral perfusion.

6. Metabolic state should be monitored with arterial blood gases, blood glucose, and serum lactate concentrations.

7. Ensure that the appropriate antibiotics are administered at appropriate doses and intervals. Determine whether intraoperative administration is needed. Broad-spectrum antibiotics should be administered until causative organisms are identified.

8. Patients with preexisting cardiac disease often are receiving long-acting β-adrenergic blockers, such as carvedilol and atenolol, reducing the effects of β-adrenergic agonists. In this situation inotropic support might require adding the phosphodiesterase inhibitor milrinone or the calcium channel sensitizer levosimendan.

9. Patients with preexisting cardiac disease may be taking cardioactive agents, such as angiotensin-converting enzyme inhibitors, angiotensin receptor blockers, and/or calcium channel blockers, which have vasodilating and negative inotropic effects. This situation increases the requirements for pharmacologic support.

10. Pulmonary edema: In patients with pulmonary edema and sepsis plus coexisting cardiac disease, especially heart failure, it is necessary to distinguish between cardiogenic and noncardiogenic causes. This is accomplished using a pulmonary artery catheter and measuring the pulmonary occlusion pressure. Echocardiography might also be useful. Hypodynamic septic shock might mimic primary heart failure and it might be impossible to distinguish between them.

PHARMACOLOGIC STRATEGIES
Etomidate

Etomidate is a popular agent for the induction of anesthesia in hemodynamically unstable patients. This popularity is caused by etomidate's rapid and predictable onset of action and recovery, its relative hemodynamic stability, limited suppression of ventilation, and favorable safety profile. The standard induction dose of etomidate

(0.2–0.3 mg/kg) predictably and rapidly (within 5–15 seconds) causes hypnosis. Patients regain consciousness within 5 to 14 minutes.

Using etomidate during induction of anesthesia in septic shock has been controversial because of the drug's tendency to induce adrenal suppression. Prolonged etomidate infusions in patients with sepsis are associated with greater mortality, with adrenal suppression as the suspected cause. Therefore, there has been much debate as to whether a single dose of etomidate is safe to use in patients with sepsis. This debate has been occasioned by the observation that some patients with sepsis have adrenal insufficiency. The CORTICUS study reported steroid suppression in 60% of patients with sepsis who received etomidate, compared with 43% who did not. Suppression continued for up to 72 hours, indicating that adverse effects are possible even with a single bolus.[21,22] Adrenal insufficiency was diagnosed in 68 of 72 patients with sepsis given etomidate within the prior 72 hours as evidenced by their lack of response to high-dose cosyntropin stimulation. The incidence and mortality of adrenal insufficiency was investigated in a retrospective study of 65 patients with severe sepsis or septic shock when induced with etomidate or midazolam.[23] Hospital mortality rate was 36% in the etomidate group and 43% in the midazolam group, which was not statistically significant. The incidence of relative adrenal insufficiency was significantly higher in the etomidate group than in the midazolam group (84% and 48%, respectively; $P = .003$).[24] Therefore, the issue is not whether to use etomidate but whether to administer corticosteroids for a few days after a single etomidate dose.

Much of the mortality during induction of anesthesia is caused by cardiovascular events.[25] The clinical significance of these cardiovascular events can be debated, but etomidate does not cause significant acute hemodynamic instability like other induction agents. Although etomidate might cause adrenal suppression, the major cause of morbidity and mortality during sepsis is cardiovascular instability, the anesthesiologist's main focus should be on maintaining hemodynamic stability. In conclusion, consensus and a recent meta-analysis favors using etomidate for anesthesia induction in severe sepsis and septic shock,[26] although it is certainly reasonable to choose an alternative induction agent with the knowledge that dosage, monitoring, and available therapy must be tailored to lessen the likelihood of cardiovascular collapse.

Vasopressors–Inotropes

Treatment of hypotension in patients with sepsis with concomitant cardiac disease is challenging. Hyperdynamic septic shock is usually treated with vasopressors to increase the low systemic vascular resistance, with the drugs of choice being norepinephrine with or without vasopressin. Among the rationales for using vasopressin in septic shock are its potential cardioprotective mechanisms. Lower heart rates, higher arterial pressures, and lower norepinephrine doses during vasopressin therapy were hypothesized to protect the heart from myocardial ischemia. In a prospective substudy of the VASST (Vasopressin in Septic Shock Trial) project, Mehta and colleagues[6] evaluated this hypothesis, but failed to find lower cardiac biomarkers or fewer ischemic electrocardiographic changes in patients receiving vasopressin compared with those receiving only norepinephrine. However, among patients with ischemic heart disease it might be advisable to add a vasopressin infusion instead of increasing the rate of a catecholamine infusion, if the catecholamine induces excessive tachycardia. In patients with sepsis with preexisting heart failure or valvular disease who need inotropic support using β-adrenergic agonists might be problematic, especially if they induce excessive tachycardia and/or vasodilation. In the latter situation, it might be prudent to add a vasoconstrictor (eg, norepinephrine or vasopressin) to increase the systemic vascular resistance and raise the blood pressure. Some have advocated using levosimendan in such situations. A meta-analysis showed that in severe sepsis and septic shock, levosimendan is associated with a significant reduction in mortality compared with standard inotropic therapy.[27]

Glucose

Glucose homeostasis in sepsis runs the gamut from hyperglycemia secondary to the secretion of counterregulatory hormones to hypoglycemia likely caused by failure of the gluconeogenic mechanism. In septic shock, hyperglycemia is associated with greater morbidity, whereas even one episode of hypoglycemia is associated with greater mortality. Therefore, during anesthesia and surgery it is essential to closely monitor blood glucose concentrations, especially to detect and treat hypoglycemia. Elevated glucose concentrations are controlled with continuous insulin infusions to achieve a target glucose concentration between 140 and 180 mg/dL. Hypoglycemia is the feared complication of this treatment and, thus, during surgery close monitoring is required. Tight control of hyperglycemia during sepsis was considered a therapeutic approach that reduces morbidity and possibly mortality. However, despite initial enthusiasm, recent studies reported that tight glycemic control (80–100 mg/dL) using intensive insulin therapy failed to have a beneficial effect on mortality of patients with severe sepsis and septic shock, in part because of increased risk of hypoglycemia.

Steroids

The routine administration of corticosteroids in severe sepsis and septic shock is not recommended. However, hypotensive patients requiring high doses of vasopressors or unresponsive to such agents who have been adequately fluid resuscitated should be treated with stress doses (eg, 50 mg of intravenous hydrocortisone every 6 hours).[21]

Antibiotics

It is imperative that intravenous antibiotics be started as early as possible after the diagnosis of severe sepsis and septic shock. Moreover, it is important that appropriate culture samples be obtained before beginning the antimicrobial therapy.[28] Antimicrobial drugs are best given intravenously and in sufficient doses to achieve therapeutic concentrations. The choice of drugs should be based on clinical history, physical examination, imaging studies, likely pathogens, optimal penetration of antimicrobial drugs into infected tissues, and the local pattern of sensitivity to antimicrobial agents. Broad-spectrum agents should be used initially with one or more agents active against all possible bacterial/fungal pathogens.[28] During the intraoperative period it is important to administer antibiotics according to the presurgery schedule so that no doses are missed.

Anesthetics

Anesthetic agents can decrease contractility and cause vasodilation, attributable to direct drug effect and the depth of anesthesia reducing sympathetic tone. Therefore, anesthesia should be induced with the lowest dose of the safest drug. Propofol, unlike etomidate, may not be the safe choice of induction agent in patients with sepsis, whereas in some cases ketamine might be a substitute for etomidate. Yet, it should not be used in patients with concomitant heart failure, because of its negative inotropic effects in patients already experiencing maximal sympathetic stimulation and/or chronic catecholamine depletion, which attenuates the sympathomimetic effects of ketamine. In patients with coexisting coronary artery disease, ketamine-induced tachycardia might trigger cardiac ischemia. Maintenance of anesthesia requires coordination between dosing anesthetic agents, administering vasoactive drugs, and giving intravenous fluids, all directed by physiologic monitoring. This coordination is especially challenging when balancing the treatment of sepsis, the treatment of underlying cardiac dysfunction, and the need to maintain anesthesia.

NONPHARMACOLOGIC STRATEGIES

Anesthesia and surgery in the patient with sepsis with concomitant cardiac dysfunction can result in further hemodynamic and respiratory deterioration. Before surgery hemodynamics may seem to have stabilized with vasopressors and inotropes, while ventilation seems stabilized with high positive end-expiratory pressure and/or other respiratory modalities. However, surgical stresses can rapidly upset this pseudostability. In patients with evidence of major cardiac dysfunction already receiving maximal or near maximal pharmacologic support, some have advocated inserting an intra-aortic balloon pump before surgery. However, in the hyperdynamic patient with sepsis the further lowering of systemic resistance by intra-aortic balloon counterpulsation could be detrimental and thus is best avoided in such patients.[29] However, in low cardiac output states perioperative balloon counterpulsation might be useful, although it is associated with complications, such as femoral/iliac artery injury, groin hematoma, and lower limb ischemia.[30] The latter is especially problematic in patients receiving vasoconstrictors.

Extracorporeal venoarterial membrane oxygenation (ECMO) has been used to support cardiac and respiratory function in hypodynamic septic shock.[31] However, experience with ECMO in adults with septic shock is limited. The major limitation to ECMO involves situations with severely reduced systemic vascular resistance plus very low cardiac output, wherein even maximal ECMO blood flow may not restore adequate arterial blood flow or perfusion pressure. Furthermore, the need to anticoagulate, might limit its use during and immediately after surgery. Complications of ECMO are frequent and include renal failure, pneumonia, sepsis, and bleeding.[32]

Another modality that has been used in patients with severe sepsis is attempting to remove toxic substances with either extracorporeal removal of cytokines with continuous venoveno hemoperfusion or endotoxin adsorption with a polymyxin B column. The latter has been used in septic shock with endotoxemia confirmed by the endotoxin activity assay. Some have combined ECMO with continuous venoveno hemoperfusion to stabilize patients until the toxins have been reduced.[33]

Ventilation Strategies

Patients with sepsis are vulnerable to developing acute respiratory distress syndrome (ARDS). Therefore, protective ventilation strategies should be used during anesthesia and surgery even if there is no evidence of ARDS. In a meta-analysis among patients without ARDS, protective ventilation with lower tidal volumes (6 mL/kg) was associated with better clinical outcomes and shorter duration of mechanical ventilation.[34] Therefore, it is recommended that patients with sepsis be ventilated with lung protective strategies, also during surgery. When using low tidal volumes, especially during thoracic and abdominal surgery, it is important to intermittently perform recruitment maneuvers to treat and prevent atelectasis. In patients who have developed ARDS, it might also be necessary to use permissive hypercapnia and inhaled nitric oxide to maintain protective ventilation and oxygenation, respectively. With cardiac and noncardiac pulmonary hypertension inhaled nitric oxide might reduce pulmonary artery pressures and improve hemodynamics.

SURGICAL TREATMENT OPTIONS

In patients with sepsis with concurrent cardiac dysfunction source control surgery should be performed as soon as possible after diagnosis and initial hemodynamic stabilization. The surgery should be short and the concept of damage control used in unstable trauma patients should be invoked.[9] Therefore, the focus should be on infection source control using resection and/or wide drainage rather than definitive repair. An example of damage control is the approach to perforated diverticular disease with generalized peritonitis, using limited resection of the diseased segment, creation of a colostomy and mucous fistula, abdominal lavage, and application of a vacuum-assisted closure dressing.[35] If necessary, the abdomen should be left open to avoid abdominal compartment syndrome. After the initial surgery the patients should be resuscitated and stabilized hemodynamically in the ICU. In patients with concomitant cardiac disease this period is critical because additional fluid "third-spacing" can occur requiring fluid resuscitation, which must be performed with caution in such patients. Treating acidosis, hypothermia, and hyperthermia is a key to improving cardiac function. Once the patient is stabilized, further surgery should be contemplated, if necessary. Subsequent surgery often focuses on further septic source control, using debridement and drainage. Definitive surgery must often wait until the sepsis has resolved and the patient has recovered. The major complications in a series of 42 nontrauma damage control laparotomies were sepsis (14 patients) and intra-abdominal collections (10 patients). There were significantly fewer postoperative complications among those undergoing early abdominal closure.[36]

TREATMENT RESISTANCE/COMPLICATIONS

Resistance to treatment with vasoactive and inotropic agents should make one consider the possibility of adrenal corticosteroid insufficiency and/or hypothyroidism. The former might be absolute (ie, adrenal shutdown) or relative (insufficient cortisol for the degree of stress). If adrenal insufficiency is suspected as causing treatment resistance then "stress" dose corticosteroid therapy should be started. Another possible cause is real hypothyroidism (not "sick" euthyroid disorder), which can be rapidly diagnosed with thyrotropin-stimulating hormone and free T4 assays. If the patient is hypothyroid, careful treatment with intravenous T3 is indicated. Another cause of resistance to vasoactive and inotropic agents is low pH (<7.2), which might reduce cardiac function and the effectiveness of administered catecholamines. Judicious therapy to increase the pH is indicated to improve the response to catecholamines.

ATRIAL FIBRILLATION

AF and other supraventricular arrhythmias are the most common arrhythmias found in adult ICU patients. Theses arrhythmias can either be new-onset or preexisting. The latter condition is not unexpected because the prevalence of chronic AF increases with age (0.7% in the 55–59 age group; 18% in the ≥85 age group). Critically ill patients who develop new-onset AF are a special group. They are divided into those with and without chest cavity pathology. After thoracic and cardiac surgery, AF occurs with regularity (eg, among 12%–45% of patients after pulmonary and esophageal surgery). Within 2 to 3 days after cardiac surgery up to 80% of patients develop AF. New-onset AF in critically ill patients without major chest cavity problem is common.

Holter monitoring of 66 medical ICU patients with septic shock revealed that 29 (44%) developed new-onset AF associated with advanced age and left ventricular ejection fraction less than 45%.[37] Besides being associated with older age, new-onset AF is associated with sepsis.[27] This association with sepsis has led to the idea that AF is a marker and not the cause of the increased mortality, that is, it is a manifestation of multiple organ system dysfunction.

Therefore, when anesthetizing patients with sepsis, especially those with cardiac disease, there is a high likelihood that new-onset AF will develop. Treatment is difficult because this AF is often resistant to cardioversion and pharmacologic treatment. Amiodarone, as opposed to β-adrenergic antagonists, is often the treatment of choice. Although β-adrenergic and calcium channel antagonists have been used in patients with sepsis, their negative inotropic effects must be considered. Moreover, patients with chronic AF, either sustained or paroxysmal, likely will need rate control because of elevated ventricular rates secondary to the sepsis or treatment with β-adrenergic agonists. Vasopressin seems to decrease the incidence of new-onset arrhythmias.[38]

ANTICOAGULATION

Another issue when managing patients with sepsis with concomitant cardiac disease is that many are receiving anticoagulant and antiplatelet therapy. Therefore, when such patients are taken for emergent or urgent surgery the consequences of this therapy must be considered. In those receiving warfarin rapid reversal of their anticoagulation is achieved with prothrombin complex concentrate (a combination of factors II, VII, IX, and X) or more slowly with low-dose intravenous vitamin K. Fresh frozen plasma can also be used but the large volume required might prove problematic in patients with heart failure. Reversal of novel oral anticoagulants (dabigatran, rivaroxaban, apixaban) is problematic, although reversal agents are in development. Timely, reversal of potent, long-acting antiplatelet agents (eg, clopidogrel and prasugrel) is not possible in emergency surgery, resulting in the need for platelet transfusions and managing increased bleeding. The consequences of stopping anticoagulation must also be considered, especially in patients with prosthetic heart valves and intracoronary stents.

EVALUATION OF OUTCOME AND LONG-TERM RECOMMENDATIONS

Mortality from serious sepsis and septic shock remains extremely high despite much effort to improve treatment regimens. Patients who survive severe sepsis and septic shock frequently have long convalescences. The metabolic effects of sepsis cause physical (critical care polymyopathy and polyneuropathy) weakness and mental fatigue that affect mobilization and activities of daily living.[39]

In the immediate period of convalescence the patient must diuresis the large volumes of intravenous fluid used in the initial resuscitation. This is especially problematic when the cardiovascular system is unable to deal with a sudden influx of fluid. Patients with underlying heart failure and/or valvular lesions are especially vulnerable to deterioration of cardiovascular homeostasis. Some of these patients need further surgery during this period so it is important to evaluate their fluid status and ability to deal with the fluid shifts during and after surgery. Furthermore, the tachycardia caused by the need to compensate for the increased intravascular volume might trigger myocardial ischemia. The stress associated with convalescing from the metabolic and hemodynamic perturbations caused by sepsis make those suffering from ischemic heart disease vulnerable to acute coronary events. Furthermore, these patients are vulnerable to repeat bouts of sepsis, especially nosocomial ones.

EVALUATION
Ultrasound/Echocardiography

The noninvasive nature and instantaneous diagnostic capability of bedside echocardiography (transthoracic and transesophageal) make its use extremely valuable in severe sepsis and septic shock, especially when there is hemodynamic compromise. Echocardiography is useful in managing the patient with septic shock (**Box 4**). In recent years, echocardiography has aided in elucidating the characteristics of sepsis-related myocardial dysfunction. Although not proven yet in terms of patient outcome, echocardiography is regarded as an important intraoperative monitoring tool in patients with sepsis with concomitant cardiac disease.

Biomarkers: Troponin and B-Type Natriuretic Peptide

The diagnostic and prognostic uses of biomarkers, such as cardiac troponins and natriuretic peptides, in critically ill patients warrant definition. Elevated troponin concentrations in sepsis, severe sepsis, or septic shock indicate a poor prognosis. However, in this population troponin release also occurs in the absence of flow-limiting coronary artery disease, suggesting mechanisms other than thrombotic coronary artery occlusion are operative, that is, possibly transient loss of membrane integrity with troponin leakage or microvascular thrombotic injury. Therefore, in sepsis with concomitant cardiac dysfunction, an elevated troponin concentration might not indicate primary cardiac problems. In contrast to troponin, the implications of elevated B-type natriuretic peptide (BNP) concentrations in sepsis are less clear. The relationship between BNP and left ventricular ejection fraction and left-sided filling pressures is weak, whereas data on the prognostic impact of high BNP levels in sepsis are conflicting. Mechanisms other than left ventricular wall stress may contribute to BNP release, including right ventricular overload, catecholamine therapy, renal failure, central nervous system disease, and cytokine up-regulation. Whereas cardiac troponins may be used in monitoring patients during severe sepsis or septic shock, to identify those requiring early and aggressive supportive therapy, routine measurement of BNP and other natriuretic peptides is currently not indicated.

SUMMARY

Anesthesia in patients with sepsis with preexisting or sepsis-induced cardiac dysfunction is challenging because the interaction of these two conditions greatly complicates management. Often therapeutic modalities that are effective in treating one of these conditions are rendered ineffective by the presence of both conditions. Therefore,

---

Box 4
Uses of echocardiography in sepsis

1. Differential diagnosis of shock and recognition of sepsis-associated myocardial dysfunction

2. Detecting preexisting cardiac pathology, thus aiding in simultaneously managing the hemodynamic effects of the sepsis and the cardiodynamic consequences of the cardiac problem

3. Hemodynamic monitoring through repeated bedside assessments

4. Complementing hemodynamic information obtained from other monitoring and diagnostic modalities

5. Screening for intracardiac sources of sepsis, such as bacterial endocarditits

during anesthesia and surgery such patients require close physiologic monitoring to guide rapid effective responses to hemodynamic perturbations and then assess the effects of such therapy. Anesthetic management usually requires multiple vasoactive drugs directed by hemodynamic and metabolic monitoring including transesophageal echocardiography. Unfortunately, such patients have increased mortality because of the difficulty in optimally and simultaneously managing both the cardiac dysfunction and sepsis.

REFERENCES

1. D'Orio V, Mendes P, Saad G, et al. Accuracy in early prediction of prognosis of patients with septic shock by analysis of simple indices: prospective study. Crit Care Med 1990;18:1339–45.
2. Merx MW, Weber C. Sepsis and the heart. Circulation 2007;116:793–802.
3. Scott EC, Ho HC, Yu M, et al. Pre-existing cardiac disease, troponin I elevation and mortality in patients with severe sepsis and septic shock. Anaesth Intensive Care 2008;36:51–9.
4. Capp R, Horton CL, Takhar SS, et al. Predictors of patients who present to the emergency department with sepsis and progress to septic shock between 4 and 48 hours of emergency department arrival. Crit Care Med 2015;43:983–8.
5. Dünser MW, Hasibeder WR. Sympathetic overstimulation during critical illness: adverse effects of adrenergic stress. J Intensive Care Med 2009;24:293–316.
6. Mehta S, Granton J, Gordon AC, et al. Vasopressin and Septic Shock Trial (VASST) Investigators. Cardiac ischemia in patients with septic shock randomized to vasopressin or norepinephrine. Crit Care 2013;17:R117.
7. Grozdanovski K, Milenkovic Z, Demiri I, et al. Early prognosis in patients with community-acquired severe sepsis and septic shock: analysis of 184 consecutive cases. Prilozi 2012;33:105–16.
8. Hsiao CY, Yang HY, Chang CH, et al. Risk factors for development of septic shock in patients with urinary tract infection. Biomed Res Int 2015;2015:717094.
9. Sheng WH, Wang JT, Lin MS, et al. Risk factors affecting in-hospital mortality in patients with nosocomial infections. J Formos Med Assoc 2007;106:110–8.
10. Degoricija V, Sharma M, Legac A, et al. Survival analysis of 314 episodes of sepsis in medical intensive care unit in university hospital: impact of intensive care unit performance and antimicrobial therapy. Croat Med J 2006;47:385–97.
11. Garnacho-Montero J, Garcia-Garmendia JL, Barrero-Almodovar A, et al. Impact of adequate empirical antibiotic therapy on the outcome of patients admitted to the intensive care unit with sepsis. Crit Care Med 2003;31:2742–51.
12. Litmanovitch M, Joynt GM, Skoularigis J, et al. Emergency percutaneous balloon mitral valvotomy in a patient with septic shock. Chest 1995;108:570–2.
13. Tsapenko MV, Herasevich V, Mour GK, et al. Severe sepsis and septic shock in patients with pre-existing non-cardiac pulmonary hypertension: contemporary management and outcomes. Crit Care Resusc 2013;15:103–9.
14. Spapen H, Vincken W. Pulmonary arterial hypertension in sepsis and the adult respiratory distress syndrome. Acta Clin Belg 1992;47:30–41.
15. Hibbert B, Kazmi M, Veinot JP, et al. Infective endocarditis presenting as ST-elevation myocardial infarction: an angiographic diagnosis. Can J Cardiol 2012;28:515.e15-7.
16. Gelsomino S, Maessen JG, van der Veen F, et al. Emergency surgery for native mitral valve endocarditis: the impact of septic and cardiogenic shock. Ann Thorac Surg 2012;93:1469–76.

17. Kollef MH, Ladenson JH, Eisenberg PR. Clinically recognized cardiac dysfunction: an independent determinant of mortality among critically ill patients. Is there a role for serial measurement of cardiac troponin I? Chest 1997;111:1340–7.
18. Tiruvoipati R, Sultana N, Lewis D. Cardiac troponin I does not independently predict mortality in critically ill patients with severe sepsis. Emerg Med Australas 2012;24:151–8.
19. Hussain N. Elevated cardiac troponins in setting of systemic inflammatory response syndrome, sepsis, and septic shock. ISRN Cardiol 2013;2013:723435.
20. Karvouniaris M, Papanikolaou J, Makris D, et al. Sepsis-associated takotsubo cardiomyopathy can be reversed with levosimendan. Am J Emerg Med 2012; 30:832.e5-e7.
21. Sprung CL, Annane D, Keh D, et al, CORTICUS Study Group. Hydrocortisone therapy for patients with septic shock. N Engl J Med 2008;358:111–24.
22. Cuthbertson BH, Sprung CL, Annane D, et al. The effects of etomidate on adrenal responsiveness and mortality in patients with septic shock. Intensive Care Med 2009;35:1868–76.
23. Tekwani KL, Watts HF, Sweis RT, et al. A comparison of the effects of etomidate and midazolam on hospital length of stay in patients with suspected sepsis: a prospective, randomized study. Ann Emerg Med 2010;56:481–9.
24. Kim TY, Rhee JE, Kim KS, et al. Etomidate should be used carefully for emergent endotracheal intubation in patients with septic shock. J Korean Med Sci 2008;23: 988–91.
25. Erdoes G, Basciani RM, Eberle B. Etomidate: a review of robust evidence for its use in various clinical scenarios. Acta Anaesthesiol Scand 2014;58:380–9.
26. Gu WJ, Wang F, Tang L, et al. Single-dose etomidate does not increase mortality in patients with sepsis: a systematic review and meta-analysis of randomized controlled trials and observational studies. Chest 2015;147:335–46.
27. Makrygiannis SS, Margariti A, Rizikou D, et al. Incidence and predictors of new-onset atrial fibrillation in noncardiac intensive care unit patients. J Crit Care 2014; 29:697.e1-5.
28. Handelsman J, Maki DG. Does combination antimicrobial therapy reduce mortality in gram-negative bacteraemia? A meta-analysis. Lancet Infect Dis 2004;4: 519–27.
29. Krishna M, Zacharowski K. Principles of intra-aortic balloon pump counterpulsation. Cont Educ Anaesth Crit Care Pain 2009;9:24–8.
30. Siu SC, Kowalchuk GJ, Welty FK, et al. Intra-aortic balloon counterpulsation support in the high-risk cardiac patient undergoing urgent noncardiac surgery. Chest 1991;99:1342–5.
31. Park TK, Yang JH, Jeon K, et al. Extracorporeal membrane oxygenation for refractory septic shock in adults. Eur J Cardiothorac Surg 2015;47:e68–74.
32. Zangrillo A, Landoni G, Biondi-Zoccai G, et al. A meta-analysis of complications and mortality of extracorporeal membrane oxygenation. Crit Care Resusc 2013; 15:172–8.
33. Bruenger F, Kizner L, Weile J, et al. First successful combination of ECMO with cytokine removal therapy in cardiogenic septic shock: a case report. Int J Artif Organs 2015;38:113–6, 37.
34. Serpa Neto A, Cardoso SO, Manetta JA, et al. Association between use of lung-protective ventilation with lower tidal volumes and clinical outcomes among patients without acute respiratory distress syndrome: a meta-analysis. JAMA 2012;308:1651–9.

35. Cirocchi R, Arezzo A, Vettoretto N, et al. Role of damage control surgery in the treatment of Hinchey III and IV sigmoid diverticulitis: a tailored strategy. Medicine (Baltimore) 2014;93:e184.
36. Khan A, Hsee L, Mathur S, et al. Damage-control laparotomy in nontrauma patients: review of indications and outcomes. J Trauma Acute Care Surg 2013;75: 365–8.
37. Guenancia C, Binquet C, Laurent G, et al. Incidence and predictors of new-onset atrial fibrillation in septic shock patients in a medical ICU: data from 7-day Holter ECG monitoring. PLoS One 2015;10(5):e0127168.
38. Reardon DP, DeGrado JR, Anger KE, et al. Early vasopressin reduces incidence of new onset arrhythmias. J Crit Care 2014;29:482–5.
39. Zhang K, Mao X, Fang Q, et al. Impaired long-term quality of life in survivors of severe sepsis: Chinese multicenter study over 6 years. Anaesthesist 2013;62: 995–1002.
40. Landesberg G, Jaffe AS, Gilon D, et al. Troponin elevation in severe sepsis and septic shock: the role of left ventricular diastolic dysfunction and right ventricular dilatation. Crit Care Med 2014;42:790–800.
41. Landesberg G, Gilon D, Meroz Y, et al. Diastolic dysfunction and mortality in severe sepsis and septic shock. Eur Heart J 2012;33:895–903.
42. Sevilla Berrios RA, O'Horo JC, Velagapudi V, et al. Correlation of left ventricular systolic dysfunction determined by low ejection fraction and 30-day mortality in patients with severe sepsis and septic shock: a systematic review and meta-analysis. J Crit Care 2014;29:495–9.

Anesthesia for Patients with Peripheral Vascular Disease and Cardiac Dysfunction

Sara E. Neves, MD*

KEYWORDS

- Vascular disease • Cardiac dysfunction • Perioperative ischemia
- Peripheral arterial disease • Coronary artery disease

KEY POINTS

- Vascular disease and cardiac dysfunction are linked in many ways. They share common risk factors and comorbidities.
- Patients with systemic vascular disease often have concomitant heart disease; the blood vessels of the heart are not spared. Poor cardiac function worsens peripheral arterial disease.
- Preoperative surgical risk stratification and workup are important steps in the care of these complicated patients.
- Many of these patients require additional monitoring such as intraarterial blood pressure monitoring, central line placement, and perioperative echocardiography.
- Early recognition and treatment of complications such as myocardial ischemia, stroke, or limb ischemia will improve outcomes.

Vascular disease and cardiac dysfunction are linked in many ways. They share common risk factors and comorbidities, and patients with systemic vascular disease often have concomitant heart disease, because the blood vessels of the heart are not spared. In patients presenting for surgery, the presence of vascular disease puts the patient at increased risk for perioperative cardiac complications, and vascular surgery poses the highest surgical risk for perioperative cardiac events. In addition, the diseased vessels supplying critical organs depend on the perfusion pressure supplied by the heart, so any cardiac dysfunction thus amplifies the effect of poor perfusion. Patients presenting with both vascular disease and cardiac dysfunction pose a particular challenge to the anesthesiologist; although treatment goals are similar, small physiologic disturbances can quickly lead to large, serious changes in clinical status.

Disclosures: No disclosures to make or conflicts of interest.
Department of Anesthesia, Critical Care, and Pain Medicine, Beth Israel Deaconess Medical Center, 330 Brookline Avenue, Boston, MA 02215, USA
* 1580 Massachusetts Avenue, Apartment 5C, Cambridge, MA 02138.
E-mail address: saraeneves@gmail.com

Anesthesiology Clin 34 (2016) 775–795
http://dx.doi.org/10.1016/j.anclin.2016.06.011
1932-2275/16/© 2016 Elsevier Inc. All rights reserved.

Vascular disease comprises a wide spectrum of afflictions, from those affecting the major arteries, to the blood supply to critical organs, to inflammation of the entire vasculature. The often systemic nature of vascular disease means that any organ with a blood supply (thus, every organ) can be compromised. Optimizing and maintaining cardiac perfusion is therefore especially critical, because cardiac function is a major factor in maintaining perfusion of every other organ.

The spectrum of cardiac disease is similarly broad. Coronary artery disease, conduction abnormalities, valvular disease, and congestive heart failure (HF) all imply impaired cardiac function, which leads to poor perfusion of organs. A brief discussion of each, with particular attention to coronary artery atherosclerosis, follows.

ISCHEMIC HEART DISEASE

Coronary artery disease, or ischemic heart disease (IHD) is characterized by atherosclerosis of coronary blood vessels. This deposition of plaques can lead to stenosis of the vessels and also put the patient at risk for sudden plaque rupture and vessel occlusion. The most common risk factors for IHD are listed below.

Risk Factors for Ischemic Heart Disease

- Male gender,
- Age,
- Dyslipidemia,
- Systemic hypertension,
- Cigarette smoking,
- Diabetes mellitus,
- Obesity,
- Sedentary lifestyle, and
- Family history of IHD.

Cardiac tissue already maximally extracts oxygen that is delivered via coronary vessels. Therefore, the only way to increase oxygen supply to the heart is by increasing perfusion, mainly through coronary artery dilatation. When atherosclerosis of the coronaries causes stenosis, the heart compensates by vasodilatation. This can balance oxygen demand and supply at rest, but with exercise, the heart can no longer compensate, leading to local ischemia and the typical exertional angina symptoms experienced by the patient. This is the same mechanism causing claudication in patients with peripheral arterial disease (PAD), who feel a dull, crushing, or aching patient in the affected extremity with exertion that is relieved by rest.

In contrast, plaque rupture causes an acute narrowing or occlusion of a coronary vessel, so that there is a sudden imbalance of oxygen demand and supply, or a complete lack of oxygen supply to the affected area of cardiac muscle. This ischemia pain will not be relieved by rest and in the case of a transmural infarction, is the most serious presentation of an acute coronary syndrome. Acute coronary syndrome is correlated with a hypercoagulable state; plaque rupture activates the coagulation cascade that then leads to partial or complete occlusion of the coronary vessel. There are 3 subtypes of acute coronary syndrome—unstable angina, non–ST-elevation myocardial infarction, or ST-elevation myocardial infarction.

Ischemic Heart Disease and Acute Coronary Syndromes

A diagnosis of IHD is made by careful history and physical examination, with specific inquiry into the presence of risk factors, angina symptoms, and assessment of the patient's exercise tolerance (**Fig. 1**). Diagnostic tests include electrocardiography (ECG)

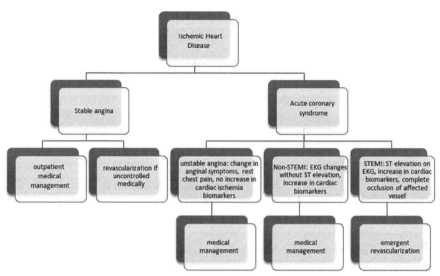

Fig. 1. Diagnosis of ischemic heart disease and acute coronary syndromes. EKG, electrocardiograph; STEMI, ST-elevation myocardial infarction.

or echocardiography, often with a functional component to examine cardiac function under stress rather than simply at rest (**Table 1**). A cardiac catheterization is the definitive test to determine the presence of coronary atherosclerosis; however, as an invasive procedure with nontrivial risks, this is usually reserved for highest risk patients.

Stress Testing

Treatment of IHD is 4-fold.
1. Treatment of associated diseases that either increase oxygen demand (such as infection, fever, thyrotoxicosis, tachycardia) or decrease oxygen delivery (severe

Table 1
Stress testing

Stress Test Type	Stress Source	Parameter Measured	Appropriate Test Subjects
ECG stress	Exercise	ECG changes	• Able to reach target heart rate with exercise • No previous ECG abnormalities (bundle branch blocks)
Nuclear stress	• Exercise • Chronotrope (dobutamine) • Coronary vasodilator (adenosine)	Uptake of nuclear tracer into active contracting cardiac muscle	• No contraindications to nuclear testing • Exercise not required
Echocardiography	• Exercise • Chronotrope (dobutamine) • Coronary vasodilator (adenosine)	Observation of regional wall motion abnormalities	• Anatomically straightforward echocardiography • Exercise not required

anemia, elevated filling pressures) will decrease ischemia by restoring oxygen supply/demand balance.
2. Lifestyle modifications such as maintaining an ideal body weight, treating dyslipidemia and hypertension, smoking cessation, and regular aerobic exercise can help slow progression of the disease.
3. Pharmacologic treatment of IHD includes beta-blockers to improve coronary perfusion (by increasing diastolic time), treatment of hypertension, and prevention of dysrhythmias, angiotensin-converting enzyme inhibitors to reduce risk of left ventricle dysfunction and remodeling, nitrates to vasodilate coronaries and reduce left ventricular afterload during an acute episode of angina, and antiplatelet agents to limit activation of coagulation cascade should a plaque rupture.
4. Revascularization is indicated when medical management cannot resolve angina, when there is flow-limiting stenosis of a coronary artery, or when left ventricular function is affected to the point that the ejection fraction is less than 40%. Revascularization is either via percutaneous coronary intervention (PCI), with or without stent placement, or with a surgical approach of coronary artery bypass grafting.

VALVULAR DISEASE

Clinical suspicion for a valvular problem is raised when patients present with exertional dyspnea, chest pain, syncope, signs of volume overload, or a new murmur on examination. Diagnosis is made with auscultation, echocardiography, cardiac MRI, or cardiac catheterization with measurements of flow velocity and gradients.

Stenotic valvular lesions typically cause pressure overload to the affected ventricle or atrium, leading to cardiac hypertrophy. Stenotic lesions require avoidance of tachycardia, which limit the time the heart has to push past the stenosis, and also limits time for coronary perfusion, which is especially important in the hypertrophied muscle. In particular, aortic stenosis limits blood flow from the left ventricle to the rest of the arterial system. Central and peripheral vasoconstriction must occur to maintain perfusion pressure to distal sites, including coronary arteries. Sudden vasodilatation, as with induction of general anesthesia, can compromise this perfusion and lead to ischemia of vital organs, most dramatically cardiac ischemia, which then leads to a decrease in cardiac function, limiting the heart's ability to push blood past the stenosis, further reducing perfusion, causing a dreaded "cycle of death" that occurs if perfusion is unable to be restored. In patients with mitral or aortic stenosis, volume overload, loss of sinus rhythm, and tachycardia can affect the left atrium's ability to eject through the stenosis and can result in pulmonary edema.

In contrast, regurgitant valvular lesions result in volume overload to the affected ventricle or atrium. Regurgitant lesions result in a loss of effective cardiac output owing to a fraction of stroke volume flowing backward through the insufficient valve. These lesions require afterload reduction and mild tachycardia to maintain forward flow and limit the regurgitant fraction.

Hypertrophied or dilated cardiac muscle can make the heart prone to arrhythmias, most often atrial fibrillation. Loss of atrial kick can reduce cardiac output dramatically in a patient with valvular disease. Maintaining sinus rhythm is an important way to compensate for cardiac dysfunction owing to a valvular lesion.

Arrhythmias and Conduction Abnormalities

An arrhythmia can be described as an abnormal path of conduction and can originate in either the atrium or the ventricle, presenting as either tachyarrhythmias or bradyarrhythmias. They are caused by increased automaticity, either in normally conducting or normally nonconducting myocytes, reentry through abnormal pathways, or abnormal cardiac potentials triggered during diastole.

Conduction abnormalities are a break or a blockage in the conduction pathway. They are described by the location and severity (degree) of the blockade. The most common arrhythmias and conduction abnormalities are described below.

Sinus Tachycardia

- Heart rate greater than 100.
- Nonpathologic; a normal physiologic response.

Sinus Bradycardia

- Heart rate of less than 60.
- Can be physiologic in patients with strong vagal tone; well-conditioned athletes.
- Can be iatrogenic owing to beta-blockade or other antiarrhythmic agents.
- Can be pathologic if the patient is unable to increase heart rate in response to physiologic demand, or has associated symptoms (dizziness, syncope).

Premature Beats

- Atrial: usually benign, abnormal P wave with narrow QRS complex, no compensatory pause, not indicative of developing malignant dysrhythmia, caused by excessive sympathetic stimulation, caffeine, alcohol, stress, and recreational drugs; can lead to supraventricular tachycardia.
- Ventricular: no P-wave, wide QRS complex, often followed by a compensatory pause, can lead to malignant arrhythmias as ventricular tachycardia or ventricular fibrillation via R-on-T phenomenon.

Atrial Fibrillation

- Most common sustained cardiac dysrhythmia.
- Rapid disordered atrial electrical activity.
- Variable conduction to ventricle, with ventricular response up to 180 bpm.
- Loss of coordinated atrial contraction.
- Typically requires anticoagulation to reduce risk of arterial emboli owing to clot from low-flow state within left atrium.
- Atrial flutter has a predictable conduction through to ventricle, in a 1:1, 1:2, 1:3, or 1:4 ratio, but association with atrial fibrillation requires prophylactic anticoagulation.

Multifocal Atrial Tachycardia

- Typically hemodynamically stable.
- Usually associated with pulmonary disease.
- Presence of 3 or more P-wave morphologies.
- No anticoagulation required.

Supraventricular Tachycardia

- Narrow QRS complex tachycardia, with heart rates of greater than 160 bpm.
- Typically caused by an accessory conducting pathway so that conduction travels anterograde through the atrioventricular (AV) node, retrograde through the accessory pathway, creating a loop of rapid conduction, called AV-node reentrant tachycardia.
- Treated with vagal maneuvers, beta-blockers, or calcium channel blockers (for patients with stable hemodynamics) or with adenosine or cardioversion (unstable hemodynamics).

- Wolf–Parkinson–White syndrome is a congenital conduction abnormality with paroxysmal episodes of supraventricular tachycardia.

Ventricular Tachycardia

- Three or more premature ventricular beats occurring together at a rate of greater than 120 bpm.
- No P-waves, wide QRS complexes.
- Can deteriorate into ventricular fibrillation.
- Can be related to myocardial ischemia (acute myocardial infarction), structural abnormalities, mechanical ventilation, central catheter insertion, or drug therapy.
- Managed pharmacologically if hemodynamically stable, with cardioversion if not.
- Torsade de Pointes: polymorphic ventricular tachycardia related to prolongation of QT interval; treated with cardioversion, intravenous magnesium, withdrawal of QT prolonging medications.

Ventricular Fibrillation

- Rapid uncoordinated depolarization of cardiac myocytes.
- No organized contraction of ventricle.
- Always associated with pulselessness and lack of cardiac output.
- Most common cause of sudden cardiac death.
- Cardiopulmonary resuscitation must be initiated immediately.
- Electrical defibrillation is only reliable method to convert to regular rhythm; best outcomes occur if defibrillation occurs within 3 to 5 minutes of event.
- Pharmacologic agents will not circulate in a no cardiac output state.

Atrioventricular Heart Block

- Disruption of the conduction signal traveling from sinus node to AV node and His-Purkinje system.
- First degree: length of PR interval of greater than 200 ms, every P wave conducts to a normal QRS, patients are typically asymptomatic, no pacemaker is required.
- Second-degree AV heart block:
  ○ Mobitz type 1: progressive prolongation of PR interval until beat is dropped; usually asymptomatic.
  ○ Mobitz type 2: sudden interruption of conduction, or dropped beat, without prolongation of PR interval, in an unpredictable manner, usually symptomatic and often progresses to third-degree heart block.
- Third-degree heart block: complete disassociation between sinus and AV node, both conducting independently. Ventricular escape rate can be 30 to 55 bpm, usually too slow for adequate cardiac output. Exogenous cardiac pacing is required; atropine or isoproterenol are administered for acute episodes of complete heart block as pacing is being instituted.

Bundle Branch Blocks

- Related to structural heart disease or myocardial ischemia.
- Right bundle branch block often of little clinical significance.
- Left bundle branch block associated with poorer prognosis.
- Both can rarely lead to complete heart block.
- Patients with left bundle branch block in whom a pulmonary artery catheter (PAC) is placed should have special precautions taken, because 2% to 5% of patients develop transient right bundle branch block during placement of a PAC; if left bundle branch block is already present, this could lead to complete heart block.

Cardiac Implanted Electronic Devices

- Can function as pacemakers, defibrillators, or both (**Table 2**).

HEART FAILURE

Congestive heart failure (HF) is the lack of cardiac output to appropriately meet tissue perfusion requirements. The ejection fraction may be preserved (diastolic HF) or reduced (systolic HF). Pathology and progression of the disease is related to structural changes in the heart and remodeling, which lead to ineffective pumping and a reduction in cardiac output. These structural abnormalities can also predispose the heart to life-threatening arrhythmias. Patients with severely reduced ejection fraction benefit from an automated implantable defibrillator and may benefit from resynchronization therapy via dual chamber pacing to resynchronize ventricular contraction between the right and left ventricles.

IHD is the most common etiology, with dilated cardiomyopathy the second most common. Patients present with progressive exercise intolerance, dyspnea, orthopnea, and signs of volume overload. The disease is classified by symptomatology and also by staging as defined by the American College of Cardiology and the American Heart Association.

New York Heart Association Classification of Heart Failure

Class I: asymptomatic
Class II: limited strenuous activity owing to dyspnea.
Class III: limited mild-moderate activity owing to dyspnea.
Class IV: dyspnea at rest.

American College of Cardiology/American Heart Association Stages of Congestive Heart Failure

Stage A: high risk but no diagnosis of heart failure (risk factors, family history, or using cardiotoxins).
Stage B: structural heart disease without symptoms of HF (valvular disease, left ventricular hypertrophy or systolic dysfunction, previous myocardial infarction).
Stage C: structural heart disease with symptoms of HF (exercise intolerance, dyspnea).
Stage D: refractory HF requiring intervention (infusions, cardiac implantable electronic device, mechanical devices).[1]

Treatment of Congestive Heart Failure

- Avoid ventricular remodeling with angiotensin-converting enzyme inhibitors.
- Loop diuretics to treat volume overload and avoid pulmonary congestion.
- Management of other risk factors (treating IHD, hypertension, valvular disease).

Table 2
Cardiac implanted electronic devices

A/V/D/O	A/V/D/O	I/T/D/O	P/M/C/R/O	P/S/D/O
Pacing chamber	Sensing chamber	Response to sensing	Programmability	Antitachycardia functions

Abbreviations: A, atrial; C, communicating; D, dual; I, inhibits; M, multiprogram; O, none; P, pacing; P, programmable; R, rate modulation; S, shock; T, triggers; V, ventricular.

- Inotropic drugs, cardiac resynchronization therapy, and possible implantation of mechanical devices (late stage disease).
- For right HF: reducing pulmonary hypertension by treating chronic alveolar hypoxia with oxygen therapy.

Hypertrophic Obstructive Cardiomyopathy

- Most common genetic cardiac disorder other than a bicuspid aortic valve.
- Sudden death caused by acute left ventricular outflow obstruction and ventricular dysrhythmias.
- Treatment focused on maintaining intravascular and intracardiac volume and avoiding tachycardia.

VASCULAR DISEASE

Vascular disease is manifest differently depending on the affected vessels. Disease of the large central vessels such as the aorta include aneurysms or aortic dissection (**Boxes 1** and **2**). An aortic aneurysm is defined as a dilation of all 3 layers of arterial wall such that the aortic diameter of the vessel is greater than 50% of normal. In contrast, a dissection is a tear in the vessel wall that results in communication of the lumen of the vessel and the potential space in between layers of the arterial wall. As blood is pumped through the vessel, a fraction of the blood flow tracks along the interior walls of the vessel, creating a false lumen. The most common risk factors associated with aortic aneurysms and dissection are male gender, age greater than 65 years, hypertension, and atherosclerosis, much like risk factors of cardiac disease and peripheral vascular disease.

Carotid Disease

The prevalence of asymptomatic carotid artery disease can be as high as 3.1%. Atherosclerosis, hypertension, tobacco use, diabetes, dyslipidemia, and age are again risk factors. Carotid disease can present asymptomatically as a systolic murmur audible at the neck, or as a cause of syncope or transient ischemic attacks. Diagnosis is made by ultrasonography of the carotid vessels. Patients with carotid artery disease are at higher risk for stroke owing to limited perfusion through stenotic vessels, ruptured plaques initialing the clotting cascade causing occlusion of cerebral vessels, or ruptured plaque resulting in an embolic occlusion of a distal cerebral vessel. Patients with severe stenosis (>70%), especially those under 75 years, greatly reduce their risk of stroke by surgical intervention via carotid endarterectomy. In patients with more mild disease, the risk of stroke in the perioperative period may outweigh the benefit of reduced stroke risk caused by the carotid disease.[3]

Peripheral Arterial Disease

PAD is insufficient perfusion of distal arteries owing to atherosclerosis of the vessels. Risk factors are the same as those of IHD: hypertension, dyslipidemia, obesity, age, family history, and tobacco use. The atherosclerosis present in PAD is systemic; therefore, patients have a higher risk of associated IHD and carotid artery stenosis. Continued tobacco use doubles the risk of progression of PAD to critical limb ischemia, and smoking cessation is strongly encouraged. Patients present with claudication of limbs as well as rest pain, physical examination may reveal faint or absent arterial pulses, absent hair and nail growth, nonhealing wounds, or coolness and pallor of the extremities. Diagnosis is made by measurement of the ankle–brachial index, a ratio of systolic blood pressure at the ankle to the systolic blood pressure at the brachial artery, with a ratio of less than 0.9 defining peripheral artery insufficiency, or by Doppler ultrasonography. Definitive diagnosis can also be made by angiogram; the invasive nature of the procedure and associate risk of renal dysfunction reserve this for higher risk patients or those in whom surgical intervention is planned.

Treatment of PAD includes smoking cessation and reduction of risk factors along with management of comorbid conditions. In those with progressive or uncontrolled disease, or with limb-threatening ischemia, revascularization is indicated, either via a surgical or endovascular approach. Surgical revascularization for PAD represents some of the highest risk surgery for perioperative myocardial morbidity and mortality, because these patients should be assumed to have concomitant coronary artery atherosclerosis.[4–6]

Box 1
Thoracic aneurysms

- Often affiliated with known genetic syndromes including Marfan's, Ehlers-Danlos, and bicuspid aortic valve, along with other non-specified familial aortic dissection and aneurysms
- Often asymptomatic, or have symptoms caused by compression of nearby structures (compression of recurrent laryngeal nerve causes hoarseness, compression of esophagus causes dysphagia) or proximal aneurysms cause aortic regurgitation
- Elective surgical repair when aneurysm greater than 5 cm, or with enlargement of greater than 10 mm per year
- Endovascular repair typically reserved for aneurysms of descending thoracic aorta

---

Box 2
Abdominal aneurysms

- Most commonly caused by severe atherosclerosis; the inflammatory state and vessel wall injury results in abnormal arterial wall structure
- Presents as an asymptomatic pulsatile abdominal mass
- Elective repair when aneurysm greater than 5.5 cm, or if enlarging by more than 0.6 cm per year
- Most often repaired endovascular graft placement
- Mortality after elective AAA repair is strongly correlated with age[2]

Peripheral Venous Disease

Surgical patients are very prone to venous disease, namely deep venous thrombosis and superficial thrombophlebitis. Virchow's triad describes the 3 conditions necessary for development of a venous thrombus: venous stasis, hypercoagulability, and disruption of vascular endothelium. All 3 are commonly encountered by the surgical patient population. Deep venous thrombosis is a life-threatening condition owing to the risk of extension and dislodgement of the clot and embolization to heart and pulmonary vasculature. Superficial thrombophlebitis occurs in a superficial vein, such as cephalic or saphenous veins, and is not associated typically with pulmonary embolism. Diagnosis of superficial thrombophlebitis is usually made clinically; diagnosis of deep vein thrombosis is made with Doppler ultrasonography or contrast venography.

Systemic Vasculitis

There are several systemic inflammatory conditions that affect the vascular system (**Table 3**). There clinical presentations are varied and there can be specific implications for anesthetic management of these patients during surgery.

Table 3 Systemic inflammatory conditions that affect the vascular system		
Systemic Vasculitis	**Vessels Affected**	**Anesthetic Implications**
Raynauds	Episodic vasospastic ischemia of digits	• Maintain normothermia (avoid hypothermia as a trigger) • Avoid invasive blood pressure management
Thromboangiitis obliterans	Inflammatory vasculitis of small and medium-sized arteries and veins	• Avoid invasive BP measurement, normothermia • Careful padding and positioning of extremities
Wegeners granulomatosis	Necrotizing granulomas in vessel walls	• Potential narrowing of airway owing to granuloma and scar formation, avoid airway trauma to limit risk of bleeding • Avoid invasive BP measurement; limit arterial punctures • Manage other affected systems (renal, pulmonary disease)
Temporal arteritis	Inflammation of arteries of head and neck; possible involvement of ophthalmic artery leading to blindness	Patients maybe on steroid therapy and require stress-dose steroids
Takayasu's arteritis	Progressive obliteration of large arterial vessels (aorta and main branches)	• Patients on steroid therapy may require stress-dose steroids • Risk of cerebral ischemia from disease carotid arteries, avoid hyperextension of neck • Difficult noninvasive BP measurement owing to obstructed upper extremity vessels

Abbreviation: BP, blood pressure.

PATIENTS WITH CARDIAC DYSFUNCTION AND VASCULAR DISEASE PRESENTING FOR SURGERY

The anesthesiologist can encounter these complex patients in any setting, but likely they will present with surgical problems related to their cardiac, vascular disease, or common comorbidities. Patients with cardiac dysfunction and peripheral arterial disease presenting for coronary artery revascularization tend to have worse outcomes and higher rates of ischemic and embolic events.[7]

Preoperative Evaluation

A thorough assessment of the patient's physiologic status is necessary to risk stratify the patient for surgery (**Boxes 3** and **4**). There are several tools available to guide management of these patients. The Revised Cardiac Risk Index provides an algorithm for the management of patients with IHD presenting for noncardiac surgery (**Fig. 2**).

> **Box 3**
> **History assessment**
>
> - IHD: previous myocardial infarction, angina symptoms, exercise tolerance, history of coronary intervention or cardiac surgery
> - Cardiac medications, particularly anticoagulants and antiplatelet regimens
> - Particular focus on comorbid conditions such as cerebrovascular disease, renal disease, diabetes mellitus, congestive heart failure, hypertension, smoking history

> **Box 4**
> **Physical assessment**
>
> - Examination of pulses
> - Neurologic exam
> - Volume status

Major Adverse Cardiac Events
- Death.
- Q-wave myocardial infarction.
- Need for revascularization (coronary artery bypass grafting, PCI).

Active Cardiac Conditions
- Acute coronary syndromes.
- Decompensated congestive HF.
- Significant arrhythmias (ventricular tachycardia, ventricular fibrillation).
- Significant valvular disease (critical aortic stenosis, severe mitral regurgitation).

Major Cardiac Risk Factors
- Ischemic cardiac disease.
- Cerebrovascular disease.
- Compensated congestive HF.
- Diabetes mellitus on insulin therapy.
- Renal Insufficiency with serum creatinine greater than 2.0.

Surgical Risk Stratification
- High risk (>5% risk of perioperative major adverse cardiac events):
  - Vascular surgery,
  - Emergency major surgery, and
  - Surgery with large blood loss/volume shifts.
- Intermediate risk (>1% but <5% risk of major adverse cardiac events):
  - Intrathoracic,
  - Intraperitoneal,
  - Orthopedic surgery,
  - Head and neck procedures, and
  - Prostate surgery.
- Low risk (<1% risk of major adverse cardiac events):
  - Breast surgery,
  - Cataract surgery,
  - Endoscopic procedures, and
  - Superficial biopsies.[8]

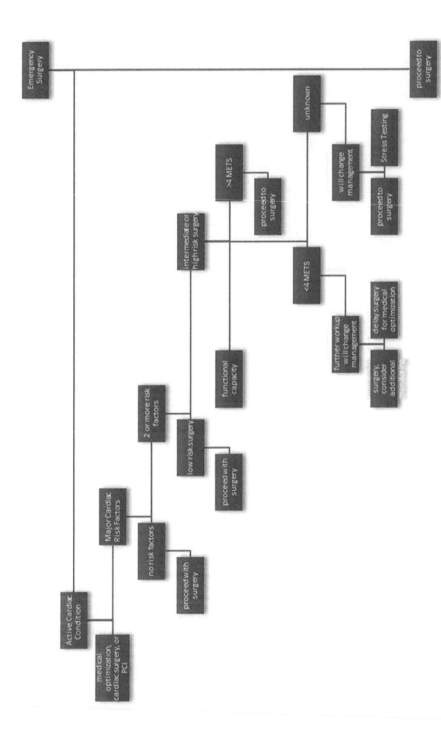

Fig. 2. The revised cardiac risk index algorithm for the management of patients with ischemic heart disease presenting for noncardiac surgery. PCI, percutaneous coronary intervention.

There is a known association with peripheral arterial insufficiency and coronary artery disease; in addition to the Revised Cardiac Risk Index independent predictors of cardiac risk, there is evidence that a low ankle-brachial index also correlates with postoperative cardiac complications.[9] There is no added benefit to coronary revascularization (either PCI or coronary artery bypass grafting) in stable coronary artery disease solely as preparation for surgery; patients should only be revascularized preoperatively if they have indications for revascularization independent of need for surgery.

Preoperative ECG testing is indicated in any patient with a history of coronary artery disease or other structural heart disease, except for low-risk surgery. For asymptomatic patients or those without risk factors undergoing intermediate or high-risk surgeries, it is reasonable to consider obtaining a baseline preoperative ECG in anticipation of potential cardiac events; however, routine preoperative ECG testing is not recommended.[10]

Laboratory testing can offer insight into comorbid conditions such as renal insufficiency, diabetes, and other electrolyte abnormalities. There is some evidence to suggest that preoperative anemia in the elderly has been associated with postoperative cardiac events.[11] Appropriate coagulation studies are important in patients on anticoagulants.

Patients should be encouraged to use the perioperative period as an impetus to quit smoking. Smoking carries a 40% increase odds of 30-day mortality and with a large increase in major morbidities such as postoperative mechanical ventilation, surgical site infection, sepsis, and pneumonia.[12] With smoking abstinence, carbon monoxide levels decrease and mucociliary clearance improves rapidly. There has been some concern that in the first few weeks of abstinence secretion production and airway irritation may in fact increase; however, the data for this are limited and the benefits of improved oxygenation and the opportunity to cease tobacco use altogether should lead the physician to encourage smoking cessation at any time, rather than trying to implement a specific deadline.[13]

There is also a growing body of literature suggesting that preoperative evaluations should be harnessed to identify patients with poorly controlled hypertension who may benefit from postoperative care coordination for long-term follow-up of this treatable disease.[14–16]

The American College of Cardiology/American Heart Association Guideline on Perioperative Cardiovascular Evaluation and Management of Patients Undergoing Noncardiac Surgery provides recommendations regarding management of patients for noncardiac surgery after PCI (**Table 4**).

Table 4
ACC/AHA recommendations regarding management of patients for noncardiac surgery after percutaneous coronary intervention

Type of PCI	Recommendation
Balloon angioplasty	Postpone elective surgery for 14 d, especially if discontinuation of antiplatelet medication is required
Bare metal stent	Postpone elective surgery for 30 d
Drug-eluting stent	Postpone elective surgery for 365 d May consider surgery after 180 d if risk of delay carries greater risk than that of ischemia and stent thrombosis

Abbreviations: ACC/AHA, American College of Cardiology/American Heart Association; PCI, percutaneous cardiac intervention.

Data from Fleisher LA, Fleischmann KE, Auerbach AD, et al. 2014 ACC/AHA guideline on perioperative cardiovascular evaluation and management of patients undergoing noncardiac surgery: a report of the American College of Cardiology/American Heart Association Task Force on Practice Guidelines. Circulation 2014;130:e278–333.

Additional Preoperative Considerations

Vascular disease is a portent of concomitant coronary artery disease. In addition, cardiac dysfunction and vascular disease share many common risk factors and comorbidities, such as dyslipidemia, hypertension, diabetes, and renal disease. Beta-blockers should be continued perioperatively, but the initiation of beta-blocker therapy immediately preoperatively for cardiovascular protection has been associated with more risk than benefit. Other cardiovascular medications should be continued perioperatively, with special consideration of diuretics and antihypertensives (**Table 5**).[17,18]

For patients with known valvular disease, it is reasonable to expect to have echocardiography within the last year, especially in patients with new or uncontrolled symptoms, or input from the cardiologist following the patient. Information regarding any valve replacements, specifically the type, location, and need for anticoagulation perioperatively, as well as any preoperative endocarditis prophylaxis required, is important to have.

Antibiotic prophylaxis against infective endocarditis is required only for 4 high-risk cardiac conditions. This balances the available evidence weighing the benefits of antibiotic prophylaxis with the risks of anaphylaxis and contributing to antibiotic resistance.

Cardiac Conditions Requiring Infective Endocarditis Prophylaxis

- Prosthetic cardiac valves,
- Previous history of infective endocarditis,
- Cardiac transplant recipients with structurally abnormal valves, and
- Congenital heart disease meeting one of following conditions:
  - ○ Unrepaired cyanotic congenital heart disease,
  - ○ Completely repaired defect using prosthetic materials, within the first 6 months, and
  - ○ Repaired congenital heart disease with residual defects at or near the site of prosthetic repair.[19–21]

Table 5 Perioperative management of medications	
Beta-blockade	Continue; only initiate if >1 wk before surgery
Calcium channel blockers	Continue
Nitrates	Hold; risk of hypotension
Statins	Continue, some advantage to initiating
Angiotensin-converting enzyme inhibitors, angiotensin receptor blockers	Consider holding 24 h preoperatively; risk of refractory hypotension
Antiarrhythmics	Continue
Antiplatelets	Balance risk of bleeding vs risk of ischemia and stent thrombosis If dual antiplatelet therapy cannot be continued, at least continue aspirin

PREOPERATIVE ASSESSMENT OF CARDIAC IMPLANTABLE INTRACARDIAC DEVICE
History

- Patient's underlying rhythm: underlying rhythm compatible with perfusion for short periods of time if necessary.

- Type of device: make, single-, dual-, or biventricular device, presence of defibrillator.
- Settings: chamber paced, chamber sensed, mode of response, programmable function, and antitachycardia response.
- Location: site of generator, location of leads may influence location of central line placement.

Surgical Requirements

Location of surgery, presence of electrocautery, physiologic stress of surgery, need for central line or PAC.

Intraoperative Management

Goals of anesthetic management of a patient with concomitant vascular disease and cardiac dysfunction are to maintain perfusion to vital organs, avoid myocardial ischemia, and avoid vascular compromise. Monitoring of heart rate, blood pressure, oxygenation and ventilation, and temperature are standard for any anesthetic. However, for the patient with cardiac disease and vascular dysfunction, additional monitoring may be beneficial.

Electrocardiographic monitoring

Electrocardiographic monitoring is usually via leads II and V. Lead II can reveal ischemia of the right coronary artery, and is helpful for diagnosing conduction abnormalities. Lead V is helpful for monitoring the distribution of the left anterior descending artery. This offers a relatively sensitive and specific monitor for cardiac ischemia. The specificity and sensitivity can be increased by monitoring a third lead.

Arterial catheterization

The 3 indications for arterial line placement are need for frequent blood gas measurements, need for frequent laboratory testing, and close monitoring of blood pressure (more frequently than every 3 minutes). Vascular and cardiac patients are likely to be at higher risk for labile hemodynamics, may have associated comorbidities such as lung disease requiring blood gas measurements, and may require frequent laboratory measurements for blood sugar, or coagulation status, or electrolyte abnormalities. It is therefore quite reasonable to consider arterial line placement in a patient with significant cardiac and/or vascular disease.

Arterial cannulation is invasive and carries risk of distal ischemia. The Allen's test is used to verify collateral circulation; however, the test has high operator variability and has not been shown to predict postcannulation digital ischemia. Some of the risk factors associated with ischemic complications of radial artery cannulation are listed below.

Risk Factors Associated with Ischemic Complications of Radial Artery Cannulation

- Documented incomplete hand collateralization.
- Circulatory failure.
- Hypotension.
- High-dose vasopressor therapy.
- Hematoma at puncture site.
- Small artery size.
- Duration of cannulation.
- Number of puncture attempts.
- Length of catheter (shorter catheters more often associated with arterial occlusion).

- Polypropylene catheter (instead of Teflon).
- Female gender.

Factors not associated with increased risk of arterial occlusion include technique (no difference between direct puncture vs the "through and through" transfixation methods), recannulation of previously cannulated artery, and reversing direction of the cannula.[22]

Central venous catheter

Patients with vascular disease often have poor peripheral intravenous access. An upper extremity may be off limits owing to an existing or planned arteriovenous fistula for dialysis access in patients with coexisting renal disease. In patients with significant vascular disease and cardiac dysfunction, hemodynamic lability during surgery may necessitate vasoactive infusions, which are best administered through central venous access. It is worth noting that a standard triple lumen central venous catheter has one 16-G lumen and two 18-G lumens, which in a 15- to 21-inch length catheter means considerable resistance to rapid, large volume infusions. If large and rapid infusion is anticipated, consider placement of a large bore, shorter length central venous catheter.

Pulmonary artery catheter

PACs offer an approximation of the left atrial pressure through measurement of the pulmonary capillary wedge pressure, measurement of the cardiac output via thermodilution, and measurement of pulmonary artery pressure. The use of PAC has been scrutinized for risks with lack of proven benefit. Increased pulmonary capillary wedge pressure is a relatively late and inaccurate sign of myocardial ischemia, making PACs an impractical intraoperative screening tool for myocardial ischemia. PACs can still be helpful in patients with history of right HF or pulmonary hypertension undergoing high-risk surgery.

Echocardiography

New regional wall motion abnormalities observed on echocardiography are the gold standard for diagnosing myocardial ischemia. This would suggest that intraoperative echocardiography would be a useful tool for monitoring for ischemia. In fact, there has been evidence to suggest that preoperative stress echocardiography is a poor predictor of the location of intraoperative new wall motion abnormalities as observed by real-time intraoperative transesophageal echocardiography (TEE). Limitations of TEE include need for specially trained staff, contraindications to TEE placement, and impracticality of constant TEE monitoring during management of anesthetic. There are likely to be more anesthesia providers qualified to perform transthoracic echocardiography, it is reasonable to consider use of transthoracic echocardiography if myocardial ischemia is suspected and the chest is out of the surgical field.[23]

Choice of anesthetic

There is little to no evidence to support one anesthetic over another for a given surgery. Most major surgeries require general anesthesia owing to the possibility of large fluid shifts, hemodynamic instability, and surgical site. Some evidence has shown that the ischemic preconditioning offered by inhalational anesthetics can be cardioprotective. Of the intravenous anesthetics, propofol can cause dose-dependent hypotension, etomidate is relatively hemodynamically stable but carries a risk of adrenal suppression, and ketamine, although also hemodynamically stable, can cause cardiac depression in a patient who is catecholamine depleted.[24] However, there is no evidence to suggest that there is a protective advantage for either total intravenous anesthetic or inhalational agent against perioperative myocardial ischemia.[10]

In appropriate cases, regional anesthesia can be the safest technique for a complex patient—a brachial plexus block for an arteriovenous fistula creation in a patient with end-stage renal disease and often several other comorbidities provides a safe and effective anesthetic. Neuraxial blockade has not been shown to be a more effective anesthetic technique in preventing intraoperative cardiac complications. However, an epidural catheter placed to help control postoperative pain can reduce the risk of postoperative myocardial infarction caused by the physiologic stress from uncontrolled pain.[10] Special consideration must be given to any anticoagulants or antiplatelet agents being administered preoperatively, intraoperatively, or postoperatively. The American Society of Regional Anesthesia publishes guidelines and advisories regarding safe use of neuraxial techniques in anticoagulated patients.

INTRAOPERATIVE MANAGEMENT
Preserving Cardiac Function

Patients with cardiac dysfunction are particularly sensitive to hemodynamic instability. Hemodynamics should be maintained within about 20% of the patient's preoperative values. Induction of and emergence from general anesthesia are particularly vulnerable periods for cardiac function; care must be taken to avoid tachycardia and large swings in blood pressure, which can increase myocardial oxygen demand and reduce oxygen supply. Maintenance of normothermia reduces the risk of postoperative shivering, another source of increased myocardial oxygen demand.

Management of Vascular Disease

Atherosclerotic vessels can no longer adapt to changes in blood pressure and can no longer constrict or dilate to maintain a stable perfusion pressure. Perfusion therefore becomes flow dependent as autoregulation of organs becomes impaired.

Avoiding hypotension will help to ensure adequate perfusion, and avoiding hypertension theoretically reduces the risk of shear forces causing plaque rupture in atherosclerotic vessels, or increased wall tension risking rupture in patients with aneurysms. Particularly high-risk events in vascular patients undergoing surgery are any points in which the vessels are clamped, entered, or manipulated, because this poses a risk of dissection, plaque rupture, or embolic events.

Care must be taken in the positioning of patients with vascular disease. There should be careful manipulation of the neck in patients with carotid artery disease, and those with peripheral vascular disease should have extra care in positioning and padding; any wounds or skin breakdown is at risk of not healing.

Management of Comorbidities

The several associated risk factors and consequential comorbidities of cardiac and vascular disease must also be managed carefully. Patients who smoke may have pulmonary disease and would benefit from bronchodilators. Diabetic patients should have a serum blood glucose of less than 180 mg/dL perioperatively to avoid surgical risks of hyperglycenia and hypoglycemia. Patients with cardiac and vascular disease are at particular risk for acute kidney injury. There is evidence that prolonged periods of hypotension (mean arterial pressure of <60 mm Hg for >10 minutes) are associated with postoperative acute kidney injury.[2,25]

COMPLICATIONS

In addition to the complications that are always possible in any anesthetic, there are particular considerations in the patient with cardiac and vascular dysfunction.

Intraoperative Myocardial Ischemia

If intraoperative myocardial ischemia is suspected, the surgical team should be notified immediately, to allow time to reasonably abort the procedure and proceed to revascularization should it become necessary.

- Note ECG changes, obtain 12-lead ECG.
- Place patient on 100% Fio_2.
- Immediately correct hemodynamic derangements (tachycardia, hypotension, hypertension).
- Consider rectal aspirin.
- Obtain intraoperative cardiac consult.
- Consider intraoperative transthoracic echocardiography or TEE, if equipment and staff available.
- Consider placement of arterial line for closer monitoring or central line placement for administration of vasoactive infusions.
- Treat significant arrhythmias (ventricular tachycardia or fibrillation) promptly, with cardiopulmonary resuscitation or defibrillation as indicated.

Critical Limb/Digit Ischemia

A ruptured plaque, vasospasm, or embolus can cause partial or total occlusion of an artery. This situation represents a vascular emergency to immediately revascularize the affected extremity. There can be many causes, such as manipulation of the vessels, particularly with clamping, with arterial cannulation, or with vasospasm from extravascular infiltration or accidental intraarterial injection of vasoactive medications.

- Place patient on 100% Fio_2.
- Avoid hypotension.
- Obtain STAT vascular consult.
- Consider cold compresses and elevation of extremity for extravascular infiltration.
- Consider regional block to induce vasodilatation (after consultation with vascular surgeon).
- Consider anticoagulation with heparin (in discussion with vascular surgeon).

Stroke

It can be difficult to recognize stroke in the perioperative setting. Patients are either under general anesthesia or are recently emerged and can be disoriented, lethargic, or not yet following instructions. Other diagnoses such as residual neuromuscular blockade, overnarcotization, nerve damage to an extremity, or hypothermia can all mask signs of stroke, leading to late diagnosis. Clinical suspicion must be high, especially in patients with previous cerebrovascular disease or known carotid stenosis. Patients may present with delayed awakening, focal neurologic deficits, or confusion.

- Avoid hypotension; if confirmed nonhemorrhagic stroke, will need mild hypertension to optimize cerebral perfusion.
- Obtain STAT computed tomography scan of the head.
- Obtain a neurology consult.
- Avoid hyperglycemia.

Table 6
Antiplatelet/Anticoagulants agents

Antiplatelet/Anticoagulant	Mechanism of Action	Reversal
Aspirin	COX-1 inhibitor	Platelet transfusion
Clopidogrel	Inhibits ADP receptor on platelet membranes	Platelet transfusion
Heparin	Antithrombin III activator	Protamine
Enoxaparin	Inactivates clotting factor Xa	Protamine
Warfarin	Inhibits vitamin K-dependent synthesis of clotting factors	Vitamin K FFP Prothrombin complex concentrate
Dabigatran	Direct thrombin inhibitor	Praxbind
Rivaroxaban	Factor Xa inhibitor	Prothrombin complex concentrate

Abbreviations: ADP, adenosine diphosphate; COX, cyclooxygenase; FFP, fresh frozen plasma.

- Maintain normothermia.
- Consider intubation in obtunded patient.

Bleeding

Patients on anticoagulants or antiplatelet agents are at an increased risk for bleeding. Antiplatelet agents can reversibly or irreversibly inactivate platelets (**Table 6**). Permanently inactivated platelets will be dysfunctional for their lifetime, so these agents need to be held for 7 days, the half-life of platelets. Platelet transfusion can help to overcome platelet dysfunction, but platelets transfused within 24 hours of last dose of clopidogrel may be inactivated by residual circulating drug.

SUMMARY

Anesthesia for patients with peripheral vascular disease and those cardiac dysfunction share common goals of anesthetic management. Cardiac and vascular pathology carry similar risk factors and therefore often occur together. Preoperative optimization reduces the risk factors a patient brings to the operating room, careful monitoring results in early detection of potential problems, and maintaining perfusion will limit the damage to the heart and distal organs.

REFERENCES

1. Groban L, Butterworth J. Perioperative management of chronic heart failure. Anesth Analg 2006;103(3):557–75.
2. Brienza N, Giglio MT, Marucci M, et al. Does perioperative hemodynamic optimization protect renal function in surgical patients? a meta-analytic study. Crit Care Med 2009;37(6):2079–90.
3. den Hartog AG, Achterberg S, Moll FL, et al. Asymptomatic carotid artery stenosis and the risk of ischemic stroke according to subtype in patients with clinical manifest arterial disease. Stroke 2013;44:1002–7.
4. Slovut DP, Lipsitz EC. Surgical technique and peripheral artery disease. Circulation 2012;126:1127–38.

5. Vartanian SM, Conte MS. Surgical intervention for peripheral arterial disease. Circ Res 2015;116:1614–28.

6. Hines RL, Marschall KE. Stoelting's anesthesia and co-existing disease. 6th edition. Philadelphia: Elsevier Saunders; 2012.

7. Kertai MD. Preparative coronary revascularization in high-risk patients undergoing vascular surgery: a core review. Anesth Analg 2008;106(3):751–8.

8. Mukherjee D, Eagle KA. Perioperative cardiac assessment for noncardiac surgery: eight steps to the best possible outcome. Circulation 2003;107:2771–4.

9. Fisher BW, Ramsay G, Majumdar SR, et al. The ankle-to-arm blood pressure index predicts risk of cardiac complications after noncardiac surgery. Anesth Analg 2008;107(1):149–54.

10. Fleisher LA, Fleischmann KE, Auerbach AD, et al. 2014 ACC/AHA guideline on perioperative cardiovascular evaluation and management of patients undergoing noncardiac surgery: a report of the American College of Cardiology/American Heart Association Task Force on Practice Guidelines. Circulation 2014;130: e278–333.

11. Gupta PK, Sundaram A, MacTaggart JN, et al. Preoperative anemia is an independent predictor of postoperative mortality and adverse cardiac events in elderly patients undergoing elective vascular operations. Ann Surg 2013; 258(6):1096–102.

12. Turan A, Mascha EJ, Roberman D, et al. Smoking and perioperative outcomes. Anesthesiology 2011;114(4):837–46.

13. Warner DO. Perioperative abstinence from cigarettes: physiologic and clinical consequences. Anesthesiology 2006;104(2):356–67.

14. Schonberger RB, Burg MM, Holt NF, et al. The relationship between day-of-surgery and primary care blood pressure among Veterans presenting from home for surgery. Is there evidence for anesthesiologist-initiated blood pressure referral? Anesth Analg 2012;114:205–14.

15. Schonberger RB, Dai F, Brandt C, et al. Balancing model performance and simplicity to predict postoperative primary care blood pressure elevation. Anesth Analg 2015;121:632–41.

16. Schonberger RB, Dai F, Brandt C, et al. Ambulatory medical follow-up in the year after surgery and subsequent survival in a national cohort of Veterans Health Administration surgical patients. J Cardiothorac Vasc Anesth 2016;30(3):671–9.

17. Shah TR, Veith FJ, Bauer SM. Cardiac evaluation and management before vascular surgery. Curr Opin Cardiol 2014;29(6):499–505.

18. Dai N, DaChun X, Zhang J, et al. Different β-blockers and initiation time in patients undergoing noncardiac surgery: a meta-analysis. Am J Med Sci 2014;347(3): 235–44.

19. Wilson W, Taubert KA, Gewitz M, et al. Prevention of infective endocarditis: guidelines from the American Heart Association. Circulation 2007;116:1736–54.

20. Hall R, Mazer CD. Antiplatelet drugs: a review of their pharmacology and management in the perioperative period. Anesth Analg 2011;112(2):292–318.

21. Schlösser FJV, Vaartjes I, van der Heijden GJMG, et al. Mortality after elective abdominal aortic aneurysm repair. Ann Surg 2010;251(1):158–64.

22. Brzezinski M, Luisetti T, London MJ. Radial artery cannulation: a comprehensive review of recent anatomic and physiologic investigations. Anesth Analg 2009; 109(6):1763–81.

23. Galal W, Hoeks SE, Flu WJ, et al. Relation between preoperative and intraoperative new wall motion abnormalities in vascular surgery patients: a transesophageal echocardiographic study. Anesthesiology 2010;112:557–66.

24. Van der Linden PJ, Dierick A, Wilmin S, et al. A randomized controlled trial comparing an intraoperative goal-directed strategy with routine clinical practice in patients undergoing peripheral arterial surgery. Eur J Anaesthesiol 2010; 27(9):788–93.

25. Sun LY, Wijeysundera DN, Tait GA, et al. Association of intraoperative hypotension with acute kidney injury after elective noncardiac surgery. Anesthesiology 2015; 123(3):515–23.

Anesthesia for Patients with Concomitant Hepatic and Pulmonary Dysfunction

Geraldine C. Diaz, DO[a],*, Michael F. O'Connor, MD[a],
John F. Renz, MD, PhD[b]

KEYWORDS

- Hepatopulmonary syndrome • Portopulmonary hypertension
- Intrapulmonary vascular dilatation • Cirrhosis • Anesthesia

KEY POINTS

- Hepatic function and pulmonary function are interrelated with failure of one organ system affecting the other.
- With improved treatments, patients with concomitant hepatic and pulmonary failure increasingly have a good quality of life and life expectancy. Therefore, more patients are presenting for elective as well as emergent surgical procedures.
- Hepatopulmonary syndrome originates from the development of intrapulmonary vascular dilatations that are common in patients with end-stage liver disease.
- Hypoxemia requires a thorough evaluation in patients with end-stage liver disease. The most common causes respond to appropriate therapy.
- Portopulmonary hypertension and hepatopulmonary syndrome are associated with high perioperative morbidity and mortality.

INTRODUCTION

The prevalence of end-stage liver disease (ESLD) has steadily increased over the past 2 decades to become a common comorbidity encountered by the practicing anesthesiologist. Dramatic improvements in the medical management of cirrhosis by gastroenterologists and liver surgeons, including the use of beta blocker prophylaxis for portal hypertension, endoscopy for the management of esophageal varices, transjugular intrahepatic portosystemic shunt, and effective medications to suppress viral replication, have increased the life expectancy and quality of life for patients with ESLD. Today, patients with ESLD are seeking emergent as well as elective surgical

[a] Department of Anesthesiology/Critical Care, University of Chicago, 5841 South Maryland Avenue, Chicago, IL 60637, USA; [b] Department of Surgery, University of Chicago, 5841 South Maryland Avenue, Chicago, IL 60637, USA
* Corresponding author.
E-mail address: gdiaz@dacc.uchicago.edu

procedures for conditions that were previously regarded as posing too high a risk for surgery. This change mandates not only a greater understanding of the physiology of cirrhosis but also the systemic manifestations of the failing liver on other organs.

This article examines anesthesia for patients with concomitant hepatic and pulmonary dysfunction. Concomitant hepatic and pulmonary dysfunction can be encountered within 3 broad scenarios. The most frequent scenario is patients with a history of independent pulmonary and hepatic diseases, for example, a patient with alcoholic liver disease and chronic obstructive pulmonary disease secondary to smoking. In this setting, the history and severity of the disease processes will be variable as will the influence of each on the other organ system's physiology. The variability in pathophysiology typically results in one organ system being the dominant source of morbidity that is accentuated by dysfunction of the other. In these situations, anesthetic management is directed toward the principally disaffected organ system. The truly concomitant scenarios of ESLD with associated pulmonary manifestations, such as portopulmonary hypertension (POPH) and hepatopulmonary syndrome (HPS), as well as inherited metabolic disorders affecting both organ systems, such as alpha-1-antitrypsin (A1AT) deficiency and cystic fibrosis (CF), require more complex medical management and are the focus of this article. Current definitions, diagnostic criteria, pathophysiology, algorithms for preoperative screening, and management for these patients in the setting of nontransplant surgery are explored.

PULMONARY FUNCTION IN THE SETTING OF LIVER DISEASE

The failing liver imposes early and significant effects on pulmonary function. The most frequently recognized restrictive pulmonary complications arise from ascites secondary to portal hypertension. Ascites expands the abdominal cavity, impedes mobility of the diaphragm, and can result in pleural effusions.[1] In addition to these restrictive changes, liver disease impairs gas exchange through ventilation-perfusion (VQ) mismatch, impedes oxygen diffusion, and facilitates intrapulmonary shunts.[1] Patients with ESLD demonstrate a widened alveolar-arterial oxygen concentration gradient (A-a gradient), impaired diffusing capacity of the lungs for carbon monoxide (DLCO), and hypoxemia that typically progress with the severity of liver disease.[2,3]

The most commonly encountered pulmonary complications associated with ESLD result from VQ mismatch. Ascites, anasarca, pleural effusions, and hepatomegaly impede chest wall motion, reduce lung recoil, and impair diaphragmatic excursion.[4] These restrictive changes reduce respiratory volumes, decrease functional residual capacity, and increase closing capacity.[5] Increased pulmonary parenchymal pressure from interstitial edema promotes small airway collapse and obstruction.[5] Therefore, hypoxemia evolves with liver disease progression from a principally restrictive process to a combination of restrictive as well as obstructive processes.[6]

Although the physiology of portal hypertension has been widely recognized, the physiologic changes induced on pulmonary vascular tone through hepatic vasoactive mediators are increasingly recognized as a significant contribution to VQ imbalance.[5] As cardiac output and circulating blood volumes increase, systemic venodilation increases blood flow through the pulmonary circulation. This increase creates a relative VQ imbalance of impaired gas exchange through physiologic shunting. Hypoxemia is accentuated by inhibition of the hypoxic pulmonary vasoconstrictive reflex observed in cirrhosis.[7]

Abnormal diffusion capacity can be an early manifestation of pulmonary dysfunction in patients with ESLD with a DLCO of less than 75% predicted observed in most liver transplant candidates.[3,4] A reduced DLCO is hypothesized to result from the increased cardiac output associated with the hyperdynamic physiology of cirrhosis, which results in a greater volume of blood rapidly transiting dilated capillaries. Greater volumes, shorter transit time, and increased vessel diameter create a central stream of blood that has insufficient time to permit adequate gas diffusion.[8] Reactive thickening of the capillary-alveolar membrane is observed and further impairs gas exchange.[9]

Intrapulmonary shunts secondary to the physiology of cirrhosis have been identified in as many as 80% of patients evaluated for liver transplantation.[10–12] Although intra-pulmonary shunts may be diagnosed by the multiple inert gas elimination technique, contrast-enhanced echocardiography is the diagnostic modality of choice.[10] The A-a gradient is increased and hypoxemia exacerbated by the development of anatomic venous shunts that completely bypass ventilating units.[13] Intrapulmonary collateral circulation has been the historic explanation of hypoxemia in cirrhosis; however, postmortem studies only occasionally describe arteriovenous communications within the lung parenchyma.[14] The most frequent pathologic finding is a marked dilation of the pulmonary vessels at the precapillary level suggesting the true physiologic contribution of anatomic shunts is less than the effects of vascular dilatation.[14]

PULMONARY COMPLICATIONS ASSOCIATED WITH CHRONIC LIVER DISEASE

There are numerous pulmonary complications associated with chronic liver disease. This discussion focuses on those pulmonary complications whereby portal hypertension is fundamental to the pathogenesis of the pulmonary disorder. These complications include HPS and POPH (**Table 1**). The occurrence and severity of HPS and POPH do not correlate to the Child-Pugh or Model for End-Stage Liver Disease (MELD) score.[15,16]

Table 1
Hepatopulmonary syndrome versus portopulmonary hypertension

	HPS	POPH
Pathophysiology	Intrapulmonary vascular dilatations Angiogenesis, increased VEGF ET-B receptor upregulation Increased NO Increased CO	Pulmonary arterial remodeling and obstruction Prostacyclin deficiency Increased ET-1 levels NO deficiency
Diagnostic criteria	Intrapulmonary vascular dilatation A-a gradient >15 mm Hg (>20 mm Hg if >64 y) or Pao_2 <80 mm Hg	mPAP >25 mm Hg PAOP <15 mm Hg PVR >3 Wood units (>240 dyne/s/cm^5)
5-y Survival	15%–23%	4%–14%[a]
Effect of LT	Resolution expected	Resolution unpredictable
Pharmacologic therapies	Supplemental oxygen	Prostacyclin analogues Endothelin receptor antagonist Phosphodiesterase-5 inhibitors
Future directions	Angiogenesis blockade	Drug effect on portal hypertension Estrogen signaling blockade

Abbreviations: CO, carbon monoxide; ET, endothelin; LT, liver transplantation; mPAP, mean pulmonary arterial pressure; NO, nitric oxide; PAOP, pulmonary arterial occlusion pressure; PVR, pulmonary vascular resistance; VEGF, vascular endothelial growth factor.
[a] Without medical therapy.

Hepatopulmonary Syndrome

HPS is the most common pulmonary complication of chronic liver disease with an incidence of up to 30% among cirrhotic patients.[16,17] HPS originates from the development of intrapulmonary vascular dilatations (IPVD) that are a common observation in autopsy series of patients with ESLD.[14] IPVDs are vascular anomalies consisting of abnormally dilated pulmonary capillaries that can coexist with pleural and pulmonary direct arteriovenous communications and are detected by contrast-enhanced transthoracic echocardiography (cTTE).[8] IPVD manifest as a delayed visualization of microbubbles in the left cardiac chambers 3 to 6 cardiac cycles after their appearance in the right atrium following injection of agitated saline.[18]

To fulfill the diagnosis of HPS, these anomalies must result in *impaired oxygenation* of blood as it passes through the pulmonary circulation.[19] Only a fraction of patients with ESLD and IPVD will fulfill the criteria for abnormal gas exchange characteristic of HPS.[20] These diagnostic criteria are age-based and include (a) the presence of liver disease and/or portal hypertension, (b) an A-a gradient $\geq$15 mm Hg in adults younger than 65 years or $\geq$20 mm Hg for adults 65 years and older, or a Pao_2 less than 80 mm Hg while breathing room air at sea level, and (c) evidence of IPVD.[19] A widened room air A-a gradient and a reduced DLCO are typical on laboratory analysis.[20] Pulse oximetry (blood oxygen saturation [Spo_2]) is emerging as a screening tool for HPS with a high sensitivity and specificity.[21,22] In a prospective study of patients undergoing liver transplant evaluation, an Spo_2 of less than 96% was 100% sensitive and 88% specific for detecting HPS patients with a Pao_2 of less than 70 mm Hg. Effective Spo_2 screening successfully limited the need for ABG testing to only 14% of the cohort.[23] Serial Spo_2 measurements are also useful for monitoring impaired oxygenation over time in HPS patients.[24]

Dyspnea on standing (platypnea) and hypoxemia exacerbated in the upright position (orthodeoxia) are present in up to 25% of patients with HPS.[25] These clinical findings result from increasing VQ mismatch in the dependent areas of the lungs where IPVDs are more concentrated and larger.[25] Patients with severe HPS may manifest digital clubbing and cyanosis.[19] Roentgenograms may be normal or demonstrate bibasilar nodular or reticulonodular opacities reflecting diffuse vascular pulmonary dilation.[8] These patients not only experience a markedly impaired quality of life but also mortality that is approximately twice that of cirrhotic patients without HPS.[15,17] The increased mortality of patients with HPS is independent of age, MELD, hypoxemia, and comorbidities.[15]

Cirrhosis is not a prerequisite for the development HPS, as HPS has been described in noncirrhotic patients with presinusoidal and postsinusoidal portal hypertension, such as Budd Chiari syndrome, as well as patients with ischemic hepatitis.[26,27] There is no established effective medical therapy currently available for HPS. In patients with Pao_2 less than 60 mm Hg at rest or with exertion, the administration of supplemental oxygen is appropriate because chronic hypoxemia may contribute to the mortality of HPS.[15,17] Liver transplant (LT) is effective therapy for HPS, resulting in complete resolution or significant improvement in gas exchange in more than 85% of patients with severe hypoxemia.[28] The United Network for Organ Sharing awards MELD exception allocation points for patients with HPS to improve pre-LT and post-LT survival.[29]

The pathogenesis of HPS remains debated but is postulated to involve nitric oxide (NO) in the development of IPVD.[20] Exhaled NO derived from the lungs is observed in cirrhotic patients with HPS that normalizes following LT.[30] Furthermore, animal models demonstrate excessive NO production through endothelial NO synthase activation.[31] Induction of NO synthase and carbon monoxide production through heme oxygenase activation in intravascular monocytes and macrophages recruited to the lungs from bacterial translocation and endotoxemia has also been demonstrated.[32] Pulmonary angiogenesis via production of vascular endothelial growth factor has also been implicated as a contributor to IPVD.[33]

General anesthesia for anything outside of LT in patients with HPS is associated with very high perioperative risk.[34] HPS is often underappreciated in patients with ESLD with abnormal gas exchange and should be suspected in any patient with a low SpO_2. If suspected, a screening cTTE or intraoperative transesophageal echocardiography (TEE) can be used to confirm the diagnosis. When recognized, aggressive weaning of mechanical ventilation to extubate as early as possible in the postoperative period is advised. Noninvasive positive pressure ventilation (NPPV) immediately following extubation to augment oxygenation can be very useful.[34]

Portopulmonary Hypertension

POPH is pulmonary arterial hypertension in the setting of portal hypertension. POPH requires only the presence of portal hypertension and can exist with or without cirrhosis.[19] The severity of POPH does not correlate with the degree of portal hypertension or the progression of liver disease.[35] The diagnostic criteria for POPH include a mean pulmonary artery pressure (mPAP) greater than 25 mm Hg, pulmonary vascular resistance (PVR) greater than 240 dyne/s/cm[5], and a pulmonary artery occlusion pressure (PAOP) less than 15 mm Hg.[19]

POPH is present in as many as 10% of patients evaluated for LT.[36] Clinical symptoms typically present late in the course of disease and include exertional dyspnea, fatigue, chest pain, syncope, and orthopnea. Electrocardiography can reveal right atrial enlargement, right ventricular hypertrophy, and a right axis deviation. Chest roentgenograms demonstrate cardiomegaly or enlarged pulmonary arteries. Transthoracic echocardiography (TTE) is mandatory in the detection and evaluation of POPH. TTE is used to evaluate right ventricular performance and estimate right ventricular systolic pressure (RVSP) that correlates well with the mPAP measured by right heart catheterization (RHC). RHC is the diagnostic gold standard for POPH that must be interpreted in the context of the TTE.[36] The transpulmonary gradient (TPG), defined as the difference between the mPAP and PAOP, has been proposed as a useful hemodynamic parameter to assess POPH. A TPG greater than 12 mm Hg indicates an elevated PVR.[37]

As no animal model currently exists, the precise pathogenesis of POPH remains unknown with most data inferred from the study of pulmonary arterial hypertension.[20] POPH has been postulated to result from an imbalance between pulmonary vasoconstrictors and vasodilators. The hyperdynamic physiology of cirrhosis, coupled with significant portal shunting, increases pulmonary blood flow and shear stress that stimulates endothelial injury, intimal proliferation, media hypertrophy, and fibrosis.[38] These changes lead to in situ thrombosis, obstruction of pulmonary arterial blood, pulmonary arterial wall thickening, and elevation of PVR.[38] The vasoconstrictive and proliferative substances involved in neurohumoral activation are not completely identified but are postulated to include endothelin 1A, thromboxane A2, interleukin-1, and interleukin-6, which reach the pulmonary circulation through anatomic shunt, inadequate hepatic clearance, or production by the failing liver.[39] Prostacyclin and NO deficiency have also been noted.[40]

POPH has a poor prognosis, with an estimated 14% 5-year survival without pharmacologic therapy.[40] Mortality is related to complications of ESLD or right heart failure. Available medical therapies target the deficiency in endothelial cell vasodilator production, vascular smooth muscle relaxation, and vascular wall remodeling through endothelin receptor antagonists, phosphodiesterase type 5 inhibitors, and prostacyclin analogues.[40]

POPH is associated with extraordinarily high perioperative morbidity and mortality.[41] A thorough understanding of pulmonary hypertension is a prerequisite to proceeding, and a TTE is invaluable in clinical management. Preoperatively, an elevated RVSP greater than 40 mm Hg, reduced right heart function, or significant tricuspid regurgitation indicate an RHC to distinguish POPH from volume overload. If mPAP is greater than 35 mm Hg or there is evidence of right heart dysfunction, elective surgery should not be performed. Patients should be optimized with pharmacologic therapy before considering elective surgery. Intraoperative management includes TEE for continuous evaluation of right heart function, pulmonary artery catheterization, acid-base optimization, and judicious volume administration.

POPH is an indication for LT, but the response to LT is unpredictable.[37] An mPAP greater than 45 mm Hg is a relative contraindication for LT because of the high perioperative risk of right heart failure; however, moderate POPH (mPAP 35–45 mm Hg) that responds to medical therapy often benefits from LT.[41]

METABOLIC DISEASES
Alpha-1-Antitrypsin Deficiency

A1AT is an autosomal codominant inherited metabolic disorder of the serine protease inhibitor superfamily of proteins.[42] A1AT deficiency was first associated with early onset emphysema in 1963 by Laurell and Eriksson.[43] Pulmonary manifestations associated with A1AT include bronchiectasis, emphysema, and pulmonary infections. Later, Sharp and colleagues[44] described the association of A1AT with liver disease in 1969. Liver disease manifests as a transaminitis (hepatitis) that progresses to cirrhosis and HCC. Pulmonary disease is the most prevalent complication of A1AT with a penetrance of greater than 80%.[42] Liver disease can be present in as many as one-third of patients, half of whom are cirrhotic at the time liver dysfunction is diagnosed. Patient with cirrhotic A1AT have a very high predisposition to develop HCC that is estimated to be as high as 36% in longitudinal follow-up studies. Among patients with A1AT who smoke, lung morbidity is 3-fold higher than morbidity from liver disease; however, pulmonary and hepatic morbidity are roughly equal among nonsmokers.[42]

Multiple variant alleles can account for the development of A1AT.[45] The disease is characterized by its phenotypic description that is noted as a protease inhibitor (PI) followed by the two codominant alleles. The M allele is the functionally normal allele, so a codominant normal would be PIMM. The Z allele is most commonly associated with morbidity, particularly the codominant PIZZ. Morbidity from A1AT deficiency can result from gain of toxic function as well as loss-of-function defects in the A1AT protein. Within the liver, "gain of toxic function" results from inappropriate protein polymerization resulting in toxic protein accumulation within hepatocytes. Dysfunctional PIZZ protein accumulation has been identified by electron microscopy, periodic acid-Schiff staining, and diastase-resistant inclusions within hepatocyte endoplasmic reticula. Protein accumulation stimulates inflammation and hepatitis with chronic hepatitis resulting in fibrosis and cirrhosis. The mechanisms responsible for protein accumulation have not been elicited but may involve impaired excretion via an intracellular chaperone (calnexin) or impaired intracellular degradation.[45]

A1AT is principally produced in liver and secreted into the systemic circulation to reach the lungs.[42] A small amount of A1AT is produced locally by macrophages and bronchial epithelial cells but is insufficient to avert morbidity. Pulmonary injury results from a loss-of-function defect where insufficient levels of circulating A1AT are present to neutralize powerful proteolytic enzymes. Chronic unopposed proteolysis results in tissue loss, bronchiectasis, and emphysema. The strong association between PIZZ phenotype and liver disease prompted the American Thoracic Society/European Respiratory Society to recommend A1AT testing for all unexplained liver disease in infants through adults.[46]

Clinical management of A1AT deficiency typically focuses on the pulmonary manifestations of bronchiectasis, chronic respiratory infection, and emphysema. These manifestations have been addressed via the traditional therapies of smoking cessation, vaccination, bronchodilators, steroids, and supplemental oxygen. The rate of forced expiratory volume in 1 second (FEV_1) deterioration is the most sensitive metric to assess the efficacy of medical therapy and risk stratification.[42]

Increasing data demonstrate the incidence of hepatic disease has been underestimated.[42] Improved medical management of pulmonary disease has increased longevity and permitted liver disease to progress such that all patients with known A1AT should now undergo a thorough evaluation for ESLD. This evaluation should include physical examination for signs of liver disease (spider nevi, caput medusae, gynecomastia, ascites), laboratory evaluation (thrombocytopenia, elevated prothrombin time), cross-sectional imaging, and biopsy or ultrasound elastography as indicated. The recent implementation of ultrasound elastography is highly accurate in the real-time assessment of hepatic fibrosis without the need for a liver biopsy.[47] Previously unrecognized liver disease should delay surgery, if possible, until optimization and complete risk stratification can be achieved.

Cystic Fibrosis

CF is an inherited metabolic disorder that affects multiple organ systems.[48] However, pulmonary and hepatic diseases are the principal causes of morbidity, with cirrhosis the second most common cause of mortality after respiratory failure. Dramatic improvements in the medical management of patients with CF have significantly increased life expectancy leading to more patients presenting for emergent and elective surgeries. Increased longevity facilitates disease progression within organ systems outside the lungs. As a result, the incidence of patients with CF presenting with advanced, concomitant pulmonary and hepatic disease is increasing.[48]

Chronic viscous mucous production, inflammation, and pulmonary infection resulting in parenchymal destruction characterize the physiology observed with CF.[48] Pulmonary function tests demonstrate an obstructive pattern of airway disease with decreased FEV_1, decreased peak expiratory flow, and increased residual volume (RV). Chronic hypoxemia and hypercarbia increase PVR that can progress to pulmonary hypertension and ultimately right heart failure.[49]

Lung-directed therapy for CF is constantly improving and currently includes aggressive chest physiotherapy, aerosolized suppressive antibiotic therapy, nebulized DNAase to reduce air trapping, and aerosolized hypertonic saline to acutely increase mucociliary clearance.[48,50] Supplemental oxygen reduces PVR and improves right ventricular performance in patients with CF, whereas beta-adrenergic agonists and glucocorticoids (oral or inhaled) may be beneficial in select patients with bronchial hyperreactivity.[49,51]

CF does manifest upper airway disease that is particularly relevant for the anesthesiologist in the setting of concomitant ESLD. Mucosal hypertrophy and hyperplasia, in addition to pedunculated nasal polyps, are observed in most patients with CF.[48] The presence of any of these findings concomitant with thrombocytopenia secondary to portal hypertension should prompt the clinician to avoid any manipulation of the naso-pharynx, either for intubation or drainage/feeding tube insertion.

Bile excretion from biliary epithelia is impaired in CF resulting in chronic malabsorption of lipid-soluble vitamins and cholelithiasis.[52] Sphincter of Oddi dysfunction secondary to pancreatic fibrosis further promotes cholelithiasis with coagulopathy and bone disease arising in the absence of appropriate vitamin supplementation. These patients typically require multiple endoscopic retrograde cholangiopancreatography procedures that are complicated by sphincter of Oddi scarring and an underlying coagulopathy. Earlier age of CF onset is associated with greater hepatobiliary and pancreatic disease. Antibiotic-induced suppression of vitamin K synthesis by intestinal bacteria exacerbates vitamin K malabsorption and promotes coagulopathy. Abnormal liver function tests and hepatic steatosis are additional features of CF occurring in up to 70% of adult patients, with progression to cirrhosis and portal hypertension occurring in as many as 10% of adults. The incidence of hepatocellular carcinoma among patients with CF with cirrhosis is increased.[52]

Anesthetic goals include minimization of ventilatory depression, optimization of pulmonary function, and avoidance of respiratory complications. Preoperative arterial blood gas and pulmonary function tests assess carbon dioxide retention and hypoxemia. Patients who require oxygen or positive pressure ventilation have advanced disease and are at risk of postoperative complications. Early extubation is critical as prolonged intubation and mechanical ventilation lead to propagation of respiratory failure, infections, and increased mortality. Humidified and warmed gases avoid worsening inspissation of airway secretions, whereas beta-adrenergic agonists may relieve bronchospasm. Reliance on muscle tone for maintenance of airway patency is characteristic of patients with CF because of the progressive destruction of airway cartilage.[48] Neuromuscular blockade may result in airway collapse and airflow obstruction; thus, the type of surgery and requirement for muscle relaxation should be discussed before administration of neuromuscular blockade. Neuraxial or regional anesthesia avoids airway manipulation with its attendant risks of pulmonary complications while also providing postoperative analgesia.

The goals of postoperative care include pain control while minimizing respiratory depression and facilitating chest physiotherapy to prevent pulmonary complications. A multimodal approach to perioperative pain control should be used to avoid respiratory depression from opioids. Patients may benefit from NPPV, and especially those who require chronic NPPV should have immediate access to their NPPV machine in the postoperative area. Patients with moderate to severe pulmonary disease may benefit from overnight continuous monitoring during their recovery from surgery and anesthesia.[48]

ALGORITHM FOR THE MANAGEMENT OF HYPOXIA IN PATIENTS WITH CHRONIC LIVER DISEASE

An algorithm for the evaluation of a patient with known liver disease and dyspnea or an asymptomatic patient with a low Spo_2 is summarized in **Fig. 1**. The evaluation begins with a thorough history and physical including exercise tolerance, positional dyspnea, and fatigue. In addition to routine laboratories, a chest roentgenogram, chest computed tomography (CT) scan, and pulmonary function testing should be considered. Abnormalities in imaging or pulmonary function testing can be further classified as intrinsic lung disease, pneumonia, or restrictive disease secondary to pleural effusions, diaphragmatic impedance, or ascites. Restrictive disease is treated with diuretics, paracentesis, or thoracentesis as indicated, whereas therapies for intrinsic lung disease and pneumonia are targeted at the cause.

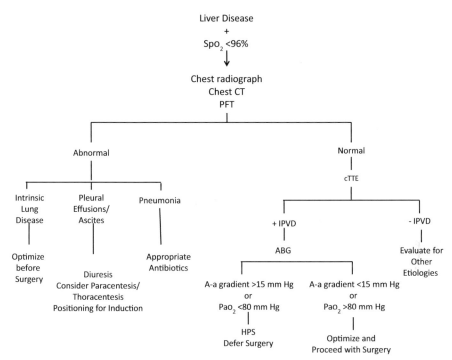

Fig. 1. Algorithm for the evaluation of patients with known liver disease and dyspnea or asymptomatic patients with a low SpO_2. ABG, arterial blood gas; CT, computed tomography.

If the imaging and pulmonary function testing do not identify the cause, the next indicated evaluation would be cTTE for the evaluation of IPVD. If IPVDs are demonstrated, then a room air arterial blood gas will differentiate true HPS from those patients with intrapulmonary shunting from chronic liver disease without hypoxemia. If IPVDs are not demonstrated on cTTE, then patients should be evaluated for other causes.

SUMMARY

Hepatic function and pulmonary function are intimately related with failure of one organ system affecting the other. As patients with ESLD or metabolic disorders that concomitantly affect hepatic and pulmonary function enjoy an improved quality of life and life expectancy, the prevalence of these patients is increasing with more presenting for elective as well as emergent surgical procedures. It is incumbent on the practicing anesthesiologist to understand the physiology of liver failure and its early effect on pulmonary function to ensure a satisfactory outcome.

REFERENCES

1. Mandell M, Masahiko T. Pulmonary complications of liver disease. In: Wagener G, editor. Liver anesthesiology and critical care medicine. 1st edition. New York: Springer; 2012. p. 255–64.
2. Hourani J, Bellamy P, Tashkin D. Pulmonary dysfunction in advanced liver disease: frequent occurrence of an abnormal diffusing capacity. Am J Med 1991; 90:693–700.

3. Scarlata S, Conte M, Cesari M, et al. Gas exchanges and pulmonary vascular abnormalities at different stages of chronic liver disease. Liver Int 2011;31:525–33.
4. Mohamed R, Freeman J, Guest P, et al. Pulmonary gas exchange abnormalities in liver transplant candidates. Liver Transpl 2002;8:802–8.
5. Agusti A, Roca J, Rodriguez-Roisin R. Mechanisms of gas exchange impairment in patients with liver cirrhosis. Clin Chest Med 1996;17:49–66.
6. Yigit I, Hacievliyagil S, Seckin Y. The relationship between severity of liver cirrhosis and pulmonary function tests. Dig Dis Sci 2008;53:1951–6.
7. Daoud F, Reeves J, Schaeffer J. Failure of hypoxic pulmonary vasoconstriction in patients with liver cirrhosis. J Clin Invest 1972;51:1076–80.
8. Rodriguez-Roisin R, Krowka M. Hepatopulmonary syndrome - a liver-induced lung vascular disorder. N Engl J Med 2008;358:2378–87.
9. Matsubara O, Nakamura T, Uchara T, et al. Histometrical investigation of the pulmonary artery in severe hepatic disease. J Pathol 1984;143:31–7.
10. Jin-Kim B, Lee S, Park S, et al. Characteristics and prevalence of intrapulmonary shunt detected by contrast echocardiography with harmonic imaging in liver transplant candidates. Am J Cardiol 2004;94:525–8.
11. Santa-Cruz R, Pearson M, Cohen M, et al. Clinical predictors and characteristics of patients with chronic liver disease and intrapulmonary shunts. Clin Cardiol 2005;28:437–41.
12. Langiulli M, Aronow W, Das M, et al. Prevalence and prognosis of intrapulmonary shunts in patients with hepatic cirrhosis. Cardiol Rev 2006;14:53–4.
13. Krowka M, Cortese D. Severe hypoxemia associated with liver disease: Mayo Clinic experience and the experimental use of almitrine bismesylate. Mayo Clin Proc 1987;62:164–73.
14. Berthelot P, Walker J, Sherlock S. Arterial changes in the lungs in cirrhosis of the liver. N Engl J Med 1966;274:291–8.
15. Swanson K, Wiesner R, Krowka M. Natural history of hepatopulmonary syndrome: impact of liver transplantation. Hepatology 2005;41:1122–9.
16. Pascasio J, Grilo I, Lopez-Pardo F, et al. Prevalence and severity of hepatopulmonary syndrome and its influence on survival in cirrhotic patients evaluated for liver transplantation. Am J Transplant 2014;14:1391–9.
17. Schenk P, Fuhrmann V, Madl C. Hepatopulmonary syndrome: prevalence and predictive value of various cut offs for arterial oxygenation and their clinical consequences. Gut 2002;51:853–9.
18. Krowka M, Tajik A, Dickerson E, et al. Intrapulmonary vascular dilatations (IPVD) in liver transplant candidates: screening by two-dimensional contrast-enhanced echocardiography. Chest 1990;97:1165–70.
19. Rodriguez-Roisin R, Krowka M, Herve P, et al, ERS Task Force Pulmonary-Hepatic Vascular Disorders (PHD) Scientific Committee. Pulmonary-hepatic vascular disorders (PHD). Eur Respir J 2004;24:861–80.
20. Machicao V, Balakrishnan M, Fallon M. Pulmonary complications in chronic liver disease. Hepatology 2014;59:1627–37.
21. Abrams G, Sanders M, Fallon M. Utility of pulse oximetry in the detection of arterial hypoxemia in liver transplant candidates. Liver Transpl 2002;8:391–6.
22. Krowka M. Hepatopulmonary syndrome: monitoring at your fingertip. Dig Dis Sci 2011;56:1599–600.
23. Arguedas M, Singh H, Faulk D, et al. Utility of pulse oximetry screening for hepatopulmonary syndrome. Clin Gastroenterol Hepatol 2007;5:749–54.
24. Kochar R, Tanikella R, Fallon M. Serial pulse oximetry in hepatopulmonary syndrome. Dig Dis Sci 2011;56:1862–8.

25. Gomez F, Martinez-Palli G, Barbera J, et al. Gas exchange mechanism of ortho-deoxia in hepatopulmonary syndrome. Hepatology 2004;40:660–6.
26. Kaymakoglu S, Kahraman T, Kudat H, et al. Hepatopulmonary syndrome in non-cirrhotic portal hypertensive patients. Dig Dis Sci 2003;48:556–60.
27. Fuhrmann V, Madl C, Mueller C, et al. Hepatopulmonary syndrome in patients with hypoxic hepatitis. Gastroenterology 2006;131:69–75.
28. Gupta S, Castell H, Rao R. Improved survival after liver transplantation in patients with hepatopulmonary syndrome. Am J Transplant 2010;10:354–63.
29. Available at: UNOS.org. Accessed January 2, 2016.
30. Rolla G, Brussino L, Colagrande P, et al. Exhaled nitric oxide and impaired oxygenation in cirrhosis patients before and after liver transplantation. Ann Intern Med 1998;129:375–8.
31. Fallon M, Abrams G, Luo B, et al. The role of endothelial nitric oxide synthase in the pathogenesis of a rat model of hepatopulmonary syndrome. Gastroenterology 1997;113:606–14.
32. Carter E, Hartsfield C, Miyazono M, et al. Regulation of heme oxygenase-1 by nitric oxide during hepatopulmonary syndrome. Am J Physiol Lung Cell Mol Physiol 2002;283:346–53.
33. Zhang J, Luo B, Tang I, et al. Pulmonary angiogenesis in a rat model of hepatopulmonary syndrome. Gastroenterology 2009;136:1070–80.
34. Fauconnet P, Klopfenstein C, Schiffer E. Hepatopulmonary syndrome: the anaesthetic considerations. Eur J Anaesthesiol 2013;30:721–30.
35. Kawut S, Krowka M, Trotter J, et al. Clinical risk factors for portopulmonary hypertension. Hepatology 2008;48:196–203.
36. Krowka M, Swanson K, Frantz R, et al. Portopulmonary hypertension: results from a 10-year screening algorithm. Hepatology 2006;44:1502–10.
37. Krowka M, Fallon M, Mulligan D, et al. Model for end-stage liver disease (MELD) exception for portopulmonary hypertension. Liver Transpl 2006;12:S114–6.
38. Dickinson M, Bartelds B, Borgdorff M, et al. The role of disturbed blood flow in the development of pulmonary arterial hypertension: lessons from preclinical animal models. Am J Physiol Lung Cell Mol Physiol 2013;305:L1–14.
39. Budhiraja R, Hassoun P. Portopulmonary hypertension: a tale of two circulations. Chest 2003;123:562–76.
40. Raevens S, Geerts A, Van Steenkiste C, et al. Hepatopulmonary syndrome and portopulmonary hypertension: recent knowledge in pathogenesis and overview of clinical assessment. Liver Int 2015;35:1646–60.
41. Ramsay M. Portopulmonary hypertension and right heart failure in patients with cirrhosis. Curr Opin Anaesthesiol 2010;23:145–50.
42. Stoller J, Aboussouan L. A review of alpha-1 antitrypsin deficiency. Am J Respir Crit Care Med 2012;185:246–59.
43. Laurell CB, Eriksson A. The electrophoretic alpha-1 globulin pattern of serum in alpha-1 antitrypsin deficiency. Scand J Clin Lab Invest 1963;73:934–9.
44. Sharp H, Bridges R, Krivit W, et al. Cirrhosis associated with alpha-1 antitrypsin deficiency: a previously unrecognized inherited disorder. J Lab Clin Med 1969;73:934–9.
45. De Serres F, Blanco I, Fernandez-Bustillo E, et al. PI S and PI Z alpha-1 antitrypsin deficiency worldwide: a review of existing genetic epidemiological data. Monaldi Arch Chest Dis 2007;67:184–208.
46. Stoller J, Sandhaus R, Turino G, et al. Delay in diagnosis of alpha-1 antitrypsin deficiency: a continuing problem. Chest 2005;128:1989–94.

47. Wong G, Espinosa W, Wong V. Personalized management of cirrhosis by non-invasive tests of liver fibrosis. Clin Mol Hepatol 2015;21:200–11.
48. Huffmyer J, Littlewood K, Nemergut E. Perioperative management of the adult with cystic fibrosis. Anesth Analg 2009;109:1949–61.
49. Fraser K, Tullis D, Sasson Z, et al. Pulmonary hypertension and cardiac function in adult cystic fibrosis: role of hypoxemia. Chest 1999;115:1321–8.
50. Fuchs H, Borowitz D, Christiansen D, et al. Effects of aerosolized recombinant human DNase on exacerbations of respiratory symptoms and on pulmonary function in patients with cystic fibrosis. N Engl J Med 1994;331:637–42.
51. Chmiel J, Konstan M. Anti-inflammatory medications for cystic fibrosis lung disease: selecting the most appropriate agent. Treat Respir Med 2005;4:255–73.
52. Sokol R, Durie P. Recommendations for management of liver and biliary tract disease in cystic fibrosis: Cystic Fibrosis Foundation Hepatobiliary Disease Consensus Group. J Pediatr Gastroenterol Nutr 1999;28:S1–13.

Index

Note: Page numbers of article titles are in **boldface** type.

A

Acute coronary syndrome, ischemic heart disease and, 776–777
Allogeneic blood transfusion, for management of anemia in perioperative setting, 717–718
Alpha-1-antitrypsin deficiency, 802–803
Anemia, anesthesia for patients with, **711–730**
    definition and controversies, 712–713
    harm from, 715–717
    management in perioperative setting, 717–723
      allogeneic blood transfusion, 717–718
      autologous transfusion techniques, 722
      erythropoietin-stimulating agents, 720–721
      iron, 720
      managing hospital-acquired anemia, 723
      optimization of hemostasis, 721–722
      patient blood management, 718–720
      supportive care, 722–723
    new frontiers, 723–724
    prevalence and significance in perioperative setting, 714–715
Anemia of chronic disease, anesthetic management of patients with, 661–662
Anesthetic management, of medically complex patients, 633–808
    with anemia, **711–730**
      definition and controversies, 712–713
      harm from, 715–717
      management in perioperative setting, 717–723
      new frontiers, 723–724
      prevalence and significance in perioperative setting, 714–715
    with cardiac and hematologic disorders, **659–668**
      anemia of chronic disease, 661–662
      anticoagulation for cardiac devices, 663–665
      heart failure with reduced ejection fraction, 665
      platelet abnormalities, 662–663
      sickle cell anemia, 660–661
    with cardiac and hepatic dysfunction, **731–745**
      anesthetic implications and management, 737–742
      pathogenesis and physiology, 732–736
    with cardiac and pulmonary disease, **633–643**
      effects of cardiovascular disease on pulmonary system, 634–639
      effects of pulmonary disease on the cardiovascular system, 639–640
    with cardiac and renal dysfunction, **697–710**
      anesthetic goals with cardiovascular disease, 699–702
      anesthetic goals with kidney disease, 698–699
      cardiorenal syndrome, 702–703

Anesthesiology Clin 34 (2016) 809–820
http://dx.doi.org/10.1016/S1932-2275(16)30091-X
1932-2275/16/$ – see front matter

anesthesiology.theclinics.com

Anesthetic (*continued*)
    intraoperative management, 705–706
    postoperative management, 706–707
    preoperative assessment, 703
    regional and neuraxial, 703–704
  with hepatic and pulmonary dysfunction, **797–808**
    algorithms for hypoxia management in chronic liver disease, 804–805
    metabolic diseases, 802–804
    pulmonary complications associated with chronic liver disease, 799–802
    pulmonary function in setting of liver disease, 798–799
  with hepatic and renal impairment, **645–648**
    evaluation, adjustment, and recurrence, 653
    hepatic disease therapies, 653–654
    management goals, 648–651
    nonpharmacologic strategies, 652–653
    patient evaluation overview, 646–648
    pharmacologic strategies, 651–652
    renal disease therapies, 654–655
    self-management strategies, 653
    surgical options, 655–656
  with peripheral vascular disease and cardiac dysfunction, **775–795**
    complications of anesthesia in, 792–793
    heart failure, 781–782
    intraoperative management, 791
    ischemic heart disease, 776–778
    in patients presenting for surgery, 784–791
    valvular disease, 778–781
    vascular disease, 782–784
  with sepsis and cardiac dysfunction, **761–774**
    anticoagulation, 770
    atrial fibrillation, 769–770
    evaluation, 770
    interactions between, 761–764
    management goals, 764–765
    nonpharmacologic strategies, 768–769
    outcome and long-term recommendations, 770
    pharmacologic strategies, 765–768
    surgical treatment options, 769
    treatment resistance/complications, 769
  with sepsis and multiple organ dysfunction, **681–696**
    diagnosis and management of organ dysfunction, 687–690
    immunologic response, 683–685
    incidence and risk factors, 682
    outcomes, 691
    pathogenic stimulus, 682–683
    prognostic indicators, 690–691
    quantifying organ dysfunction, 685–686
    SIRS and sepsis spectrum, 685
    treatment of sepsis, 686–687
    withdrawal of support and end-of-life care, 691
  in trauma patients with cardiac disease, **669–680**

management goals, 671–678
with traumatic brain injury, **747–759**
classification, 748–749
intracranial pressure/cerebral perfusion pressure management, 750–752
intraoperative management, 753–754
monitoring devices, 752–753
pathophysiology, 749–750
patients with multiple traumatic injuries, 755–756
perioperative care, 754–755
prevention of secondary injury, 750
Anesthetics, in concomitant sepsis and cardiac dysfunction, 767–768
Antibiotics, in concomitant sepsis and cardiac dysfunction, 767
Anticoagulation, for cardiac devices, in patients with concomitant cardiac and hematologic disorders, 663–665
artificial valves, 663–664
ventricular assist device, 664–665
in patients with concomitant sepsis and cardiac dysfunction, 770
Arrhythmias, surgery in patients with, 778–779
in trauma patients with cardiac disease, 677–678
Artificial valves, anticoagulation in patients with concomitant cardiac and hematologic disorders, 663–664
Atrial fibrillation, in patients with concomitant sepsis and cardiac dysfunction, 769–770
surgery in patients with, 779
Atrioventricular heart block, surgery in patients with, 780
Autologous blood transfusions, for anemia in perioperative setting, 722

B

B-type natriuretic protein (BNP), in patients with concomitant sepsis and cardiac dysfunction, 771
Biomarkers, in patients with concomitant sepsis and cardiac dysfunction, 771
Bleeding, in surgical patients with peripheral vascular disease and cardiac dysfunction, 793
Blood management, patient, for anemia in perioperative setting, 717–723, 718–723
allogeneic blood transfusion, 717–718
autologous transfusion techniques, 722
erythropoietin-stimulating agents, 720–721
iron, 720
managing hospital-acquired anemia, 723
optimization of hemostasis, 721–722
patient blood management, 718–720
supportive care, 722–723
Blunt cardiac injury, in trauma patients with cardiac disease, 676–677
Brain injury, traumatic. See Traumatic brain injury.
Bundle branch block, surgery in patients with, 780

C

Cardiac disease, anesthesia for patients with peripheral vascular disease and, **775–795**
complications of anesthesia in, 792–793
bleeding, 793
critical limb/digit ischemia, 792

Cardiac (*continued*)
  intraoperative myocardial infarction, 792
  stroke, 792–793
 heart failure, 781–782
  classification, 781
  congestive, 781–782
  hypertrophic obstructive cardiomyopathy, 782
  staging, 781
 intraoperative management, 791
  of comorbidities, 791
  preserving cardiac function, 791
  of vascular disease, 791
 ischemic heart disease, 776–778
  acute coronary syndrome and, 776–777
  risk factors, 776
  stress testing, 777–778
 in patients presenting for surgery, 784–791
  with cardiac implanted intracardiac device, 788
  infective endocarditis prophylaxis, 788
  preoperative evaluation, 784–788
 valvular disease, 778–781
  arrhythmias and conduction abnormalities, 778–779
  atrial fibrillation, 779
  atrioventricular heart block, 780
  bundle branch block, 780
  cardiac implanted electronic devices, 781
  multifocal atrial tachycardia, 779
  premature beats, 779
  sinus bradycardia, 779
  sinus tachycardia, 779
  supraventricular tachycardia, 779–780
  ventricular fibrillation, 780
  ventricular tachycardia, 780
 vascular disease, 782–784
  carotid disease, 782
  peripheral arterial disease, 782–783
  peripheral venous disease, 783
  systemic vasculitis, 784
 with concomitant hematologic disorders and, **659–668**
  anemia of chronic disease, 661–662
  anticoagulation for cardiac devices, 663–665
   artificial valves, 663–664
   ventricular assist device, 664–665
  heart failure with reduced ejection fraction, 665
  platelet abnormalities, 662–663
   idiopathic thrombotic purpura, 662–663
   thrombocytosis, 662
   thrombotic thrombocytopenic purpura, 663
  sickle cell anemia, 660–661
   sickle cell disease, 660–661
   sickle cell trait, 661

with concomitant hepatic dysfunction, **731–745**
    anesthetic implications and management, 737–742
        intraoperative management, 738–741
        postoperative management, 741–742
        preoperative considerations and testing, 737–738
    pathogenesis and physiology, 732–736
        cirrhotic cardiomyopathy, 733–734
        coronary artery disease, 735
        electrophysiologic abnormalities, 734–735
        hyperdynamic state, 732–733
        liver cirrhosis and cardiovascular system, 732
        portopulmonary hypertension, 736
with concomitant pulmonary disease and, **633–643**
    heart failure, 634–637
    obstructive lung disease, 639–641
    obstructive sleep apnea and obesity hypoventilation syndrome, 641–642
    restrictive lung disease, 641
    valvular disease, 637–639
with concomitant renal dysfunction, **697–710**
    anesthetic goals with cardiovascular disease, 699–702
    anesthetic goals with kidney disease, 698–699
    cardiorenal syndrome, 702–703
    intraoperative management, 705–706
    postoperative management, 706–707
    preoperative assessment, 703
    regional and neuraxial, 703–704
concomitant sepsis and, **761–774**
    anticoagulation, 770
    atrial fibrillation, 769–770
    evaluation, 770
    interactions between, 761–764
    management goals, 764–765
    nonpharmacologic strategies, 768–769
        ventilation, 768–769
    outcome and long-term recommendations, 770
    pharmacologic strategies, 765–768
        anesthetics, 767–768
        antibiotics, 767
        etomidate, 765–766
        glucose, 767
        steroids, 767
        vasopressors-inotropes, 766–767
    surgical treatment options, 769
    treatment resistance/complications, 769
surgical critical care for trauma patients with, **669–680**
    effects of aging on cardiac performance, 670–671
    evolution of trauma epidemiology in the US, 669–670
    management goals, 671–678
        identification of shock state and relationship to cardiac dysfunction, 671–672
        managing the cardiac dysfunction, 674–676
        targeted assessment of perfusion and resuscitation, 672–673

Cardiogenic shock, in trauma patients with cardiac disease, 675–676
Cardiorenal syndrome, 702–703
Cerebral perfusion pressure management, management of, in traumatic brain injury,
    750–752
Chronic obstructive pulmonary disease, with concomitant cardiac disease, 639–641
Cirrhosis, of liver, impact on cardiovascular system, 732
Cirrhotic cardiomyopathy, 733–734
Congestive heart failure, 781–782
Coronary artery disease, effects on liver, 735
Critical care. See Surgical critical care.
Cystic fibrosis, 803–804

E

Echocardiography, in patients with concomitant sepsis and cardiac dysfunction, 771
Endocarditis, infective, prophylaxis in surgical patients with heart disease, 788
Erythropoietin-stimulating agents, in patient blood management for anemia in perioperative
    setting, 720–721
Etomidate, in concomitant sepsis and cardiac dysfunction, 765–766

G

Geriatric patients, surgical critical care for trauma patients with cardiac disease, **669–680**
Glucose, in concomitant sepsis and cardiac dysfunction, 767

H

Heart failure, with concomitant pulmonary disease and, 634–637
        diastolic dysfunction, 635–636
        left heart systolic dysfunction, 634–635
        lung-protective ventilation and right heart dysfunction/failure, 636–637
        right ventricular dysfunction, 636
    in patients with peripheral vascular disease, 781–782
        classification, 781
        congestive, 781–782
        hypertrophic obstructive cardiomyopathy, 782
        staging, 781
    with reduced ejection fraction, in patients with concomitant hematologic disorders, 665
Hematologic disorders, with concomitant cardiac disorders and, **659–668**
        anemia of chronic disease, 661–662
        anticoagulation for cardiac devices, 663–665
            artificial valves, 663–664
            ventricular assist device, 664–665
        heart failure with reduced ejection fraction, 665
        platelet abnormalities, 662–663
            idiopathic thrombotic purpura, 662–663
            thrombocytosis, 662
            thrombotic thrombocytopenic purpura, 663
        sickle cell anemia, 660–661
            sickle cell disease, 660–661
            sickle cell trait, 661

Hemostasis, in patient blood management for anemia in perioperative setting, 721–722
Hepatic disease, with concomitant cardiac dysfunction, **731–745**
    anesthetic implications and management, 737–742
        intraoperative management, 738–741
        perioperative considerations and testing, 737–738
        postoperative management, 741–742
    pathogenesis and physiology, 732–736
        cirrhotic cardiomyopathy, 733–734
        coronary artery disease, 735
        electrophysiologic abnormalities, 734–735
        hyperdynamic state, 732–733
        liver cirrhosis and cardiovascular system, 732
        portopulmonary hypertension, 736
    with concomitant pulmonary dysfunction, **797–808**
        algorithms for hypoxia management in chronic liver disease, 804–805
        metabolic diseases, 802–804
            alpha-1-antitrypsin deficiency, 802–803
            cystic fibrosis, 803–804
        pulmonary complications associated with chronic liver disease, 799–802
            hepatopulmonary syndrome, 800–801
            portopulmonary hypertension, 801–802
        pulmonary function in setting of liver disease, 798–799
    with concomitant renal impairment, **645–648**
        evaluation, adjustment, and recurrence, 653
        hepatic disease therapies, 653–654
        management goals, 648–651
        nonpharmacologic strategies, 652–653
        patient evaluation overview, 646–648
        pharmacologic strategies, 651–652
        renal disease therapies, 654–655
        self-management strategies, 653
        surgical options, 655–656
Hepatopulmonary syndrome, 800–801
Hospital-acquired anemia, 723
Hyperdynamic state, in liver disease, effects on cardiovascular system, 732–733
Hypertrophic obstructive cardiomyopathy, 782
Hypoxia, algorithm for management in chronic liver disease, 804–805

I

Idiopathic thrombotic purpura, with concomitant cardiac disease and, 662–663
Implanted intracardiac devices, surgery in patients with, 788
Inotropes, in concomitant sepsis and cardiac dysfunction, 766–767
Intracranial pressure, management of, in traumatic brain injury, 750–752
Iron, in patient blood management for anemia in perioperative setting, 720
Ischemia, of critical limb/digit, in surgical patients with peripheral vascular disease and
    cardiac dysfunction, 793
Ischemic heart disease, 776–778
    acute coronary syndrome and, 776–777
    risk factors, 776
    stress testing, 777–778

K

Kidney disease. *See* Renal disease.
Kidney transplantation, in patients with concomitant hepatic and renal disease, 656–657

L

Liver disease. *See* Hepatic disease.
Liver transplantation, in patients with concomitant hepatic and renal disease, 656–657

M

MODS. *See* Multiple organ dysfunction syndrome.
Multiple organ dysfunction syndrome (MODS), surgical critical care for patient with sepsis
    and, **681–696**
        diagnosis and management of, 687–690
            cardiovascular, 687–688
            endocrine, 690
            gastrointestinal, 688–689
            hematologic, 689–690
            renal, 689
            respiratory, 688–689
        immunologic response, 683–685
        incidence and risk factors, 682
        outcomes, 691
        pathogenic stimulus, 682–683
        prognostic indicators, 690–691
        quantifying organ dysfunction, 685–686
        SIRS and sepsis spectrum, 685
        treatment of sepsis, 686–687
        withdrawal of support and end-of-life care, 691
Myocardial infarction, intraoperative, in patients with peripheral vascular disease and
    cardiac dysfunction, 793
    in trauma patients with cardiac disease, 674–675
Myocardial ischemia, in trauma patients with cardiac disease, 674–675

O

Obesity hyperventilation syndrome, with concomitant cardiac disease, 641–642
Obstructive lung disease, with concomitant cardiac disease, 639–641
Obstructive sleep apnea, with concomitant cardiac disease, 641–642
Organ dysfunction, multiple. *See* Multiple organ dysfunction syndrome (MODS).
Organ protection, intraoperative, with concomitant hepatic and renal impairment, 650

P

Patient blood management. *See* Blood management, patient.
Peripheral vascular disease, anesthesia for patients with cardiac dysfunction and, **775–795**
        complications of anesthesia in, 792–793
            bleeding, 793
            critical limb/digit ischemia, 792

   intraoperative myocardial infarction, 792
   stroke, 792–793
  heart failure, 781–782
   classification, 781
   congestive, 781–782
   hypertrophic obstructive cardiomyopathy, 782
   staging, 781
  intraoperative management, 791
   of comorbidities, 791
   preserving cardiac function, 791
   of vascular disease, 791
  ischemic heart disease, 776–778
   acute coronary syndrome and, 776–777
   risk factors, 776
   stress testing, 777–778
  in patients presenting for surgery, 784–791
   with cardiac implanted intracardiac device, 788
   infective endocarditis prophylaxis, 788
   preoperative evaluation, 784–788
  valvular disease, 778–781
   arrhythmias and conduction abnormalities, 778–779
   atrial fibrillation, 779
   atrioventricular heart block, 780
   bundle branch block, 780
   cardiac implanted electronic devices, 781
   multifocal atrial tachycardia, 779
   premature beats, 779
   sinus bradycardia, 779
   sinus tachycardia, 779
   supraventricular tachycardia, 779–780
   ventricular fibrillation, 780
   ventricular tachycardia, 780
  vascular disease, 782–784
   carotid disease, 782
   peripheral arterial disease, 782–783
   peripheral venous disease, 783
   systemic vasculitis, 784
Platelet abnormalities, with concomitant cardiac disorders, 662–663
 idiopathic thrombotic purpura, 662–663
 thrombocytosis, 662
 thrombotic thrombocytopenic purpura, 663
Portopulmonary hypertension, 736, 801–802
Premature beats, surgery in patients with, 779
Pulmonary dysfunction, with concomitant cardiac disease, **633–643**
 heart failure, 634–637
 obstructive lung disease, 639–641
 obstructive sleep apnea and obesity hypoventilation syndrome, 641–642
 restrictive lung disease, 641
 valvular disease, 637–639
 concomitant with hepatic disease, **797–808**
 algorithms for hypoxia management in chronic liver disease, 804–805

Pulmonary (*continued*)
        metabolic diseases, 802–804
            alpha-1-antitrypsin deficiency, 802–803
            cystic fibrosis, 803–804
        pulmonary complications associated with chronic liver disease, 799–802
            hepatopulmonary syndrome, 800–801
            portopulmonary hypertension, 801–802
        pulmonary function in setting of liver disease, 798–799

    R

Renal disease, with concomitant cardiac dysfunction, **697–710**
        anesthetic goals with cardiovascular disease, 699–702
        anesthetic goals with kidney disease, 698–699
        cardiorenal syndrome, 702–703
        intraoperative management, 705–706
        postoperative management, 706–707
        preoperative assessment, 703
        regional and neuraxial, 703–704
    with concomitant hepatic impairment, **645–648**
        evaluation, adjustment, and recurrence, 653
        hepatic disease therapies, 653–654
        management goals, 648–651
        nonpharmacologic strategies, 652–653
        patient evaluation overview, 646–648
        pharmacologic strategies, 651–652
        renal disease therapies, 654–655
        self-management strategies, 653
        surgical options, 655–656
Restrictive lung disease, anesthesia in patients with concomitant cardiac disease, 641
RIFLE criteria, for renal disease, 646

    S

Sepsis, concomitant cardiac dysfunction and, **761–774**
        anticoagulation, 770
        atrial fibrillation, 769–770
        evaluation, 770
        interactions between, 761–764
        management goals, 764–765
        nonpharmacologic strategies, 768–769
            ventilation, 768–769
        outcome and long-term recommendations, 770
        pharmacologic strategies, 765–768
            anesthetics, 767–768
            antibiotics, 767
            etomidate, 765–766
            glucose, 767
            steroids, 767
            vasopressors-inotropes, 766–767
        surgical treatment options, 769

treatment resistance/complications, 769
surgical critical care for patient with MODS and, **681–696**
    diagnosis and management of organ dysfunction, 687–690
        cardiovascular, 687–688
        endocrine, 690
        gastrointestinal, 688–689
        hematologic, 689–690
        renal, 689
        respiratory, 688–689
    immunologic response, 683–685
    incidence and risk factors, 682
    outcomes, 691
    pathogenic stimulus, 682–683
    prognostic indicators, 690–691
    quantifying organ dysfunction, 685–686
    SIRS and sepsis spectrum, 685
    treatment of sepsis, 686–687
    withdrawal of support and end-of-life care, 691
Shock, in trauma patients with cardiac disease, 671–673
Sickle cell anemia, anesthesia in patients with, 660–661
    sickle cell disease, 660–661
    sickle cell trait, 661
Sinus bradycardia, surgery in patients with, 779
Sinus tachycardia, surgery in patients with, 779
Sleep apnea, obstructive, with concomitant cardiac disease, 641–642
Steroids, in concomitant sepsis and cardiac dysfunction, 767
Stroke, in surgical patients with peripheral vascular disease and cardiac dysfunction,
    792–793
Supraventricular tachycardia, surgery in patients with, 779–780
Surgical critical care, for patients with sepsis and MODS, **681–696**
    for trauma patient with cardiac disease, **669–680**

T

Targeted resuscitation, in trauma patients with cardiac disease, 674–675
Temperature management, in patients with traumatic brain injury, 755
Thrombcytosis, with concomitant cardiac disease and, 662
Thrombotic thrombocytopenic purpura, with concomitant cardiac disease and, 663
Transjugular intrahepatic portosystemic shunt (TIPS), 635–636
Transplantation, liver or renal, in patients with concomitant hepatic and renal disease,
    656–657
Trauma patients, with cardiac disease, surgical critical care for, **669–680**
    effects of aging on cardiac performance, 670–671
    evolution of trauma epidemiology in the US, 669–670
    management goals, 671–678
        identification of shock state and relationship to cardiac dysfunction, 671–672
        managing the cardiac dysfunction, 674–676
        targeted assessment of perfusion and resuscitation, 672–673
Traumatic brain injury, anesthesia for patients with, **747–759**
    classification, 748–749
    intracranial pressure/cerebral perfusion pressure management, 750–752

Traumatic (*continued*)
    intraoperative management, 753–754
    monitoring devices, 752–753
    pathophysiology, 749–750
    patients with multiple traumatic injuries, 755–756
    perioperative care, 754–755
        endocrine, 754
        hematological, 754–755
        pharmacy, 755
        seizures, 754
        temperature management, 755
    prevention of secondary injury, 750
Troponin, in patients with concomitant sepsis and cardiac dysfunction, 771

U

Ultrasound, in patients with concomitant sepsis and cardiac dysfunction, 771

V

Valvular disease, anesthesia for patients with peripheral vascular disease and, 778–781
    arrhythmias and conduction abnormalities, 778–779
    atrial fibrillation, 779
    atrioventricular heart block, 780
    bundle branch block, 780
    cardiac implanted electronic devices, 781
    multifocal atrial tachycardia, 779
    premature beats, 779
    sinus bradycardia, 779
    sinus tachycardia, 779
    supraventricular tachycardia, 779–780
    ventricular fibrillation, 780
    ventricular tachycardia, 780
  with concomitant pulmonary disease, 637–639
    aortic regurgitation, 638–639
    aortic stenosis, 638
    mitral regurgitation, 638
    mitral stenosis, 637–638
    tricuspid regurgitation, 639
Vascular disease. *See also* Peripheral vascular disease.
  carotid disease, 782
  peripheral arterial disease, 782–783
  peripheral venous disease, 783
  systemic vasculitis, 784
Vasopressors, in concomitant sepsis and cardiac dysfunction, 766–767
Ventilation strategies, in concomitant sepsis and cardiac dysfunction, 768–769
Ventricular assist device, anticoagulation in patients with concomitant cardiac and
    hematologic disorders, 664–665
Ventricular fibrillation, surgery in patients with, 780
Ventricular tachycardia, surgery in patients with, 780

UNITED STATES POSTAL SERVICE® Statement of Ownership, Management, and Circulation (All Periodicals Publications Except Requester Publications)

1. Publication Title	2. Publication Number	3. Filing Date
ANESTHESIOLOGY CLINICS	000 – 277	9/18/2016

4. Issue Frequency	5. Number of Issues Published Annually	6. Annual Subscription Price
MAR, JUN, SEP, DEC	4	$313.00

7. Complete Mailing Address of Known Office of Publication (Not printer) (Street, city, county, state, and ZIP+4®)

ELSEVIER INC.
360 PARK AVENUE SOUTH
NEW YORK, NY 10010-1710

Contact Person
STEPHEN R. BUSHING

Telephone (Include area code)
215-239-3688

8. Complete Mailing Address of Headquarters or General Business Office of Publisher (Not printer)

ELSEVIER INC.
360 PARK AVENUE SOUTH
NEW YORK, NY 10010-1710

9. Full Names and Complete Mailing Addresses of Publisher, Editor, and Managing Editor (Do not leave blank)

Publisher (Name and complete mailing address)

ADRIANNE BRIGIDO, ELSEVIER INC.
1600 JOHN F KENNEDY BLVD. SUITE 1800
PHILADELPHIA, PA 19103-2899

Editor (Name and complete mailing address)

KATIE PFAFF, ELSEVIER INC.
1600 JOHN F KENNEDY BLVD. SUITE 1800
PHILADELPHIA, PA 19103-2899

Managing Editor (Name and complete mailing address)

PATRICK MANLEY, ELSEVIER INC.
1600 JOHN F KENNEDY BLVD. SUITE 1800
PHILADELPHIA, PA 19103-2899

10. Owner (Do not leave blank. If the publication is owned by a corporation, give the name and address of the corporation immediately followed by the names and addresses of all stockholders owning or holding 1 percent or more of the total amount of stock. If not owned by a corporation, give the names and addresses of the individual owners. If owned by a partnership or other unincorporated firm, give its name and address as well as those of each individual owner. If the publication is published by a nonprofit organization, give its name and address.)

Full Name	Complete Mailing Address
WHOLLY OWNED SUBSIDIARY OF REED/ELSEVIER, US HOLDINGS	1600 JOHN F KENNEDY BLVD. SUITE 1800 PHILADELPHIA, PA 19103-2899

11. Known Bondholders, Mortgagees, and Other Security Holders Owning or Holding 1 Percent or More of Total Amount of Bonds, Mortgages, or Other Securities. If none, check box ▶ ☐ None

Full Name	Complete Mailing Address
N/A	

12. Tax Status (For completion by nonprofit organizations authorized to mail at nonprofit rates) (Check one)
The purpose, function, and nonprofit status of this organization and the exempt status for federal income tax purposes:
☐ Has Not Changed During Preceding 12 Months
☐ Has Changed During Preceding 12 Months (Publisher must submit explanation of change with this statement)

13. Publication Title	14. Issue Date for Circulation Data Below
ANESTHESIOLOGY CLINICS	JUNE 2016

15. Extent and Nature of Circulation		Average No. Copies Each Issue During Preceding 12 Months	No. Copies of Single Issue Published Nearest to Filing Date
a. Total Number of Copies (Net press run)		495	397
b. Paid Circulation (By Mail and Outside the Mail)	(1) Mailed Outside-County Paid Subscriptions Stated on PS Form 3541 (Include paid distribution above nominal rate, advertiser's proof copies, and exchange copies)	133	143
	(2) Mailed In-County Paid Subscriptions Stated on PS Form 3541 (Include paid distribution above nominal rate, advertiser's proof copies, and exchange copies)	0	0
	(3) Paid Distribution Outside the Mails Including Sales Through Dealers and Carriers, Street Vendors, Counter Sales, and Other Paid Distribution Outside USPS®	134	145
	(4) Paid Distribution by Other Classes of Mail Through the USPS (e.g., First-Class Mail®)	0	0
c. Total Paid Distribution (Sum of 15b (1), (2), (3), and (4))	▶	267	288
d. Free or Nominal Rate Distribution (By Mail and Outside the Mail)	(1) Free or Nominal Rate Outside-County Copies Included on PS Form 3541	52	59
	(2) Free or Nominal Rate In-County Copies Included on PS Form 3541	0	0
	(3) Free or Nominal Rate Copies Mailed at Other Classes Through the USPS (e.g., First-Class Mail)	0	0
	(4) Free or Nominal Rate Distribution Outside the Mail (Carriers or other means)	0	0
e. Total Free or Nominal Rate Distribution (Sum of 15d (1), (2), (3) and (4))	▶	58	59
f. Total Distribution (Sum of 15c and 15e)	▶	319	347
g. Copies not Distributed (See Instructions to Publishers #4 (page #3))	▶	176	50
h. Total (Sum of 15f and g)	▶	495	397
i. Percent Paid (15c divided by 15f times 100)		84%	83%

* If you are claiming electronic copies, go to line 16 on page 3. If you are not claiming electronic copies, skip to line 17 on page 3.

16. Electronic Copy Circulation	Average No. Copies Each Issue During Preceding 12 Months	No. Copies of Single Issue Published Nearest to Filing Date
a. Paid Electronic Copies ▶	0	0
b. Total Paid Print Copies (Line 15c) + Paid Electronic Copies (Line 16a) ▶	267	288
c. Total Print Distribution (Line 15f) + Paid Electronic Copies (Line 16a) ▶	319	347
d. Percent Paid (Both Print & Electronic Copies) (16b divided by 16c × 100) ▶	84%	83%

☒ I certify that 50% of all my distributed copies (electronic and print) are paid above a nominal price.

17. Publication of Statement of Ownership
☒ If the publication is a general publication, publication of this statement is required. Will be printed in the DECEMBER 2016 issue of this publication. ☐ Publication not required.

18. Signature and Title of Editor, Publisher, Business Manager, or Owner

STEPHEN R. BUSHING - INVENTORY DISTRIBUTION CONTROL MANAGER

Date 9/18/2016

I certify that all information furnished on this form is true and complete. I understand that anyone who furnishes false or misleading information on this form or who omits material or information requested on the form may be subject to criminal sanctions (including fines and imprisonment) and/or civil sanctions (including civil penalties).

PS Form 3526, July 2014 (Page 3 of 4)   PRIVACY NOTICE: See our privacy policy on www.usps.com.

PS Form 3526, July 2014 (Page 1 of 4 (see instructions page 4))   PSN: 7530-01-000-9931   PRIVACY NOTICE: See our privacy policy on www.usps.com.

Moving?

Make sure your subscription moves with you!

To notify us of your new address, find your **Clinics Account Number** (located on your mailing label above your name), and contact customer service at:

Email: journalscustomerservice-usa@elsevier.com

800-654-2452 (subscribers in the U.S. & Canada)
314-447-8871 (subscribers outside of the U.S. & Canada)

Fax number: 314-447-8029

Elsevier Health Sciences Division
Subscription Customer Service
3251 Riverport Lane
Maryland Heights, MO 63043

*To ensure uninterrupted delivery of your subscription, please notify us at least 4 weeks in advance of move.

Printed and bound by CPI Group (UK) Ltd, Croydon, CR0 4YY

11/05/2025

01866603-0002